FIFTH EDITION

CASE FILES®
Pediatrics

Eugene C. Toy, MD
Assistant Dean for Educational Programs
Professor and Vice Chair of Medical Education
Department of Obstetrics and Gynecology
University of Texas Medical School at Houston
Houston, Texas

Mark D. Hormann, MD
Associate Professor of Pediatrics
Vice Chair for Education and Training
Division of Community and General Pediatrics
Department of Pediatrics
University of Texas Medical School at Houston
Houston, Texas

Robert J. Yetman, MD
Professor of Pediatrics
Vice Chair of Clinical Operations
Director, Division of Community and General
    Pediatrics
Department of Pediatrics
University of Texas Medical School at Houston
Houston, Texas

Margaret C. McNeese, MD
Professor of Pediatrics
Vice Dean for Admissions and Student Affairs
Division of Community and General Pediatrics
Department of Pediatrics
University of Texas Medical School at Houston
Houston, Texas

Sheela L. Lahoti, MD
Associate Professor of Pediatrics
Associate Dean for Admissions and
    Student Affairs
Division of Community and General Pediatrics
Department of Pediatrics
University of Texas Medical School at Houston
Houston, Texas

Mark Jason Sanders, MD
Assistant Professor of Pediatrics
Division of Community and General Pediatrics
Department of Pediatrics
University of Texas Medical School at Houston
Houston, Texas

Abby M. Geltemeyer, MD
Assistant Professor of Pediatrics
Division of Community and General Pediatrics
Department of Pediatrics
University of Texas Medical School at Houston
Houston, Texas

McGraw Hill Education

New York   Chicago   San Francisco   Athens   London   Madrid
Mexico City   Milan   New Delhi   Singapore   Sydney   Toronto

Case Files®: Pediatrics, Fifth Edition

1 2 3 4 5 6 7 8 9 0   DOC/DOC   19 18 17 16 15

ISBN 978-0-07-183995-2
MHID 0-07-183995-X

Notice

Medicine is an ever-changing science. As new research and clinical experience broaden our knowledge, changes in treatment and drug therapy are required. The authors and the publisher of this work have checked with sources believed to be reliable in their efforts to provide information that is complete and generally in accord with the standards accepted at the time of publication. However, in view of the possibility of human error or changes in medical sciences, neither the authors nor the publisher nor any other party who has been involved in the preparation or publication of this work warrants that the information contained herein is in every respect accurate or complete, and they disclaim all responsibility for any errors or omissions or for the results obtained from use of the information contained in this work. Readers are encouraged to confirm the information contained herein with other sources. For example and in particular, readers are advised to check the product information sheet included in the package of each drug they plan to administer to be certain that the information contained in this work is accurate and that changes have not been made in the recommended dose or in the contraindications for administration. This recommendation is of particular importance in connection with new or infrequently used drugs.

This book was set in Adobe Jenson Pro by Cenveo® Publisher Services.
The editors were Catherine A. Johnson and Cindy Yoo.
The production supervisor was Catherine Saggese.
Project management was provided by Anupriya Tyagi, Cenveo Publisher Services.
RR Donnelley was printer and binder.

This book is printed on acid-free paper.

Library of Congress Cataloging-in-Publication Data

Toy, Eugene C., author.
    Case files. Pediatrics / Eugene C. Toy, Robert J. Yetman, Mark D. Hormann, Margaret C. McNeese, Sheela L. Lahoti, Mark Jason Sanders, Abby M. Geltemeyer.—Fifth edition.
        p. ; cm.
    Pediatrics
    Preceded by Case files. Pediatrics / Eugene C. Toy ... [et al.]. 4th ed. c2013.
    Includes bibliographical references and index.
    ISBN 978-0-07-183995-2 (pbk. : alk. paper)—ISBN 0-07-183995-X
    I. Title.   II. Title: Pediatrics.
    [DNLM: 1. Pediatrics—methods—Case Reports.   2. Pediatrics—methods—Problems and Exercises.   WS 18.2]
    RJ48.2
    618.92—dc23   2015016252

McGraw-Hill Education books are available at special quantity discounts to use as premiums and sales promotions or for use in corporate training programs. To contact a representative, please visit the Contact Us pages at www.mhprofessional.com.

To our most precious and youngest pediatric patients,
the newborn babies, and to their mothers;

To the Honorable Senator Lois Kolkhorst of Brehnam, Texas,
whose passion and dedication to our patients gave birth to the Perinatal
Advisory Council, charged with elevating the healthcare of Texans;

To my colleagues of the Perinatal Advisory Council: the talented doctors,
Drs. Briggs, Cho, Guillory, Harvey, Honrubia, Hollier, Patel, Saade, Speer,
Stanley, and Xenakis; the super-nurses, Ms. Greer, Perez, Stelly, and Torvik; and our
two brilliant hospital administrators, Mr. Harrison and Woerner;

To our amazing state staff David Williams and Matt Ferrera, and Jane Guerrero
and Elizabeth Stevenson, without whom we could not succeed;

You are all the unselfish members of a team that beats as the heart
and soul of perinatal medicine in our great state of Texas.

—Eugene C. Toy

CONTENTS

Subha Amatya, MD
Pediatric Resident
University of Texas Medical School at Houston
Houston, Texas
Slipped Capital Femoral Epiphysis

Michelle Bailey, MD
Pediatric Resident
University of Texas Medical School at Houston
Houston, Texas
Nursemaid's Elbow (Subluxation of Radial Head)

Natasha Bhagwandin, MD
Pediatric Resident
University of Texas Medical School at Houston
Houston, Texas
Cerebral Palsy
Rectal Bleeding

Kelly Casteel, MD
Pediatric Resident
University of Texas Medical School at Houston
Houston, Texas
Klinefelter Syndrome
Megaloblastic Anemia

Nitish Chourasia, MD
Pediatric Resident
University of Texas Medical School at Houston
Houston, Texas
Child Abuse
Esophageal Atresia

Mary Kate Claiborne, MD
Pediatric Resident
University of Texas Medical School at Houston
Houston, Texas
Inflammatory Bowel Disease

Meghan Dupre, MD
Pediatric Resident
University of Texas Medical School at Houston
Houston, Texas
Rickets

Kristin Ernest, MD
Pediatric Resident
University of Texas Medical School at Houston
Houston, Texas
Concussion

Edward Espineli, MD
Pediatric Resident
University of Texas Medical School at Houston
Houston, Texas
Attention Deficit Hyperactivity Disorder
Muscular Dystrophy

Brittany Faron, MD
Pediatric Resident
University of Texas Medical School at Houston
Houston, Texas
Rhabdomyolysis

Keely Fitzgerald, DO
Pediatric Resident
University of Texas Medical School at Houston
Houston, Texas
Group B Streptococcal Infection
Growth Hormone Deficiency

Charisma Garcia, MD
Pediatric Resident
University of Texas Medical School at Houston
Houston, Texas
Acute Lymphoblastic Leukemia
Lead Ingestion (Microcytic Anemia)

Hunaid Gurji, DO, PhD
Pediatric Resident
University of Texas Medical School at Houston
Houston, Texas
Appendicitis
Ventricular Septal Defect

Sadiya Jamal, DO
Pediatric Resident
University of Texas Medical School at Houston
Houston, Texas
Cystic Fibrosis
Infant of a Diabetic Mother

Annie Joleen Kayanickupuram, DO
Pediatric Resident
University of Texas Medical School at Houston
Houston, Texas
Macrocytic Anemia (B12 Deficiency due to Short Gut Syndrome)
Pneumonia

Ana Lacarra, MD
Pediatric Resident
University of Texas Medical School at Houston
Houston, Texas
Abnormal Uterine Bleeding
Subdural Hematoma

Marcelino Latina, DO
Pediatric Resident
University of Texas Medical School at Houston
Houston, Texas
Ambiguous Genitalia
Precocious Puberty

Farah McCorvey, MD
Pediatric Resident
University of Texas Medical School at Houston
Houston, Texas
Malrotation
Posterior Urethral Valves

William Miller, MD
Pediatric Resident
University of Texas Medical School at Houston
Houston, Texas
Immunodeficiency

Stacy Nayes, MD
Pediatric Resident
University of Texas Medical School at Houston
Houston, Texas
Asthma Exacerbation
Sudden Infant Death Syndrome

Thao Nguyen, DO
Pediatric Resident
University of Texas Medical School at Houston
Houston, Texas
Acute Otitis Media
Neonatal Resuscitation

Raymond Parlar-Chun, MD
Pediatric Resident
University of Texas Medical School at Houston
Houston, Texas
Truncus Arteriosus

Minal Patel, MD
Pediatric Resident
University of Texas Medical School at Houston
Houston, Texas
Neuroblastoma
Retropharyngeal Abscess

Heather Peto, MD
Pediatric Resident
University of Texas Medical School at Houston
Houston, Texas
Acne Vulgaris
Failure to Thrive

Christopher Reinhackel, MD
Pediatric Resident
University of Texas Medical School at Houston
Houston, Texas
Adolescent Substance Use Disorder

Rebecca Sabates, MD
Pediatric Resident
University of Texas Medical School at Houston
Houston, Texas
Neonatal Hyperbilirubinemia

Anita Priya Shankar, MD
Pediatric Resident
University of Texas Medical School at Houston
Houston, Texas
Migraine without Aura

Mauricio Smart, MD
Pediatric Resident
University of Texas Medical School at Houston
Houston, Texas
Systemic Lupus Erythematosus

Jeanene Smith, MD
Pediatric Resident
University of Texas Medical School at Houston
Houston, Texas
Acute Poststreptococcal Glomerulonephritis
Bacterial Meningitis

Claudia Soler-Alfonso, MD
Fellow in Pediatric Genetics
University of Texas Medical School at Houston
Houston, Texas
Acute Epstein-Barr Virus Infection (Infectious Mononucleosis)
Bacterial Enteritis

Jane A. Stones, MD
Pediatric Resident
University of Texas Medical School at Houston
Houston, Texas
Turner Syndrome

Yen X. Tran, MD
Pediatric Resident
University of Texas Medical School at Houston
Houston, Texas
Obstructive Sleep Apnea Syndrome

Stephanie Treme, MD
Pediatric Resident
University of Texas Medical School at Houston
Houston, Texas
Diabetic Ketoacidosis
Sickle Cell Disease with Vaso-occlusive Crisis

Shaun S. Varghese, MD
Pediatric Resident
University of Texas Medical School at Houston
Houston, Texas
Complex Febrile Seizures

Jennifer Variste, MD
Pediatric Resident
University of Texas Medical School at Houston
Houston, Texas
Stevens-Johnson Syndrome

Michael Wang, DO
Pediatric Resident
University of Texas Medical School at Houston
Houston, Texas
Kawasaki Disease
Neonatal Herpes Simplex Virus Infection

Aravind Yadav, MD
Fellow in Pediatric Pulmonology
University of Texas Medical School at Houston
Houston, Texas
Transient Tachypnea of the Newborn

Yaxi Zeng, MD
Pediatric Resident
University of Texas Medical School at Houston
Houston, Texas
Congenital Cataracts

We appreciate all the kind remarks and suggestions from the many medical students over the past 3 years. Your positive reception has been an incredible encouragement, especially in light of the short life of the *Case Files®* series. In this fifth edition of *Case Files®: Pediatrics,* the basic format of the book has been retained. Improvements were made in updating many of the sections, including grouping of the cases in a more logical order for students to more easily cross-reference cases. We have also used case correlations to assist further. We reviewed the clinical scenarios and revised several of them, keeping their "real-life" presentations patterned after actual clinical experience. The multiple-choice questions have been carefully reviewed and rewritten to ensure that they comply with the National Board and USMLE format, and added an entire new section of Review Questions (Section IV) for the student to test their knowledge after reading the book. Through this fifth edition, we hope that the reader will continue to enjoy learning how to diagnose and manage patients through the simulated clinical cases. It certainly is a privilege to be teachers for so many students, and it is with humility that we present this edition.

The Authors

The clerkship curriculum that evolved into the ideas for this edition was inspired by two talented and forthright students, Philbert Yao and Chuck Rosipal, who have since graduated from medical school. It has been a tremendous joy to work with the excellent pediatricians at the University of Texas Medical School at Houston. I am greatly indebted to my editor, Catherine Johnson, whose exuberance, experience, and vision helped to shape this series. I appreciate McGraw-Hill's believing in the concept of teaching through clinical cases, and I would like to especially acknowledge Catherine Saggese for her production expertise, Cindy Yoo for her editorial guidance, and Anupriya Tyagi for her excellent production skills. At the University of Texas Medical School at Houston, we appreciate Giuseppe N. Colasurdo, MD and president of the University of Texas Health Sciences Center for his support and dedication to student education. Without the encouragement from my chairman Dr. Sean Blackwell, a wonderful clinician, administrator, scientist, and leader, and Dr. Patricia Butler, Vice Dean for Educational Programs, who inspires us all to be excellent educators, I could not have succeeded in this endeavor. Most of all, I appreciate my ever-loving wife Terri, and my four wonderful children Andy, Michael, Allison, and Christina, for their patience and understanding in the writing process.

Eugene C. Toy, MD

Mastering the cognitive knowledge within a field such as pediatrics is a formidable task. It is even more difficult to draw on that knowledge, procure and filter through the clinical and laboratory data, develop a differential diagnosis, and finally form a rational treatment plan. To gain these skills, the student often learns best at the bedside, guided and instructed by experienced teachers, and inspired toward self-directed, diligent reading. Clearly, there is no replacement for education at the bedside. Unfortunately, clinical situations usually do not encompass the breadth of the specialty. Perhaps, the best alternative is a carefully crafted patient case designed to stimulate the clinical approach and decision making. In an attempt to achieve that goal, we have constructed a collection of clinical vignettes to teach diagnostic or therapeutic approaches relevant to pediatrics. Most importantly, the explanations for the cases emphasize the mechanisms and underlying principles, rather than merely rote questions and answers. This book is organized for versatility. It allows the student "in a rush" to go quickly through the scenarios and check the corresponding answers, while allowing the student who wants more thought-provoking explanations to go at a more measured pace. The answers are arranged from simple to complex: a summary of the pertinent points, the bare answers, an analysis of the case, an approach to the topic, a comprehension test at the end for reinforcement and emphasis, and a list of references for further reading. The clinical vignettes are purposely placed in random order to simulate the way that real patients present to the practitioner. A listing of cases is included in Section III to aid the student who desires to test his or her knowledge of a specific area or who wants to review a topic, including basic definitions. Finally, we intentionally did not primarily use a multiple-choice question format in our clinical case scenarios because clues (or distractions) are not available in the real world. Nevertheless, several multiple-choice comprehension questions are included at the end of each case discussion to reinforce concepts or introduce related topics.

HOW TO GET THE MOST OUT OF THIS BOOK

Each case is designed to simulate a patient encounter with open-ended questions. At times, the patient's complaint is different from the most concerning issue, and sometimes extraneous information is given. The answers are organized into four different parts:

PART I

1. **Summary:** The salient aspects of the case are identified, filtering out the extraneous information. Students should formulate their summary from the case before looking at the answers. A comparison to the summation in the answer will help to improve their ability to focus on the important data while appropriately discarding the irrelevant information—a fundamental skill in clinical problem solving.

2. A straightforward **Answer** is given to each open-ended question.
3. The Analysis of the case is composed of two parts:
   a. **Objectives:** A listing of the two or three main principles that are crucial for a practitioner to manage the patient. Again, the students are challenged to make educated "guesses" about the objectives of the case upon initial review of the case scenario, which helps to sharpen their clinical and analytical skills.
   b. **Considerations:** A discussion of the relevant points and brief approach to the specific patient.

PART II

Approach to the disease process consists of two distinct parts:
   a. **Definitions:** Terminology pertinent to the disease process.
   b. **Clinical Approach:** A discussion of the approach to the clinical problem in general, including tables, figures, and algorithms.

PART III

Comprehension Questions: Each case contains several multiple-choice questions, which reinforce the material or introduce new and related concepts. Questions about material not found in the text have explanations in the answers.

PART IV

Clinical Pearls: Several clinically important points are reiterated as a summation of the text. This allows for easy review, such as before an examination.

How to Approach Clinical Problems

Part 1. Approach to the Patient

The transition of information from the textbook or journal article to the clinical situation is perhaps the most challenging in medicine. Retention of information is difficult; organization of the facts and recall of myriad data to apply to the patient are crucial. This text aids in the process. The first step is gathering information, otherwise known as establishing the database. This consists of taking the history (asking questions), performing the physical examination, and obtaining selective laboratory and/or imaging tests.

The history is the single most important method of establishing a diagnosis. Depending on the age of the child, the information may be gathered solely from the parent, from both the parent and the child, or solely from the adolescent. The student should remember not to be misled by the diagnosis of another physician or by a family member. A statement such as "Johnnie has pneumonia and needs antibiotics" may or may not be correct; an astute clinician will keep an open mind and consider other possibilities, such as upper respiratory tract infection, aspirated foreign body, reactive airway disease, or even cystic fibrosis. The art of seeking the information in a nonjudgmental, sensitive, and thorough method cannot be overemphasized.

HISTORY

1. **Basic information:**
   a. **Age, gender, and ethnicity** are important because some childhood illnesses occur with increased regularity at various ages, with higher frequency in one gender or more commonly in one ethnic group. For instance, anorexia nervosa is more common in white adolescent females, whereas complications of sickle cell anemia are more common in African American children of both genders.

2. **Chief complaint:** This is usually the response that the patient or the patient's family member gives to the question: "Why are you seeing the doctor today?"

3. **History of present illness:** The onset, duration, and intensity of the primary complaint, as well as associated symptoms, exacerbating and relieving factors, and previous attempts at therapy should be determined. For children, especially adolescents, a hidden agenda must be considered; **it is not uncommon for the adolescent to actually have questions about sexuality when the stated reason for the office visit is totally unrelated.** Both positive findings (the stool was loose, voluminous, and foul smelling) and negative findings (without blood or mucus) are appropriate.

4. **Past history:**
   a. **Pregnancy and delivery:** The age of the mother, the number of pregnancies, the route of delivery, and the gestational age of the infant often can provide clues as to the etiology of pediatric conditions. For instance, a large, full-term infant born by cesarean delivery who then develops an increased

respiratory rate and streakiness on chest radiograph is more likely to have **transient tachypnea of the newborn** than is an infant born vaginally at 28-week gestation with similar symptoms where a diagnosis of surfactant deficiency is the more likely cause of respiratory symptoms. Similarly, a history of drug use (including over-the-counter, prescription, and illicit drugs) or infections during pregnancy should be obtained.

b. **Neonatal history:** Any problems identified in the neonatal period, such as severe jaundice, infections, feeding difficulties, and prolonged hospitalization, should be reviewed, especially for the younger pediatric patients in whom residua of these problems may remain.

c. **Surgical history:** When, where, and for what reason the surgery was performed should be explored. Complications should be noted.

d. **Medical history:** Whereas minor illnesses (such as occasional upper respiratory infections) can be reviewed quickly, more serious illnesses (such as diabetes mellitus) should be investigated fully. The age at diagnosis, treatments prescribed, and response to therapies can be reviewed. The number and nature of hospitalizations and complications are often important. For instance, a diabetic patient with frequent hospitalizations for ketoacidosis may indicate a lack of education of the family or underlying psychosocial issues complicating therapy. A child with a history of frequent, serious accidents should alert the physician of possible child abuse.

e. **Developmental history:** For preschool children, a few questions about **language and fine motor, gross motor, and psychosocial skills** will provide good clues about development. For school-aged children, school performance (grades) and areas of strength and weaknesses are helpful.

5. **Allergies:** Reactions to medications should be recorded, including severity and temporal relationship to medications.

6. **Immunizations:** Dates for primary and booster series of immunizations should be recorded, preferably by reviewing the immunization cards or accessing the state's immunization registry. If the child is in school, a presumption about state laws regarding immunization completion can be made while the immunization card is being retrieved.

7. **Medications:** List the names of current medications, dosages, routes of administration and frequency, and durations of use. Prescription, over-the-counter, and herbal remedies are relevant.

8. **Sexual history of adolescents:** Details of an adolescent's sexual habits, contraceptive use, pregnancies, and sexually transmitted diseases should be determined.

CLINICAL PEARL

▶ The adolescent must be treated with sensitivity, respect, and confidentiality to foster the optimal environment for medical care.

9. **Family history:** Because many conditions are inherited, the ages and health of siblings, parents, grandparents, and other family members can provide important diagnostic clues. For instance, an obese child with a family history of adult-onset diabetes is at high risk for developing diabetes; early intervention is warranted.

10. **Social history:** Living arrangements, economic situations, type of insurance, and religious affiliations may provide important clues to a puzzling diagnostic case or suggest important information about the acceptability of therapeutic options.

11. **Review of systems:** A few questions about each of the major body systems allows the practitioner to ensure that no problems are overlooked and to obtain crucial history about related and unrelated medical conditions.

Physical Examination

1. **General appearance:** Well versus poorly nourished; evidence of toxemia, including lethargy (defined as poor or absent eye contact and refusal to interact with environment), signs of poor perfusion, hypo- or hyperventilation, and cyanosis; or stigmata of syndromes (such as Down or Turner).

2. **Skin:** In smaller children, checking the color of the skin for evidence of pallor, plethora, jaundice, or cyanosis is important. Abnormalities such as capillary hemangiomas (eg, "stork bites" in a newborn), café-au-lait spots, pigmented nevi (eg, "Mongolian spots"), erythema toxicum, or pustular melanosis can be identified. In older children, macules, papules, vesicles, pustules, wheals, and petechiae or purpura should be described, and evidence of excoriation, crust formation, desquamation, hyperpigmentation, ulceration, scar formation, or atrophy should be identified.

3. **Vital signs:** Temperature, blood pressure (generally begin routine measurement after 3 years), heart rate, respiratory rate, height, weight, and head circumference (generally measured until age 3 years). Measurements are plotted and compared to normals for age.

4. **Head, eyes, ears, nose, mouth and throat:**
   a. **Head:** For the neonate, the size of fontanelles and presence of overriding sutures, caput succedaneum (superficial edema or hematoma that crosses suture lines, usually located over crown), or cephalohematoma (hematoma that does not cross suture lines) should be noted. For the older child, the size and shape of the head as well as abnormalities such as swellings, depressions, or abnormal hair quality or distribution may be identified.
   b. **Eyes:** For infants, abnormalities in the size, shape, and position of the orbits, the color of the sclera (blue sclera, for instance, may indicate osteogenesis imperfecta), conjunctival hemorrhages, or the presence of iris defects (such as coloboma) may be found. The visual acuity of older children should be determined.

c. **Ears:** For all children, abnormalities in the size, shape, and position of the ears can provide important diagnostic clues. Whereas tympanic membranes are difficult to assess in newborns, their integrity should be assessed in older children. For all children, the quality and character of discharge from the ear canal should be documented.

d. **Nose:** The size, shape, and position of the nose (in relation to the face and mouth) can provide diagnostic clues for various syndromes, such as a small nose in Down syndrome. Patency of the nostrils, especially in neonates who are obligate nose breathers, is imperative. Abnormalities of the nasal bridge or septum, integrity of the mucosa, and the presence of foreign bodies should be noted. A butterfly rash around the nose can be associated with systemic lupus erythematosus (SLE), and a transverse crease across the anterior portion of the nose is seen with allergic rhinitis.

e. **Mouth and throat:** The size, shape, and position of the mouth and lips in relation to other facial structures should be evaluated. In infants, common findings of the mouth include disruption of the palate (cleft palate syndrome), Epstein pearls (a tiny white papule in the center of the palate), and short frenulum ("tongue-tied"). For all children, the size, shape, and position of the tongue and uvula must be considered. The number and quality of teeth for age should be assessed, and the buccal mucosa and pharynx should be examined for color, rashes, exudate, size of tonsils, and symmetry.

5. **Neck:** The neck in infants usually is short and sometimes hard to evaluate. Nonetheless, the size, shape, and preferred position of the neck can be evaluated for all children. The range of motion can be evaluated by gentle movement. Symmetry of the muscles, thyroid gland, veins, and arteries is important. An abnormal mass, such as a thyroglossal duct cyst (midline above the level of the thyroid) or brachial cleft cyst (along the sternomastoid muscle), or unusual findings, such as webbing in Turner syndrome, can be identified.

6. **Chest:** General examination of the chest should include an evaluation of the size and shape of the structures along with identification of obvious abnormalities (such as supernumerary nipples) or movement with respirations. **Respiratory rate varies according to age** and ranges from 40 to 60 breaths/min in the neonate to 12 to 14 breaths/min in the toddler. **The degree of respiratory distress can be stratified, with increasing distress noted when the child moves from subcostal to intercostal to supraclavicular to suprasternal retractions.** Palpation of the chest should confirm the integrity of the ribs and clavicles, and any swelling or tenderness in the joints. Percussion in older children may reveal abnormalities, especially if asymmetry is noted. The chest should be auscultated for air movement, vocal resonance, rales, rhonchi, wheezes, and rubs. In adolescent girls, symmetry of breast development and presence of masses or nipple discharge should be evaluated.

7. **Cardiovascular:** The precardium should be inspected for abnormal movements. The chest should be palpated for the location and quality of the cardiac impulse, and to determine if a thrill is present. The presence and quality of the

first and second heart sounds, including splitting with respirations, should be noted. Murmurs, clicks, rubs, and abnormalities in the heart rate (which vary by age) or rhythm should be identified. The peripheral perfusion, pulses, and color should be assessed.

8. **Abdominal examination:** The abdomen should be inspected to determine whether it is flat or protuberant, if masses or lesions such as striae are obvious, or if pulsations are present. In older children, the abdomen usually is flat, but in the neonate a very flat abdomen in conjunction with respiratory distress may indicate diaphragmatic hernia. The umbilicus, especially for neonates, should be evaluated for defects, drainage, or masses; a small umbilical hernia often is present and is normal. In the newborn, one umbilical vein and two umbilical arteries are normal. **In the neonate, palpation of the abdomen may reveal a liver edge about 2 cm below the coastal margin, a spleen tip, and using deep pressure, kidneys.** In older children, these structures are not usually palpable except in pathology. Depending on the history, other masses must be viewed with suspicion for a variety of conditions. Bowel sounds are usually heard throughout the abdomen except in pathology. In adolescent girls, the lower abdomen should be palpated for uterine enlargement (pregnancy).

9. **Genitalia:** Examination of the male for the size and shape of the penis, testicles, and scrotum is important. The position of the urethral opening should be assessed. In newborn girls, the labia majora usually is large and completely encloses the labia minora; the genitalia usually is highly pigmented and swollen with an especially prominent clitoris. A white discharge is usually present in the first days of life, and occasionally a blood-tinged fluid is also seen. In toddlers, examination of the genitalia can be challenging. Placing the toddler in a frog-leg position while the toddler sits in the parent's lap (or on the examination table) often allows successful viewing of external genitalia. In older girls, the knee-chest position affords an excellent view of the external genitalia. In girls outside the newborn period, the labia minora are smaller compared to the remainder of the external genitalia, and the vaginal mucosa is red and appears thin. The hymen, which is just inside the introitus, should be inspected. Abnormalities of the hymen, such as imperforation or tags, vaginal discharge, foreign bodies, and labial adhesions, may be noted. A speculum examination should be performed for sexually active adolescent girls. Tanner staging for pubertal development should be done for both boys and girls. Inguinal hernias should be identified; normalcy of anus should be confirmed.

10. **Extremities:** For all children, the size, shape, and symmetry of the extremities should be considered; muscle strength should be evaluated. Joints may be investigated for range of motion, warmth, tenderness, and redness. Normalcy of gait for age should be reviewed. For infants, recognition of dislocated hips is of critical importance, because lifelong growth abnormalities may result. For adolescents, identification of significant scoliosis is important to prevent the debilitating complications of that condition. Athletes require evaluation of the integrity of their joints, especially those joints that will be used in sporting activities.

11. **Neurologic:** Neurologic evaluation of the older child is similar to that in adults. Consciousness level and orientation are determined as a starting point. The cranial nerves should be assessed. The motor system should be evaluated (including strength, tone, coordination, and involuntary movements). Superficial and deep sensory systems, and deep tendon reflexes should be reviewed. **In younger infants, a variety of normal primitive reflexes (Moro, parachute, suck, grasp) can be found, but ensuring that these reflexes have extinguished by the appropriate age is equally important.**

LABORATORY ASSESSMENT

The American Academy of Pediatrics recommends a few laboratory screening tests be accomplished for pediatric patients. These tests vary according to the child's age and risk factors.

1. **Newborn metabolic screening** is done in all states, usually after 24 hours of age, but the exact tests performed vary by state. Conditions commonly screened for include hypothyroidism, phenylketonuria, galactosemia, hemoglobin type, and adrenal hyperplasia. Other conditions that may be assessed include maple syrup urine disease, homocystinuria, biotinidase deficiency, cystic fibrosis, tyrosinemia, and toxoplasmosis. Some states require a second newborn screen be performed after 7 days of age.

2. **Measurement of oxygen saturation** in all newborn infants is accomplished to assess for critical congenital heart defects.

3. **Hemoglobin or hematocrit levels** are recommended for high-risk infants (especially premature infants and those with low birth weight), at about 12 months of age, and as needed yearly if the risk of blood loss (such as menstruating adolescents) is high.

4. **Lead screening** is done, especially in high-risk areas, at 9 to 12 months of age and again at 2 years of age.

5. **Cholesterol screening** is performed in high-risk patients (those with positive family histories) older than 24 months.

6. **Sexually transmitted disease screening** is performed yearly on all sexually active patients.

Other specialized testing is accomplished depending on the child's age, risk factors, chief complaint, and conditions included in the differential diagnosis.

IMAGING PROCEDURES

1. **Plain radiographs** offer the advantage of inexpensive testing that reveals global views of the anatomy. Unfortunately, fine organ detail sometimes is not revealed which requires further radiographic study. Bone films for fracture, chest films for pneumonia, and abdomen films for ileus are common uses of this modality.

2. **Ultrasonography** is a fairly inexpensive modality that requires little or no sedation and has no radiation risks. It offers good organ and anatomic detail, but it can be operator dependent. Not all organs are accessible to sonography. Common examinations include the head for intraventricular hemorrhage (IVH) in the premature infant, the abdomen for conditions such as pyloric stenosis or appendicitis, and the kidneys for abnormal structure.

3. **Computerized tomography** (CT) provides good organ and anatomic detail and is quick, but it is fairly expensive, may require contrast, and does involve radiation. Some children require sedation to complete the procedure. This test is often performed on the abdomen or head in trauma victims.

4. **Magnetic resonance imaging** (MRI) is expensive but does not involve radiation. Because it is a slow procedure, sedation is often needed for younger children, and contrast is sometimes required. It allows for superb tissue contrast in multiple planes, and excellent anatomic and functional imaging. It is frequently used to provide detail of the brain in patients with seizures or developmental delay, or to provide tissue detail on a mass located virtually anywhere in the body.

5. **Nuclear scan** is moderately expensive and invasive. It provides functional information (usually organ specific) but poor anatomic detail. Radiation is involved. Common uses include bone scans for infection and renal scans for function.

Part 2. Approach to Clinical Problem Solving

There are generally **four steps** to the systematic solving of clinical problems:

1. Make the diagnosis.

2. Assess the severity of the disease.

3. Render a treatment based on the stage of the disease.

4. Follow the response to the treatment.

MAKING THE DIAGNOSIS

This is achieved with careful sifting of the database, analysis based on the risk factors present, and development of a list of possibilities (the differential diagnosis). The process includes knowing which pieces of information are more meaningful and which can be discarded. Experience and knowledge from reading help to guide the physician to key in on the most important concerns. **A good clinician also knows how to ask the same question in several different ways and using different terminology,** because patients at times will deny having been treated for asthma but will answer affirmatively to being hospitalized for wheezing. A diagnosis can be reached by systematically reviewing each possible cause and reading about each disease. The patient's presentation is then matched up against each of these possibilities and either placed higher up on the list as a potential etiology or lower down because of the disease frequency, the patient's presentation, or other clues. A patient's risk factors may influence the probability of a diagnosis. Usually a long list of possible diagnoses can be pared down to two or three top suspicions, based on key laboratory or imaging tests. For example, an adolescent presenting with a fever as the chief complaint can have an extensive differential diagnosis reduced to far fewer possibilities when the history reveals an uncle in the home with cough that contains blood, weight loss, and night sweats, and the physical examination shows an increased respiratory rate, lymphadenopathy, and right lower lobe lung crackles. In this case, the patient likely has tuberculosis.

ASSESSING THE SEVERITY OF THE DISEASE

The next step is to characterize the severity of the disease process. In asthma, this is done formally based on guidelines promulgated by the National Heart, Lung, and Blood Institute (NHLBI). Asthma categories range from mild intermittent (least severe) to severe persistent (most severe). For some conditions, such as syphilis, the staging depends on the length of time and follows along the natural history of the infection (ie, primary, secondary, or tertiary syphilis).

RENDERING TREATMENT BASED ON THE STAGE OF THE DISEASE

Many illnesses are stratified according to severity because prognosis and treatment vary based on the severity. If neither the prognosis nor the treatment was affected by the stage of the disease process, it would not make much sense to subcategorize something as mild or severe. As an example, mild intermittent asthma poses less danger than does severe persistent asthma (particularly if the patient has been intubated for asthma in the past). Accordingly, with mild intermittent asthma, the management would be intermittent short-acting β-agonist therapy while watching for any worsening of the disease into more serious categories (more severe disease). In contrast, a patient with severe persistent asthma would generally require short-acting β-agonist medications as well as long-acting β-agonists, inhaled steroids, and potentially oral steroids.

Group A β-hemolytic streptococcal pharyngeal infection ("strep throat") is associated with complications including poststreptococcal glomerulonephritis and rheumatic fever. The presence of group A β-hemolytic streptococcus confers an increased risk of problems, but neither the prognosis nor the treatment is affected by "more" group A β-hemolytic streptococcus or "less" group A β-hemolytic streptococcus. Hence, **the student should approach new disease by learning the mechanism, clinical presentation, how it is staged, and how the treatment varies based on stage.**

FOLLOWING THE RESPONSE TO TREATMENT

The final step in the approach to disease is to follow the patient's response to the therapy. **Whatever the "measure" of response, it should be recorded and monitored.** Some responses are clinical, such as a change in the patient's pain level or temperature, or results of pulmonary examination. Obviously the student must work on being more skilled in eliciting the data in an unbiased and standardized manner. Other patients may be followed by imaging, such as CT scan of a retroperitoneal (RP) node size in a patient receiving chemotherapy for neuroblastoma, or a marker such as the platelet count in a patient recovering from Kawasaki syndrome. For syphilis, it may be the nonspecific treponemal antibody test rapid plasma reagin (RPR) titer every month. The student must know what to do if the measured marker does not respond according to the expected. Is the next step to treat further, or to repeat the metastatic workup, or to follow up with another more specific test?

Part 3. Approach to Reading

The student must approach reading differently than the classic "systematic" review of a particular disease entity. Patients rarely arrive to their health care provider with a clear diagnosis; hence, the student must become skilled in applying the textbook information to the clinical setting. Everyone retains more when the reading is performed with a purpose. Experience teaches that with reading; there are several crucial questions to consider thinking clinically. They are as follows:

1. What is the most likely diagnosis?

2. What should be your next step?

3. What is the most likely mechanism for this process?

4. What are the risk factors for this condition?

5. What are the complications associated with this disease?

6. What is the best therapy?

WHAT IS THE MOST LIKELY DIAGNOSIS?

Establishing the diagnosis was discussed in the previous part. This is a difficult task to give to the medical student; however, it is the basic problem that will confront clinicians for the rest of their careers. One way of attacking this problem is to develop standard "approaches" to common clinical problems. It is helpful to memorize the most common causes of various presentations, such as "the most common cause of mild respiratory distress in a term infant born by cesarean section is retained amniotic fluid (transient tachypnea of the newborn)."

The clinical scenario would entail something such as the following:

"A 3-hour-old infant is noted to have a mildly increased respiratory rate and slight subcostal retractions. The infant is term, large for gestation age, and was born by repeat cesarean section. The pregnancy was uncomplicated. What is the most likely diagnosis?"

With no other information to go on, the student would note that this baby has respiratory distress. Using the "most common cause" information, the student would guess transient tachypnea of the newborn. If, instead, the gestational age "term" is changed to "preterm at 30 weeks' gestation," a phrase can be added, such as the following:

"The mother did not receive prophylactic steroids prior to birth."

Now, the student would use the "most common cause of respiratory distress in a preterm child whose mother did not receive prenatal steroids" is surfactant deficiency (respiratory distress syndrome).

WHAT SHOULD BE YOUR NEXT STEP?

This question in many ways is even more difficult than the most likely diagnosis, because insufficient information may be available to make a diagnosis and the next step may be to pursue more diagnostic information. Another possibility is that the diagnosis is clear, but the subsequent step is the staging of the disease. Finally, the next step may be to treat. Hence, from clinical data, a judgment needs to be rendered regarding how far along one is on the road of:

**Make diagnosis → Stage disease →
Treatment based on the stage → Follow response**

In particular, the student is accustomed to regurgitating the same information that someone has written about a particular disease but is not skilled at giving the next step. This talent is optimally learned at the bedside, in a supportive environment, with freedom to take educated guesses, and with constructive feedback. The student in assessing a child in the hospital should go through the following thinking process:

1. Based on the information I have, I believe that Cedric Johnson (a 3-month-old child with a positive respiratory syncytial virus nasal washing) has bronchiolitis.

2. I don't believe that this is severe disease (such as significant oxygen requirement, severe retractions, or carbon dioxide retention on blood gas analysis). A chest radiograph shows no lobar consolidation (I believe this is important because a lobar consolidation would suggest a bacterial etiology).

3. Therefore, the treatment is supportive care with supplemental oxygen and intravenous fluids as needed.

4. I want to follow the treatment by assessing Cedric's respiratory status (I will follow the oxygen saturation and degree of retractions), his temperature, and his ability to maintain his hydration orally without intravenous fluids. Also, if in the next few days Cedric does not get better or if he worsens, I think he will need a repeat chest radiograph to assess whether he has an evolving bacterial pneumonia.

In a similar patient, when the clinical presentation is not so clear, perhaps the best "next step" may be diagnostic in nature such as blood cultures to determine if bacteremia is present. This information is sometimes tested by the dictum, "the gold standard for the diagnosis and treatment of a bacterial infection is a culture."

Sometimes the next step is therapeutic.

WHAT IS THE MOST LIKELY MECHANISM FOR THIS PROCESS?

This question goes further than requiring the student to make the diagnosis; it also requires the student to understand the underlying mechanism for the process. For example, a clinical scenario may describe a 5-year-old child with Henoch-Schönlein purpura (HSP) who develops abdominal pain and heme-positive stools a week after diagnosis. The student first must diagnose the heme-positive stools associated with HSP, which occur in approximately 50% of patients. Then, the student must understand that the edema and damage to the vasculature of the gastrointestinal (GI) tract can cause bleeding along with colicky abdominal pain, sometimes progressing to intussusception. The mechanism of the pain and bleeding is, therefore, vasculitis causing enlarged mesenteric lymph nodes, bowel edema, and hemorrhage into the bowel. Answers that a student may speculate, but would not be as likely, include appendicitis, bacterial gastroenteritis, or volvulus.

The student is advised to learn the mechanisms for each disease process and not merely to memorize a constellation of symptoms. In other words, rather than trying to commit to memory the classic presentation of HSP (typical rash, abdominal pain, and arthritis), the student should also understand that vasculitis of the small vessels is the culprit. The vasculitis causes edema, mainly in the dependent areas, that precedes the palpable purpura. This vasculitis is responsible not only for edema in the joints (mainly in dependent areas such as the knees and ankles) causing the arthritis found in approximately two-thirds of patients, but also damage to the vasculature of the GI tract leading to the intermittent, colicky abdominal pain that can manifest as heme-positive stools or even intussusception.

WHAT ARE THE RISK FACTORS FOR THIS CONDITION?

Understanding the risk factors helps to establish the diagnosis and interpret test results. For example, understanding the risk factor analysis may help to manage a 1-year-old child with anemia found on routine screening. If the child had no risk factors for lead poisoning or thalassemia, the practitioner may choose to treat with supplemental iron because the likelihood for more serious pathology is low. On the other hand, if the same 1-year-old child was a recent immigrant from an endemic area, lived in a older home with peeling paint, had a father who worked at a battery smelting plant, and ate meals from unglazed pottery, a practitioner should presumptively diagnose lead poisoning until proven otherwise. The physician may want to obtain a serum lead level and a complete blood count with differential (looking for basophilic stippling and microcytosis), and thoroughly evaluate the child for developmental delay. Thus, the number of risk factors helps to categorize the likelihood of a disease process.

WHAT ARE THE COMPLICATIONS ASSOCIATED WITH THIS DISEASE?

A clinician must understand the complications of a disease so that the patient can be monitored. Sometimes, the student will have to make the diagnosis from clinical clues and then apply his or her knowledge of the sequelae of the pathologic process. For example, a child diagnosed with high fever, rash, lymphadenopathy, and oral and conjunctival changes is diagnosed with Kawasaki syndrome. Complications of this condition include arthritis, vasculitis of the medium-sized arteries, hydrops of the gall-bladder, urethritis, and aseptic meningitis. Understanding the types of complications helps the clinician to assess the patient. For example, one life-threatening complication of Kawasaki syndrome is coronary artery aneurysm and thrombosis. **The clinical presentation in the subacute phase is desquamation, thrombocytosis, and the development of coronary aneurysms with a high risk of sudden death.** The appropriate therapy is intravenous immunoglobulin in the acute phase and high-dose aspirin as soon as possible after the diagnosis is made. Nonrecognition of the risk of coronary artery aneurysm and appropriate therapy for thrombosis can lead to the patient's death. Students apply this information when they see on rounds a patient with Kawasaki syndrome and monitor for new murmurs, thrombocytosis, myocarditis, and development of coronary artery aneurysms. The clinician communicates to the team to watch the patient for any of these signs or symptoms so that appropriate therapy can be considered.

WHAT IS THE BEST THERAPY?

This is perhaps the most difficult question, not only because the clinician needs to reach the correct diagnosis, and assess the severity of the condition, but also because he or she must weigh the situation to reach the appropriate intervention. The student does not necessarily need to memorize exact dosages, but the medication, the route of delivery, and possible complications are important. It is important for the student to verbalize the diagnosis and the rationale for the therapy. A common error is for the student to "jump to a treatment," almost like a random guess, and therefore be given a "right or wrong" feedback. In fact, the student's guess may be correct but for the wrong reason; conversely, the answer may be a very reasonable one, with only one small error in thinking. It is crucial instead to give the steps so that feedback can be given for each step.

For example, what is the best therapy for a 15-year-old sexually active girl with severe, cystic acne? The incorrect manner of response is for the clinician to blurt out "Accutane." Rather, the student should reason it as follows:

"Severe, cystic acne can be treated with a variety of modalities. Side effects of the medications must be considered in a sexually active teenager who is statistically at high risk for pregnancy. Accutane causes severe birth defects and is absolutely contraindicated in pregnancy. Therefore, the best treatment for this adolescent may be a combination of oral antibiotics and topical medications that present a much lower chance of devastating side effects."

REFERENCES

Athreya BH, Pearlman SA, Zitelli B. *Pediatric Physical Diagnosis*. 2nd ed. Kent, UK: Anshan Publishers; 2010.

Barness LA. Pediatric history and physical examination. In: McMillan JA, DeAngelis CD, Feigin RD, eds. *Oski's Pediatrics: Principles and Practice*. 4th ed. Philadelphia, PA: Lippincott Williams & Wilkins; 2006:39-51.

Bates LS. *Pocket Guide to Physical Examination and History Taking*. 7th ed. Philadelphia, PA: Lippincott Williams & Wilkins; 2012.

Blickman JG, Parker BR, Barnes PD. *Pediatric Radiology: The Requisites*. 3rd ed. Philadelphia, PA: Mosby Publishers; 2009.

Listing of Cases

Listing by Case Number

Listing by Disorder (Alphabetical)

Clinical Cases

You are called to the delivery room because a now 2-minute-old male infant was born floppy and blue; his Apgar scores were 4 and 5. He has not responded well to stimulation and blow-by oxygen. The obstetrician who is resuscitating the infant informs you that the child was born by a spontaneous vaginal delivery to a 24-year-old primigravida. Her pregnancy was uncomplicated. Fetal heart tones were stable throughout the labor. Spinal epidural anesthesia was administered but was only partially effective; the obstetrician supplemented her labor analgesia with intravenous meperidine (Demerol) and promethazine (Phenergan). The amniotic fluid was not meconium stained, and the mother had no evidence of intraamniotic infection.

▶ What is the next best step in managing this infant?

ANSWER TO CASE 1:
Neonatal Resuscitation

Summary: A newborn is born floppy, blue, and has responded poorly to initial resuscitation efforts of warming, drying, and stimulation.

- **Next management step:** Evaluate heart rate (HR) and respirations. If no respirations are found or if HR is less than 100 beats/min, initiate positive-pressure ventilation (PPV) by bag and mask. Because this mother received meperidine during the labor process, naloxone (Narcan) administration may transiently reverse the effect of the narcotic. Because the half-life of narcotics is usually longer than naloxone, providing adequate ventilation is the key to resuscitation until the newborn regains spontaneous respirations. The newborn should be transitioned in a high-risk setting and observed closely for recurrent respiratory depression as the effect of naloxone subsides.

ANALYSIS

Objectives

1. Understand the steps of newborn delivery room resuscitation.
2. Become familiar with use of the Apgar score.
3. Become familiar with conditions causing newborn transition problems.

Considerations

This depressed infant was born to a healthy mother without prenatal or delivery complications other than the partially effective epidural anesthesia, which was supplemented with meperidine and promethazine. PPV was initiated and naloxone administered. The provider must appreciate the timing of maternal meperidine administration and its continued effects on the neonate.

> # APPROACH TO:
> ## Neonatal Resuscitation

DEFINITIONS

NARCOSIS: The condition of deep stupor or unconsciousness produced by a chemical substance such as a drug or anesthesia.

PERINATAL HYPOXIA: Inadequate oxygenation of a neonate that, if severe, can lead to brainstem depression and secondary apnea unresponsive to stimulation.

POSITIVE-PRESSURE VENTILATION (PPV): Mechanically breathing using a bag and mask.

CLINICAL APPROACH

Delivery room resuscitation follows the **ABC** rules of resuscitation for patients of all ages: establish and maintain the **A**irway, control the **B**reathing, and maintain the **C**irculation with medications and chest compressions (if necessary).

In this case, the meperidine given during labor probably is responsible for the infant's apnea and poor respiratory effort. Neonates with narcosis usually have a good HR response but poor respiratory effort in response to bag-and-mask ventilation. The first and most important corrective action is to provide effective PPV. The therapy for narcotic-related depression can then be instituted in the form of intravenous (IV), intramuscular (IM), subcutaneous (SQ), or endotracheal administration of naloxone (Narcan); repeated doses may be required should respiratory depression recur.

The **Apgar score** (Table 1–1) is widely used to evaluate a neonate's transition from the intra- to extrauterine environment. Scores of 0, 1, or 2 are given at 1 and 5 minutes of life for the listed signs. The 1-minute score helps to determine an infant's well-being in the period just prior to delivery, and scores less than 3 historically have been used to indicate the need for immediate resuscitation. In current practice, HR, color, and respiratory rate (RR) rather than the 1-minute Apgar score are used to determine this need. The 5-minute score is one indicator of how successful the resuscitation efforts were. Some continue to measure Apgar scores

Table 1–1 • APGAR EVALUATION OF A NEWBORN			
Sign	0	1	2
Heart rate	Absent	<100 beats/min	>100 beats/min
Respiratory effort	Absent	Slow, irregular	Good, crying
Muscle tone	Limp	Some flexion of extremities	Flexed, active motion
Reflex irritability (response to catheter in nose)	No response	Grimace	Cough or sneeze
Color	Blue, pale	Body pink, acrocyanosis (extremities blue)	Completely pink

beyond the 5-minute period to determine the continued response to resuscitation efforts. The Apgar score alone cannot determine neonatal morbidity or mortality.

COMPREHENSION QUESTIONS

1.1   A female infant is born through emergency cesarean section to a 34-year-old mother whose pregnancy was complicated by hypertension and abnormal fetal heart monitoring. At delivery she is covered in thick, green meconium and is limp, apneic, and bradycardic. Which of the following is the best first step in her resuscitation?

   A.   Administer IV bicarbonate.

   B.   Administer IV naloxone.

   C.   Initiate bag-and-mask ventilation.

   D.   Initiate chest compressions immediately.

   E.   Intubate with an endotracheal tube and suction meconium from the trachea.

1.2   A term male infant is delivered vaginally to a 22-year-old mother. Immediately after birth he is noted to have a scaphoid abdomen, cyanosis, and respiratory distress. Heart sounds are heard on the right side of the chest, and the breath sounds seem to be diminished on the left side. Which of the following is the most appropriate next step in his resuscitation?

   A.   Administer IV bicarbonate.

   B.   Administer IV naloxone.

   C.   Initiate bag-and-mask intubation.

   D.   Initiate chest compressions immediately.

   E.   Intubate with an endotracheal tube.

1.3   A 37-week gestation boy is born after an uncomplicated pregnancy to a 33-year-old mother. At birth he was lethargic and had an HR of 40. Oxygen was administered via bag and mask, and he was intubated; his HR remained at 40 beats/min. Which of the following is the most appropriate next step?

   A.   Administer IV bicarbonate.

   B.   Administer IV atropine.

   C.   Administer IV epinephrine.

   D.   Administer IV calcium chloride.

   E.   Begin chest compressions.

1.4 A term female infant is born vaginally after an uncomplicated pregnancy. She appears normal but has respiratory distress when she stops crying. When crying she is pink; when not she makes vigorous respiratory efforts but becomes dusky. Which of the following is the likely explanation for her symptoms?

A. Choanal atresia

B. Diaphragmatic hernia

C. Meconium aspiration

D. Neonatal narcosis

ANSWERS

1.1 **E.** If meconium is present during delivery, a decision whether to intubate and suction the trachea will depend on the newborn's degree of vigor (vigorous is defined as strong respiratory efforts, good muscle tone, and a heart rate greater than 100 beats/min). If the baby is nonvigorous as in this scenario, direct suctioning of the trachea is indicated before many breaths occur which will reduce the chance of forcing meconium into the lower airways and the development of meconium aspiration syndrome (obstructed airways by meconium, gas exchange impairment, and respiratory failure). When meconium is present and the baby is vigorous, a simple bulb syringe or large-bore suction catheter can be used to clear the airway and routine care can proceed.

1.2 **E.** The case describes diaphragmatic hernia. Because of herniated bowel in the chest, these children often have pulmonary hypoplasia. Bag-and-mask ventilation will cause accumulation of bowel gas (which is located in the chest) and further respiratory compromise. Therefore, endotracheal intubation is the best course of action.

1.3 **E.** Based on the neonatal resuscitation algorithm, if the HR is still less than 60 beats/min despite positive-pressure ventilation (PPV) with 100% oxygen, then chest compressions are given for 30 seconds. If the HR is still less than 60 beats/min, then drug therapy (usually epinephrine) is indicated.

1.4 **A.** Infants are obligate nose breathers until about 4 months of age. When crying they can breathe through their mouth, but they must have a patent nose when quiet. Choanal atresia is identified by passing a feeding tube through each nostril or by identification of clouding on cold metal held under the infant's nose. Should choanal atresia be diagnosed, endotracheal intubation bypasses the airway obstruction until surgical repair can be completed.

CLINICAL PEARLS

▶ An infant with slow heart rate, poor color, and inadequate respiratory effort requires immediate resuscitation.

▶ The therapy for narcosis (newborn respiratory depression because of maternal pain control) is adequate PPV followed by intravenous, intramuscular, subcutaneous, or endotracheal administration of naloxone (Narcan).

▶ A child with diaphragmatic hernia often presents with immediate respiratory distress, scaphoid abdomen, cyanosis, and heart sounds displaced to the right side of the chest.

▶ Choanal atresia results in respiratory distress when a child stops crying; immediate treatment is intubation until surgical correction can be completed.

REFERENCES

Carlo WA. Delivery room emergencies. In: Kleigman RM, Stanton BF, St. Geme JW, Schor NF, Behrman RE, eds. *Nelson Textbook of Pediatrics*. 19th ed. Philadelphia, PA: WB Saunders; 2011:575-579.

Carlo WA. Routine delivery room and initial care. In: Kleigman RM, Stanton BF, St. Geme JW, Schor NF, Behrman RE, eds. *Nelson Textbook of Pediatrics*. 19th ed. Philadelphia, PA: WB Saunders; 2011:536-538.

Ekrenkranz RA. Newborn resuscitation. In: McMillan JA, Feigin RD, DeAngelis CD, Jones MD, eds. *Oski's Pediatrics: Principles and Practice*. 4th ed. Philadelphia, PA: Lippincott Williams & Wilkins; 2006:207-213.

Kattwinkel J, Perlman JM, Aziz, K, et al. Neonatal resuscitation: 2010 American Heart Association Guidelines for Cardiopulmonary Resuscitation and Emergency Cardiovascular Care. *Pediatrics*. 2010;126;e1400-e1413.

Initial steps of resuscitation. In: Kattwinkel J, ed. *Textbook of Neonatal Resuscitation*. 6th ed. Elk Grove, IL: American Academy of Pediatrics-American Heart Association; 2011:37-69.

Special considerations. In: Kattwinkel J, ed. *Textbook of Neonatal Resuscitation*. 6th ed. Elk Grove, IL: American Academy of Pediatrics-American Heart Association; 2011:237-264.

Thilo EH, Rosenberg AA. Diaphragmatic hernia. In: Hay WW, Levin MJ, Sondheimer JM, Deterding RR, eds. *Current Diagnosis & Treatment: Pediatrics*. 20th ed. New York, NY: McGraw-Hill; 2011: 46-47.

Thilo EH, Rosenberg AA. Perinatal resuscitations. In: Hay WW, Levin MJ, Sondheimer JM, Deterding RR, eds. *Current Diagnosis & Treatment: Pediatrics*. 20th ed. New York, NY: McGraw-Hill; 2011: 25-30.

Wyckoff MH. Delivery room resuscitation. In: Rudolph CD, Rudolph AM, Lister G, First LR, Gershon AA, eds. *Rudolph's Pediatrics*. 22nd ed. New York, NY: McGraw-Hill; 2011:164-170.

Yoon PJ, Kelley PE, Friedman NR. Choanal atresia. In: Hay WW, Levin MJ, Sondheimer JM, Deterding RR, eds. *Current Diagnosis & Treatment: Pediatrics*. 20th ed. New York, NY: McGraw-Hill; 2011:473.

Zenel JA. Nose. In: Rudolph CD, Rudolph AM, Lister G, First LR, Gershon AA, eds. *Rudolph's Pediatrics*. 22nd ed. New York, NY: McGraw-Hill; 2011:177.

You are called to the nursery by the postpartum nurse to evaluate a 3-hour-old female infant with tachypnea. She was born at 36 weeks of gestation to a 38-year-old woman whose pregnancy was complicated by type 2 diabetes, initially treated with metformin but due to inadequate glycemic control, insulin was added during the second trimester. The mother was noncompliant with blood glucose monitoring and insulin therapy, and her hemoglobin A1C at delivery was 12%. Labor began spontaneously and rupture of membranes occurred 2 hours before delivery. The infant is on the warmer, weighs 4200 g, has a pulse of 140 beats/min, and respirations of 72 breaths/min with intercostal retractions and nasal flaring. She is jittery and plethoric. A capillary glucose measured with the bedside glucometer is 30 mg/dL.

▶ What is the next step in the evaluation of this infant?
▶ What is the treatment for this infant?
▶ What are other possible causes of this infant's tachypnea?

ANSWERS TO CASE 2:

Infant of a Diabetic Mother (IDM)

Summary: A macrosomic neonate is born to a diabetic mother with poor glucose control. The infant has symptomatic hypoglycemia, a medical emergency.

- **Next step:** Send a *stat* serum glucose to confirm the presence of hypoglycemia. Bedside glucometers measure the glucose in whole blood and tend to be 10% lower than serum values. The range of difference is greater at lower glucose values.

- **Treatment:** Administer intravenous (IV) glucose.

- **Other causes of tachypnea in the IDM:** Respiratory distress syndrome (RDS) hypertrophic cardiomyopathy, hypocalcemia, polycythemia, and clavicle fracture.

ANALYSIS

Objectives

1. Recognize the clinical features that may occur in the IDM (Figure 2–1).

2. Know the management of complications occurring in the IDM, the most common of which is neonatal hypoglycemia.

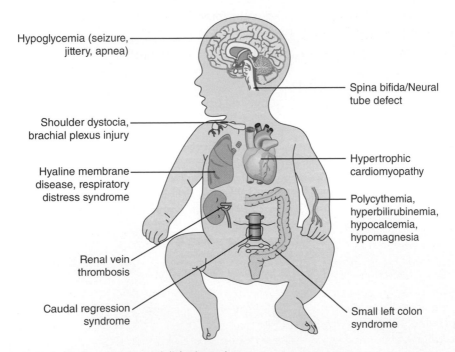

Hypoglycemia (seizure, jittery, apnea)

Spina bifida/Neural tube defect

Shoulder dystocia, brachial plexus injury

Hyaline membrane disease, respiratory distress syndrome

Hypertrophic cardiomyopathy

Polycythemia, hyperbilirubinemia, hypocalcemia, hypomagnesia

Renal vein thrombosis

Caudal regression syndrome

Small left colon syndrome

Figure 2–1. Findings in infants of diabetic mothers.

Considerations

Maternal hyperglycemia very early in gestation can cause significant birth defects, including neural tube defects and congenital heart disease. Later, in response to poorly controlled maternal hyperglycemia, **fetal hyperinsulinism begins in the second trimester resulting in fetal macrosomia and increased fetal oxygen requirements.**

Fetal insulin production causes increased glycogen production which is deposited in the fetal liver, heart, kidneys, and skeletal muscle. The large shoulders and abdomen of such infants make delivery difficult and the infant may sustain shoulder dystocia, clavicle fracture, or brachial plexus injury. Hypertrophic cardiomyopathy results from glycogen deposition in the myocardium. Increased fetal oxygen requirements cause polycythemia. Insulin appears to interfere with cortisol's ability to induce surfactant production, which predisposes the neonate to RDS. **After delivery** and removal from the high-sugar *in utero* environment, the infant's hyperinsulinism can cause **hypoglycemia**, which must be managed immediately. If the hypoglycemia is left untreated, seizures, obtundation, and respiratory arrest can occur.

APPROACH TO:
Infant of a Diabetic Mother

DEFINITIONS

GESTATIONAL DIABETES MELLITUS (GDM): Persistent hyperglycemia during pregnancy, with serum glucose levels greater than 95 mg/dL in the fasting state and above the thresholds for the oral glucose tolerance test.

HYPOGLYCEMIA: A blood glucose level less than 40 mg/dL is the usual definition, although other definitions exist. Symptoms include lethargy, listlessness, poor feeding, temperature instability, apnea, cyanosis, jitteriness, tremors, seizure activity, and respiratory distress.

MACROSOMIA: Larger than normal baby with the birth weight exceeding the 90th percentile for gestational age, or any birth weight more than 4 kg.

CLINICAL APPROACH

Diabetes affects an average of 7% of pregnancies. For most women, the condition is transient, occurring during pregnancy and disappearing after delivery. **Women are screened for gestational diabetes between 24 and 28 weeks of pregnancy** (but can be screened earlier if considered high risk). If **hyperglycemia is present in the first trimester, an increased risk for congenital anomalies** of the central nervous system, heart, kidneys, and the skeletal system (such as caudal regression syndrome in which there is hypoplasia of the sacrum and lower extremities) is noted. Women who require insulin therapy are at higher risk for a poor perinatal outcome as compared to those whose carbohydrate intolerance can be managed by diet alone. The better the glycemic control, the lower the rates of malformations, macrosomia, and hypoglycemia.

Hypoglycemia develops in about 25% to 50% of infants born to mothers with pregestational diabetes and in about 25% of infants born to mothers with gestational diabetes. Therefore, all IDM should feed within the first hour of life and have a bedside glucose measurement approximately 30 minutes after the feed. A blood **glucose level of less than 40 mg/dL with any symptom of hypoglycemia requires IV glucose. If no symptoms of hypoglycemia are present, the infant is refed and the glucose is remeasured 30 minutes after the feeding.** Glucose levels in the first 4 hours of life that do not increase above 25 mg/dL despite feeding will also require IV glucose. Monitoring of glucose typically continues for the first 12 hours of life and until three consecutive preprandial measurements are normal. Feeding patterns are monitored closely as poor feeding in the IDM can represent a metabolic or cardiac abnormality. **Hypocalcemia** is another metabolic abnormality commonly seen in IDM and presents as irritability, sweating, or seizures. Symptomatic infants will require IV calcium replacement.

Infants who are large for gestational age should be examined closely for signs of birth trauma, such as cephalohematoma, clavicle fracture, and brachial plexus injury. Macrosomia *in utero* creates an increase in the intrauterine oxygen requirement, and the relative placental insufficiency leads to increased production of erythropoietin. The resultant **polycythemia,** defined as a central hematocrit greater than 65 in a neonate, may give a ruddy or plethoric hue to the infant's skin. Polycythemia **contributes to elevated bilirubin** levels and **can cause hyperviscosity syndrome with resultant venous thrombosis** in the renal veins, cerebral venous sinus, or mesenteric veins. Polycythemia is treated with increased hydration and in rare instances partial exchange transfusion.

COMPREHENSION QUESTIONS

2.1 A 36-week gestation infant is delivered via cesarean section because of macrosomia and fetal distress. The mother has class D pregestational diabetes (insulin dependent, with vascular disease); her hemoglobin A1c is 15% (normal 7%). This infant is at risk for hypocalcemia, cardiomyopathy, polycythemia, and which of the following?

    A. Congenital dislocated hip

    B. Dacryostenosis

    C. Respiratory distress syndrome

    D. Hyperglycemia

    E. Pneumothorax

2.2 A term infant weighing 4530 g is born without complication to a mother with gestational diabetes. At 12 hours of life, he appears mildly jaundiced. Vital signs are stable, he is eating well, and his blood type is the same as his mother's blood type. Which of the following serum laboratory tests are most likely to help you evaluate this infant's jaundice?

A. Total protein, serum albumin, and liver transaminases

B. Total and direct bilirubin, liver transaminases, and a hepatitis panel

C. Total bilirubin and a hematocrit

D. Total bilirubin and a glucose

E. Total and direct bilirubin and a calcium

2.3 Which of the following is NOT a symptom of hypoglycemia?

A. Tachypnea

B. Hypothermia

C. Poor feeding

D. Vomiting

E. Jitteriness

2.4 A term boy born to a mother with insulin-dependent pregestational diabetes has a bedside capillary glucose of 32 mg/dL at 1 hour of life. He is awake and has normal vital signs. Which of the following is the most appropriate next step in management?

A. Instruct the mother to breast-feed him and recheck the glucose in 30 minutes.

B. Place an IV and administer glucose.

C. Recheck the glucose in 1 hour.

D. Measure his serum insulin level.

E. Take him to the nursery for observation.

ANSWERS

2.1 **C.** Infants born to mothers with poorly controlled diabetes are at risk for respiratory distress syndrome (surfactant deficiency) even at near-term gestational ages. The maternal hyperglycemia stimulates fetal hyperinsulinism, which has an antagonistic effect on surfactant production.

2.2 **C.** This baby most likely has hyperbilirubinemia due to polycythemia. Total bilirubin and hematocrit should be measured to determine if phototherapy is needed. The polycythemia warrants close monitoring of the infant's hydration in order to avoid worsening the hyperviscosity.

2.3 **D.** Vomiting typically is not a symptom of hypoglycemia.

2.4 **A.** Infants of diabetic mothers are at risk for hypoglycemia and should feed within the first hour of birth and glucose should be measured 30 minutes later. In this infant's case, he has not fed yet, so he should breast-feed and have the glucose remeasured. IV glucose would be needed at this time only if he has symptoms of hypoglycemia. Rechecking the glucose in an hour without feeding is withholding treatment and not appropriate; the latter choices also do not include providing the appropriate treatment.

CLINICAL PEARLS

▶ Infants of diabetic mothers are at risk for congenital malformations and perinatal complications, including hypoglycemia, polycythemia, hyperbilirubinemia, hypocalcemia, and birth trauma.

▶ Hypoglycemia manifests with nonspecific symptoms; any alteration in the infant's vital signs or general state should prompt immediate glucose measurement.

REFERENCES

Adamkin DH. Committee on Fetus and Newborn. Postnatal glucose homeostasis in late-preterm and term infants. *Pediatrics.* 2011:127;575-579.

American Diabetes Association. Standards of medical care in diabetes–2014. *Diabetes Care.* 2014; 37(1):S18-20.

Carlo WA. Infants of diabetic mothers. In: Kliegman RM, Stanton BF, St. Geme III J, Schor N, Behrman R, eds. *Nelson Textbook of Pediatrics.* 19th ed. Philadelphia, PA: WB Saunders; 2011:627-629.

French HM, Simmons RA. Infant of a diabetic mother. In: Rudolph CD, Rudolph AM, Lister GE, First LR, Gershon AA, eds. *Rudolph's Pediatrics.* 22nd ed. New York, NY: McGraw-Hill; 2011:195-198.

A mother is concerned that her 4-day-old son's face and chest are turning yellow. This Asian infant was delivered vaginally after an uncomplicated term pregnancy to a 19-year-old gravida 1 mother. The family history is unremarkable. With the exception of a large cephalohematoma, his physical examination is normal. He is breast-feeding well and shows no signs of illness.

▶ What is the most likely diagnosis?
▶ What is the next step in evaluating this patient?

ANSWERS TO CASE 3:

Neonatal Hyperbilirubinemia

Summary: A healthy, 4-day-old jaundiced, breast-feeding Asian male infant has a cephalohematoma.

- **Most likely diagnosis:** Neonatal hyperbilirubinemia

- **Next step:** Serum or transcutaneous bilirubin level

ANALYSIS

Objectives

1. Understand the etiology of physiologic neonatal jaundice.

2. Identify the causes of pathologic jaundice in a newborn.

3. Know the treatment for neonatal jaundice.

Considerations

Neonatal hyperbilirubinemia (Table 3–1) results from higher rates of bilirubin production (ie, red blood cells [RBCs] are lysed at too rapid a rate) and a limited ability to excrete it (ie, transmission of unconjugated bilirubin to the liver is interrupted; liver enzyme deficiencies preclude appropriate metabolism of the unconjugated material). This infant has several risk factors for neonatal physiologic jaundice: male gender, cephalohematoma, Asian ancestry, and breast-feeding. Other possible risk factors to be considered for neonatal jaundice are maternal diabetes, prematurity, polycythemia, trisomy 21, delayed bowel movement, upper gastrointestinal obstruction, hypothyroidism, swallowed maternal blood, and a sibling with physiologic jaundice.

Table 3–1 • DIFFERENTIAL DIAGNOSIS OF NEONATAL HYPERBILIRUBINEMIA

Unconjugated or Indirect Hyperbilirubinemia
- Hemolytic disease
  - ABO incompatibility
  - Rh incompatibility
  - Other minor blood group incompatibility
- Structural or metabolic abnormalities of RBCs
  - Hereditary spherocytosis
  - G6PD deficiency
- Hereditary defects in bilirubin conjugation
  - Crigler-Najjar—Types I and II
  - Gilbert disease
- Bacterial sepsis
- Breast milk jaundice
- Physiologic jaundice

Conjugated or Direct Hyperbilirubinemia
- Conjugated biliary atresia
- Extrahepatic biliary obstruction
- Neonatal hepatitis
  - Bacterial
  - Viral
  - Nonspecific
  - TPN related
- Short bowel related
- Inspissated bile syndrome
- Postasphyxia
- α_1-Antitrypsin deficiency
- Neonatal hemosiderosis

Revised and adapted from Cashore WJ. Neonatal hyperbilirubinemia. In: McMillan JA, DeAngelis CD, Feigin RD, Jones MD, eds. *Oski's Pediatrics: Principles and Practice.* 4th ed. Philadelphia, PA: Lippincott Williams & Wilkins; 2006:235-245.

APPROACH TO:

Neonatal Jaundice

DEFINITIONS

CONJUGATED (DIRECT) BILIRUBIN: Bilirubin chemically attached to a glucuronide by an enzymatic process in the liver; elevated levels are not neurotoxic (do not cross blood brain barrier) but may be indicative of a more serious underlying illness.

UNCONJUGATED (INDIRECT) BILIRUBIN: Bilirubin yet to be enzymatically attached to a glucuronide in the liver; elevated levels can cause neurotoxicity.

ERYTHROBLASTOSIS FETALIS: Increased RBC destruction due to transplacental maternal antibody passage active against the infant's RBC antigens.

HEMOLYSIS: Rapid breakdown of RBCs. Clinical and laboratory findings might include a rapid rise of serum bilirubin level (>0.5 mg/dL/h), anemia, pallor, reticulocytosis, and hepatosplenomegaly.

KERNICTERUS: A neurologic syndrome resulting from unconjugated bilirubin deposition in brain cells, especially the basal ganglia, globus pallidus, putamen, and caudate nuclei. Less mature or sick infants have greater susceptibility. Lethargy, poor feeding, and loss of Moro reflex are common initial signs.

POLYCYTHEMIA: A central hematocrit of 65% or higher, which can lead to blood hyperviscosity.

TRANSCUTANEOUS BILIRUBINOMETER (TcB): A device that is placed on infant's skin and produces light at several wavelengths that then measures its reflection after interacting with the serum bilirubin in the microcirculation beneath the skin. The device is used to noninvasively measure serum bilirubin as an alternative to serum bilirubin measurement.

END-TIDAL CO CONCENTRATION (ETCO): ETCO corrected for ambient CO; provides a noninvasive assessment of bilirubin production.

CLINICAL APPROACH

Physiologic jaundice comprises primarily unconjugated hyperbilirubinemia observed during the first week of life in approximately 60% of full-term infants and 80% of preterm infants. Physiologic jaundice is established by precluding known jaundice causes through history, clinical and laboratory findings. Newborn infants have a limited ability to conjugate bilirubin and cannot readily excrete unconjugated bilirubin. Jaundice usually begins on the face and then progresses to the chest, abdomen, and feet. Full-term newborns with physiologic jaundice usually have peak bilirubin concentrations of 5 to 6 mg/dL between the second and fourth days of life.

Findings suggestive of *nonphysiologic jaundice* include (1) appearance in the first 24 to 36 hours of life, (2) bilirubin rate of rise greater than 5 mg/dL/24 h, (3) bilirubin greater than 12 mg/dL in a full-term infant without other physiologic jaundice risk factors listed, and (4) jaundice that persists after 10 to 14 days of life. Nonphysiologic etiologies are commonly diagnosed in a jaundiced infant who has a family history of hemolytic disease or in an infant with concomitant pallor, hepatomegaly, splenomegaly, failure of phototherapy to lower bilirubin, vomiting, lethargy, poor feeding, excessive weight loss, apnea, or bradycardia. Causes of nonphysiologic jaundice include septicemia, biliary atresia, hepatitis, galactosemia, hypothyroidism, cystic fibrosis, congenital hemolytic anemia (eg, spherocytosis, maternal Rh, or blood type sensitization), or drug-induced hemolytic anemia.

Jaundice presenting within the first 24 hours of life requires immediate attention; causes include erythroblastosis fetalis, hemorrhage, sepsis, cytomegalic inclusion disease, rubella, and congenital toxoplasmosis. Unconjugated hyperbilirubinemia can cause kernicterus, the signs of which mimic sepsis, asphyxia, hypoglycemia, and intracranial hemorrhage. Lethargy and poor feeding are common initial signs, followed by a gravely ill appearance with respiratory distress and diminished tendon reflexes.

Approximately 2% of breast-fed full-term infants develop significant unconjugated bilirubin elevations (*breast milk jaundice*) after the seventh day of life; concentrations up to 30 mg/dL during the second to third week can be seen. If breast-feeding is continued, the levels gradually decrease. Formula substitution for breast milk for 12 to 24 hours results in a rapid bilirubin level decrease; breast-feeding can be resumed without return of hyperbilirubinemia.

The American Academy of Pediatrics recommends establishing protocols in all low-risk nurseries to assess the risk of severe hyperbilirubinemia in all newborns prior to their discharge home. This assessment can be done by measuring total serum bilirubin (TsB) levels or by using a noninvasive, TcB. The TcB bilirubin measured at the newborn's sternum correlates with serum levels and is reliable in newborns of different ethnicities and at different gestational ages. The TcB measurements are not reliable after the infant has undergone phototherapy.

The infant's serum or transcutaneous bilirubin should be charted on a bilirubin nomogram which plots bilirubin level versus hour of life to assess the patient's risk of developing severe hyperbilirubinemia. The nomogram categorizes infant's bilirubin levels as low risk, low intermediate risk, high intermediate risk, and high risk to estimate likelihood of bilirubin toxicity and the need for further evaluation or intervention. Online nomograms, such as BiliTool (www.bilitool.org), are easy to use for risk designation and to minimize medical error while also considering other risk factors that lower the threshold for initiating phototherapy.

Significant hyperbilirubinemia requires a *diagnostic evaluation*, including the measurement of indirect and direct bilirubin concentrations, hemoglobin level, reticulocyte count, blood type, Coombs test, and peripheral blood smear examination.

Phototherapy is often used to treat unconjugated hyperbilirubinemia, with the unclothed infant placed under a bank of phototherapy lights, the eyes shielded, and hydration maintained. The phototherapy light converts the skin's bilirubin isomerization into a more easily excreted form.

Exchange transfusion is needed in a small number of jaundiced infants who do not respond to conservative measures. Small aliquots of the infant's blood are removed via a blood vessel catheter and replaced with similar aliquots of donor blood. Risks of this procedure include air embolus, volume imbalance, arrhythmias, acidosis, respiratory distress, electrolyte imbalance, anemia or polycythemia, blood pressure fluctuation, infection, and necrotizing enterocolitis.

CASE CORRELATION

- See also Case 2 (Infant of Diabetic Mother). One of the complications of an infant born to a mother who has diabetes is polycythemia, a known cause of hyperbilirubinemia because the excessive red cells breakdown.

COMPREHENSION QUESTIONS

3.1 Which of the following decreases the risk of neurologic damage in a jaundiced newborn?

A. Acidosis

B. Displacement of bilirubin from binding sites by drugs such as sulfisoxazole

C. Hypoalbuminemia

D. Sepsis

E. Maternal ingestion of phenobarbital during pregnancy

3.2 An 8-day-old infant continues to have jaundice which was first noted on the second day of life; his latest total and direct bilirubin levels are 12.5 and 0.9 mg/dL, respectively. The baby and the mother have type O positive blood, the direct and indirect Coombs tests are negative, the infant's reticulocyte count is 15%, and a smear of his blood reveals no abnormally shaped cells. He is bottle-feeding well, produces normal stools and urine, and has gained weight well. Which of the following remains in the differential diagnosis?

A. Gilbert syndrome

B. Disseminated intravascular coagulation (DIC)

C. Spherocytosis

D. Polycythemia

E. An undiagnosed blood group isoimmunization

3.3 Hyperbilirubinemia associated with Crigler-Najjar syndrome type I is caused by which of the following?

A. Increased production of bilirubin

B. Impaired conjugation of bilirubin

C. Deficient hepatic uptake of bilirubin

D. Severe deficiency of uridine diphosphate glucuronosyltransferase

E. Glucose-6-phosphate dehydrogenase deficiency

3.4 A 30-hour-old full-term infant has facial and chest jaundice. He is breast-feeding well and has an otherwise normal examination. His bilirubin level is 15.5 mg/dL. Which of the following is the most appropriate course of action?

A. Recommend cessation of breast-feeding for 48 hours and supplement with formula.

B. Start phototherapy.

C. Wait for 6 hours and retest the serum bilirubin level.

D. Start an exchange transfusion.

E. No action is needed.

3.5 A 12-day-old male infant presents to clinic for well-child check. His mother is concerned because she has noticed that "his eyes are turning yellow." She reports that he is a "good eater" and is proud to report that he is exclusively breast-fed. The patient has gained weight since birth and is voiding and stooling appropriately. What is the most likely cause of his jaundice?

    A. Physiologic jaundice

    B. Crigler-Najjar

    C. Breast-feeding jaundice

    D. Breast milk jaundice

    E. TORCH infection

3.6 An infant is born at term, via prolonged spontaneously vaginal delivery requiring vacuum assisted device. He is noted to be jaundiced at 24 hours of life. Serum bilirubin is measured and shows indirect hyperbilirubinemia. All of the following should be obtained to evaluate the patient EXCEPT?

    A. Blood typing

    B. Coombs test

    C. Complete blood count (CBC) with reticulocyte count

    D. Peripheral smear

    E. TORCH panel

ANSWERS

3.1 **E.** Administration of phenobarbital induces glucuronyl transferase, thus reducing neonatal jaundice. Sepsis and acidosis increase the risk of neurologic damage by increasing the blood-brain barrier's permeability to bilirubin. Hypoalbuminemia reduces the infant's ability to transport unconjugated bilirubin to the liver, and similarly drugs that displace bilirubin from albumin elevate free levels of unconjugated bilirubin in the serum.

3.2 **A.** Gilbert syndrome would present with a negative Coombs test, a normal (or low) hemoglobin, a normal (or slightly elevated) reticulocyte count, and prolonged hyperbilirubinemia. Red cell morphology would be abnormal in DIC and spherocytosis, polycythemia would present with an elevated hemoglobin level (that listed above is normal for a newborn), and blood group isoimmunization would present with a positive Coombs test.

3.3 **D.** Although all infants are relatively deficient in uridine diphosphate glucuronosyltransferase, those with Crigler-Najjar syndrome type I have a severe deficiency, causing high bilirubin levels and encephalopathy. Treatment is phototherapy. Encephalopathy is rare with Crigler-Najjar syndrome type II, in which bilirubin levels rarely exceed 20 mg/dL.

3.4 **B.** Although the etiology of the hyperbilirubinemia must be investigated, phototherapy should be started.

3.5 **D.** Patient is above birth weight and is exclusively breast-fed.

3.6 **E.** Infection should be considered, based on maternal history; however, the other options are more important in the initial investigation.

CLINICAL PEARLS

▶ Physiologic jaundice, observed during the first week of life in the majority of infants, results from higher bilirubin production rates and a limited ability of excretion. The diagnosis is established by precluding known causes of jaundice based on history and clinical and laboratory findings.

▶ Nonphysiologic jaundice is caused by septicemia, biliary atresia, hepatitis, galactosemia, hypothyroidism, cystic fibrosis, congenital hemolytic anemia, drug-induced hemolytic anemia, or antibodies directed at the fetal RBC.

▶ High levels of unconjugated bilirubin may lead to kernicterus, an irreversible neurologic syndrome resulting from brain cell bilirubin deposition, especially in the basal ganglia, globus pallidus, putamen, and caudate nuclei. Less mature or sick infants are at greater risk. The signs and symptoms of kernicterus may be subtle and similar to those of sepsis, asphyxia, hypoglycemia, and intracranial hemorrhage.

▶ It is important to plot patient's bilirubin on a nomogram that plots hours of age against bilirubin level to categorize patient's risk for severe hyperbilirubinemia and to determine the need for phototherapy or exchange transfusion.

REFERENCES

Ambalavanan N, Carlo WA. Jaundice and hyperbilirubinemia in the newborn. In: Kliegman RM, Stanton BF, St. Geme JW, Schor NF, Behrman RE, eds. *Nelson Textbook of Pediatrics*. 19th ed. Philadelphia, PA: WB Saunders; 2011:603-608.

American Academy of Pediatrics. Management of hyperbilirubinemia in the newborn infant 35 or more weeks of gestation. *Pediatrics*. 2004;114:297-316.

Cashore WJ. Neonatal hyperbilirubinemia. In: McMillan JA, DeAngelis CD, Feigin RD, Jones MD, eds. *Oski's Pediatrics: Principles and Practice*. 4th ed. Philadelphia, PA: Lippincott Williams & Wilkins; 2006:235-245.

Lee GC, Madan A. Jaundice. In: Rudolph CD, Rudolph AM, Lister G, First LR, Siegel NJ, eds. *Rudolph's Pediatrics*. 22nd ed. Philadelphia, PA: WB Saunders; 2011:229-233.

A 2800-g male infant is born at 36 weeks of gestation to a 19-year-old mother through vaginal delivery. Delivery occurred 19 hours after membrane rupture. The mother's pregnancy was uncomplicated, but her prenatal records are not available at delivery. At 6 hours of age he is "breathing hard" and refusing to breast-feed. His respiratory rate is 60 breaths/min with "grunting." His temperature is 96.5°F (35.8°C), and his blood pressure is lower than normal. You ask the nurses to obtain a complete blood count (CBC) while you drive to the hospital from home. Upon arrival you confirm that he is in respiratory distress and that his perfusion is poor. The CBC demonstrates a white blood cell (WBC) count of 2500 cells/mm³ with 80% bands. His radiograph is shown in the figure below.

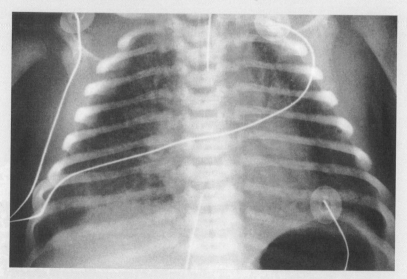

► What is the most likely diagnosis?
► What is the best therapy?

ANSWERS TO CASE 4:

Group B Streptococcal Infection

Summary: A 2800-g infant born by vaginal delivery at 36 weeks of gestation is found to have poor feeding, tachypnea, hypothermia, and poor perfusion at 6 hours of age.

- **Most likely diagnosis:** Group B *Streptococcus* (GBS) infection.

- **Best therapy:** Intravenous (IV) antibiotics (after addressing "ABCs" of resuscitation [Airway, Breathing, and Circulation]).

ANALYSIS

Objectives

1. Understand the common presentations of neonatal sepsis.

2. Understand the maternal risk factors for neonatal GBS infection.

3. Appreciate the variety of organisms responsible for neonatal infections.

4. Learn treatment options for the common neonatal infections.

Considerations

The rapid symptom onset, the low WBC count with left shift, and the chest x-ray findings are typical for GBS pneumonia. At this point, management would include rapid application of the ABCs (maintain Airway, control Breathing, and ensure adequate Circulation) of resuscitation, followed by rapid institution of appropriate antibiotics once cultures are obtained. Despite these measures, mortality from this infection is high.

APPROACH TO:
Group B Streptococcal Infection

DEFINITIONS

EARLY-ONSET NEONATAL SEPSIS SYNDROME: Neonatal sepsis occurring in the first 6 days of life. The majority of infections (~85%) occur in the first 24 hours of life, an additional 5% by approximately 48 hours, and the remainder throughout the next 4 days. The infection source usually is microorganism acquisition from the mother's genitourinary tract.

GROUP B *STREPTOCOCCUS* (GBS) COLONIZATION: Infection with GBS limited to mucous membrane sites in a healthy adult; the gastrointestinal (GI) tract is the most common colonization reservoir.

LATE-ONSET NEONATAL SEPSIS SYNDROME: Neonatal sepsis usually occurring after approximately 7 days but before approximately 90 days of life. The infection source often is the caregiver's environment.

INTRAPARTUM ANTIBIOTIC PROPHYLAXIS: Intravenous penicillin or ampicillin given during labor to prevent early-onset GBS disease.

CLINICAL APPROACH

Signs and Symptoms of Sepsis

The signs and symptoms of neonatal sepsis can be subtle and nonspecific, often overlapping with findings in other conditions, such as respiratory distress syndrome, metabolic disorders, intracranial hemorrhages, and traumatic deliveries. Temperature instability, tachypnea, hypotension, and bradycardia are common findings in sepsis and meningitis. **Overwhelming shock is manifested as pallor and poor capillary refill.** Neurologic findings of impaired level of consciousness, coma, seizures, bulging anterior fontanelle, focal cranial nerve signs, and nuchal rigidity are unusual, but when present hint at meningitis, a condition more commonly seen in late-onset disease. Examination findings seen frequently with pneumonia (more commonly seen in early-onset disease) include tachypnea, grunting, nasal flaring, retractions (costal or substernal), decreased breath sounds, and cyanosis.

Evaluation of the Potentially Septic Child

Some neonatal sepsis laboratory findings can be nonspecific, including hypoglycemia, metabolic acidosis, and jaundice. The CBC often is used to help guide therapy, although the sensitivity and specificity of this test are low. Evidence of infection on CBC includes the following:

- Markedly elevated or low WBC counts

- Increased neutrophil count

- Increased immature to total neutrophil (I/T) ratios

- Thrombocytopenia with platelet counts less than $100,000/mm^3$

The C-reactive protein (an acute phase protein increased with tissue injury) can be elevated in septic infants; some use it as an adjunct to assess for neonatal sepsis.

A blood culture is crucial for patients with suspected sepsis. Some argue that the low meningitis incidence, especially in early-onset disease, does not warrant routine cerebral spinal fluid testing; rather, the test should be reserved for documented (positive cultures) or presumed (patients so sick that a full antibiotic course is to be given regardless of culture results) sepsis. Urine cultures usually are included for late-onset disease evaluation. Urinary tract infection is uncommon in the first few days of life, and urinalysis or culture is usually not included in early-onset disease workup. Chest radiologic findings include segmental, lobar, or diffuse reticulogranular patterns, the latter easily confused with respiratory distress syndrome (lack of surfactant).

Pathogens

The organisms that commonly cause early-onset sepsis colonize in the mother's genitourinary tract and are acquired transplacentally, from an ascending infection or as the infant passes through the birth canal. **Specific organisms include GBS, *Escherichia coli*, *Haemophilus influenzae*, and *Listeria monocytogenes.*** Late-onset disease occurs when the infant becomes infected in the postnatal environment, such as from the skin, respiratory tract, conjunctivae, GI tract, and umbilicus. For the hospitalized infant, bacteria sources include vascular or urinary catheters or contact with health care workers. Organisms commonly seen to cause late-onset disease include coagulase-negative staphylococci, *Staphylococcus aureus*, *E coli*, *Klebsiella* sp, *Pseudomonas* sp, *Enterobacter* sp, *Candida*, GBS, *Serratia* sp, *Acinetobacter* sp, and anaerobes.

Group B *Streptococcus* is the most common cause of neonatal sepsis from birth to 3 months. Approximately 80% of cases occur as early-onset disease (septicemia, pneumonia, and meningitis) resulting from vertical transmission from mother to infant during labor and delivery. Respiratory signs (apnea, grunting respirations, tachypnea, or cyanosis) are the initial clinical findings in more than 80% of neonates, regardless of the site of involvement, whereas hypotension is an initial finding in approximately 25% of cases. Other signs are similar to those associated with other bacterial infections described earlier.

Neonates with GBS meningitis rarely have seizures as a presenting sign, yet 50% develop seizures within 24 hours of infection. The median age at diagnosis of early-onset GBS infection is 13 hours, earlier than for the other bacterial infections described previously. Clinical history and findings suggestive of early-onset GBS disease (rather than of a noninfectious etiology for pulmonary findings) include prolonged rupture of membranes, apnea, hypotension in the first 24 hours of life, a 1-minute Apgar score less than 5, and rapid progression of pulmonary disease.

Factors associated with increased risk for early-onset GBS disease are rupture of membranes more than 18 hours before delivery, chorioamnionitis or intrapartum temperature greater than 100.4°F (38°C), previous infant with GBS infection, mother younger than 20 years, **and low birth weight or prematurity (<37 weeks of gestation).** Mortality because of GBS disease is close to 10%. Major neurologic sequelae (cortical blindness, spasticity, and global mental retardation) occur in 12% to 30% of infants who survive meningitis.

The incidence of early-onset GBS infection decreased from 1.7 per 1000 live births in 1993 to 0.34 to 0.37 per 1000 live births in 2008. The decline is largely attributed to the widespread use of GBS risk–reduction guidelines. These guidelines recommend **screening women at 35 to 37 weeks of gestation and offering intrapartum antibiotic prophylaxis to those with risk factors or positive GBS cultures at 35 to 37 weeks of gestation.** Infants born at less than 35 weeks of gestation or born to women who received inadequate intrapartum prophylaxis sometimes undergo a limited evaluation that often includes a CBC and blood culture. Intrapartum antibiotic prophylaxis does not prevent late-onset GBS disease. The association of early antibiotic use with increased risk of late-onset serious bacterial infections remains under study.

Late-onset GBS disease is often more subtle in presentation than early-onset disease. Symptoms often occur between 7 and 30 days of life but can occur up to 3 to 4 months of age. Most commonly, late-onset GBS disease presents as bacteremia without a focus. Meningitis occurs in 20% to 30% of late-onset GBS cases, and the presenting symptom may be seizure. Other manifestations of late-onset GBS disease include focal infections such as pneumonia, septic arthritis, osteomyelitis, or cellulitis. The major risk factor for late-onset GBS disease is prematurity. Diagnostic testing for late-onset GBS disease should include CBC, blood and urine cultures, as well as CSF culture if the patient has symptoms concerning for meningitis and for the febrile neonate less than 28 days of life.

Treatment

Initial antibiotic treatment for neonatal sepsis is broad. Antibiotics are directed at the most common pathogens previously listed, often consisting of a combination of IV aminoglycosides (such as gentamicin and tobramycin) and penicillin (usually ampicillin). When GBS is identified by culture as the sole causative organism, antibiotic coverage can be narrowed to penicillin G if the patient has improved and is clinically stable. Gentamicin may be added to penicillin G for synergy but is not always required. Other antibiotics often chosen that will also provide coverage for GBS include ampicillin, first- and second-generation cephalosporins, and vancomycin.

Antibiotics are continued for at least 48 to 72 hours. If cultures are negative and the patient is well, antibiotics often are stopped. **For infants presenting with convincing signs and symptoms of sepsis, antibiotics may be continued even with negative cultures.** For infants with positive cultures, therapy continues for 10 to 21 days depending on the organism and the infection site. Close observation for signs of antibiotic toxicity is important for all infants.

CASE CORRELATION

- See also Case 3 (Neonatal Hyperbilirubinemia). One of the signs of infection in the newborn population is hyperbilirubinemia, along with other findings of temperature instability, poor feeding, lethargy, etc.

COMPREHENSION QUESTIONS

4.1 An infant was born at 36 weeks of gestation to a 30-year-old G3P2 mother via spontaneous vaginal delivery. Rupture of membranes occurred 15 hours prior to delivery. Birth weight is 4000 g, and Apgar scores were 6 and 9 at 1 and 5 minutes, respectively. Which of the following factors places this infant at greatest risk for sepsis?

   A. Maternal age
   B. Gestational size
   C. Apgar score
   D. Length of time membranes were ruptured
   E. Gestational age

4.2 A 25-day-old female infant is brought to the emergency department for fever of 101°F (38.3°C) at home. The baby was born vaginally at full term and was appropriate for gestational age. Maternal GBS was negative. Apgar scores were 8 and 9. The mother noticed the baby has had decreased feeding over the previous few days and has been sleeping more. Which of the following is the most appropriate initial choice of antibiotics for this infant?

   A. Oral amoxicillin
   B. Vancomycin
   C. Ampicillin
   D. Ampicillin and cefotaxime
   E. Ampicillin and gentamicin

4.3 A 12-hour-old infant who has been feeding poorly becomes tachypneic with grunting. Which of the following initial tests has the lowest diagnostic yield?

   A. Chest radiograph
   B. Complete blood count
   C. Urine culture
   D. Blood culture
   E. Glucose level

4.4 A 7-day-old infant is seen in the emergency department for fever and poor feeding. The baby was delivered vaginally 2 hours after the mother arrived to hospital. The delivery was a 36 weeks of gestation and the birth weight was 2900 g. Maternal laboratory test results were negative. The most likely organism causing this patient's symptoms is:

   A. Group B *Streptococcus* (GBS)
   B. *Listeria monocytogenes*
   C. *Staphylococcus aureus*
   D. *Streptococcus pneumoniae*
   E. *Haemophilus influenza*

ANSWERS

4.1 **E.** Prematurity places this baby at greater risk for sepsis. Young maternal age, low birth weight, rupture of membranes greater than 18 hours, initial Apgar less than 5, and maternal fever are additional risk factors for sepsis.

4.2 **D.** This patient may have late-onset bacterial infection, likely GBS; she should be admitted for sepsis evaluation and IV antibiotics. The best initial treatment in this age group is broad-spectrum antibiotics such as ampicillin and cefotaxime. If cultures are positive for GBS, antibiotic therapy can be narrowed to penicillin G.

4.3 **C.** Urine cultures are not usually obtained in the workup of early onset sepsis. Urinary tract infections are rare in the first few days of life.

4.4 **A.** GBS is the most common pathogen to cause neonatal sepsis in infants aged 0 to 3 months.

CLINICAL PEARLS

▶ Sepsis in the neonate can present with nonspecific findings of temperature instability, tachypnea, poor feeding, bradycardia, hypotension, and hypoglycemia.

▶ Early-onset neonatal infection (occurring in the first 6 days of life) usually is caused by organisms of the maternal genitourinary system, including GBS, *E coli*, *H influenzae*, and *L monocytogenes*. Pneumonia and sepsis are common presentations; GBS is the leading cause.

▶ Late-onset neonatal infection (occurring between 7 and 90 days of life) is often caused by organisms found in the infant's environment, including coagulase-negative staphylococci, *S aureus*, *E coli*, *Klebsiella* sp, *Pseudomonas* sp, *Enterobacter* sp, *Candida*, GBS, *Serratia* sp, *Acinetobacter* sp, and anaerobic bacteria.

▶ Treatment of early-onset neonatal infection usually includes penicillin and an aminoglycoside, whereas the treatment of late-onset disease consists of a β-lactamase–resistant antibiotic (such as vancomycin) and often a third-generation cephalosporin.

▶ The incidence of early-onset GBS infection is decreasing, likely because of the widespread implementation of GBS risk–reduction guidelines.

REFERENCES

Brady MT. Human immunodeficiency virus type 1 infection. In: Rudolph CD, Rudolph AM, Lister G, First LR, Gershon AA, eds. *Rudolph's Pediatrics*. 22nd ed. New York, NY: McGraw-Hill; 2011: 1164-1170.

Braverman RS. Ophthalmia neonatorum. In: Hay WW, Levin MJ, Sondheimer JM, Deterding RR. *Current Diagnosis & Treatment: Pediatrics*. 20th ed. New York, NY: McGraw-Hill; 2011:418-419.

Centers for Disease Control and Prevention. Prevention of perinatal group B streptococcal disease. Revised guidelines from CDC. MMWR Recomm Rep. 2010;59 (RR-10):1-32.

Edwards MS. Group B streptococcal infections. In: Rudolph CD, Rudolph AM, Lister G, First LR, Gershon AA, eds. *Rudolph's Pediatrics.* 22nd ed. New York, NY: McGraw-Hill; 2011:1097-1099.

Gallagher PG, Baltimore RS. Sepsis neonatorum. In: McMillan JA, Feigin RD, DeAngelis CD, Jones MD, eds. *Oski's Pediatrics: Principles and Practice.* 4th ed. Philadelphia, PA: Lippincott Williams & Wilkins; 2006:482-492.

Guinn AG. Red eye. In: Rudolph CD, Rudolph AM, Lister G, First LR, Gershon AA, eds. *Rudolph's Pediatrics.* 22nd ed. New York, NY: McGraw-Hill; 2011:2300-2304.

Lachenauer CS, Wessels MR. Group B *Streptococcus.* In: Kleigman RM, Stanton BF, St. Geme JW, Schor NF, Behrman RE, eds. *Nelson Textbook of Pediatrics.* 19th ed. Philadelphia, PA: WB Saunders; 2011:925-928.

McFarland EJ. Human immunodeficiency virus infection. In: Hay WW, Levin MJ, Sondheimer JM, Deterding RR. *Current Diagnosis & Treatment: Pediatrics.* 20th ed. New York, NY: McGraw-Hill; 2011:1148-1158.

Moylett EH, Shearer WT. Pediatric human immunodeficiency virus infection. In: McMillan JA, Feigin RD, DeAngelis CD, Jones MD, eds. *Oski's Pediatrics: Principles and Practice.* 4th ed. Philadelphia, PA: Lippincott Williams & Wilkins; 2006:942-952.

Ogle JW, Anderson MS. Group B streptococcal infections. In: Hay WW, Levin MJ, Sondheimer JM, Deterding RR. *Current Diagnosis & Treatment: Pediatrics.* 20th ed. New York, NY: McGraw-Hill; 2011:1163-1166.

Olitsky SE, Hug D, Plummer LS, Stass-Isern M. Disorders of the conjunctiva. In: Kleigman RM, Stanton BF, St. Geme JW, Schor NF, Behrman RE, eds. *Nelson Textbook of Pediatrics.* 19th ed. Philadelphia, PA: WB Saunders; 2011:2166-2169.

Thilo EH, Rosenberg AA. Infections in the newborn infant. In: Hay WW, Levin MJ, Sondheimer JM, Deterding RR. *Current Diagnosis & Treatment: Pediatrics.* 20th ed. New York, NY: McGraw-Hill; 2011:48-56.

Traboulsi EI. Ophthalmia neonatorum. In: McMillan JA, Feigin RD, DeAngelis CD, Jones MD, eds. *Oski's Pediatrics: Principles and Practice.* 4th ed. Philadelphia, PA: Lippincott Williams & Wilkins; 2006:811-812.

Yogev R, Chadwick E. Acquired immunodeficiency syndrome (human immunodeficiency virus). In: Kleigman RM, Stanton BF, St. Geme JW, Schor NF, Behrman RE, eds. *Nelson Textbook of Pediatrics.* 19th ed. Philadelphia, PA: WB Saunders; 2011:1157-1177.

A 3740-g infant is delivered vaginally after an uncomplicated 38-week gestation. Health care providers have immediate difficulty in determining whether the infant is a boy or girl. There appear to be small scrotal sacs that resemble enlarged labia and no palpable testes, with either a microphallus and hypospadias or an enlarged clitoris. No vaginal opening is apparent. The remainder of the examination is normal.

► What is the most likely diagnosis?
► What is the next step in evaluation?

ANSWERS TO CASE 5:

Ambiguous Genitalia

Summary: A full-term newborn has ambiguous genitalia.

- **Most likely diagnosis:** Congenital adrenal hyperplasia (CAH).
- **Next step in evaluation:** Karyotype, serum electrolyte levels, and serum 17-hydroxyprogesterone level.

ANALYSIS

Objectives

1. Understand the underlying causes of ambiguous genitalia.
2. Describe factors that influence gender assignment in infants with ambiguous genitalia.
3. Describe the treatment and follow-up of infants after gender assignment.
4. Understand the importance of timely diagnosis and treatment of CAH.

Considerations

This neonate with sexual ambiguity represents a psychosocial emergency. Upon proper gender assignment for rearing and appropriate medical management, individuals born with ambiguous genitalia should be able to lead well-adjusted lives and satisfactory sex lives. Making a correct diagnosis as early as possible is critical. **Gender assignment** in the neonate born with sexual ambiguity should be influenced by the possibility of achieving **unambiguous and sexually useful genital structures.** Clear and comprehensive discussions with the parents, focusing on their understanding, anxieties, and religious, social, and cultural beliefs, are critical for an appropriate gender assignment. Once gender is assigned, it should be reinforced by appropriate surgical, hormonal, and psychological measures.

APPROACH TO:

Child with Ambiguous Genitalia

DEFINITIONS

CONGENITAL ADRENAL HYPERPLASIA (CAH): Autosomal recessive disorder of adrenal steroid production with an enzymatic deficiency (majority 21-hydroxylase) causing inadequate production of cortisol, excessive production of androgenic intermediary metabolites, and virilization; may be associated with electrolyte disturbance and hemodynamic instability.

HERMAPHRODITISM: Discrepancy between gonad morphology and external genitalia.

INTERSEX STATE: Infant with ambiguous genitalia.

MICROPHALLUS: Penis size below the fifth percentile for age; neonate with a stretched penile length of less than 2 cm.

VIRILIZATION: Masculinization where infant girls exhibit clitoromegaly, labial fusion, and labial pigmentation; infant boys usually appear normal.

CLINICAL APPROACH

Evaluation of the infant with ambiguous genitalia must occur rapidly to alleviate family anxiety. An endocrinologist, clinical geneticist, urologist, and psychiatrist are essential members of the intersex evaluation team. The **goals of the evaluation** are to determine the **etiology** of the intersex problem, **assign gender,** and **intervene with surgical or other treatment** as soon as possible. Intersex abnormalities include the following:

Female pseudohermaphroditism: 46,XX karyotype; largest neonatal group with ambiguous genitalia; predominant etiology is CAH; rarer etiologies include exposure to maternal androgens or progestins and congenital vaginal absence with uterine absence or abnormality; degree of masculinization depends on stage of development at time of androgenic stimulation and potency and duration of exposure.

Male pseudohermaphroditism: 46,XY karyotype; primary etiology is decreased androgen binding to target tissues (androgen insensitivity syndrome); other etiologies include testosterone dyssynthesis and 5α-reductase or dihydrotestosterone deficiency; phenotypically normal females with functioning testicular tissue, variable incomplete virilization of genitalia, and short, pouch-like vaginas; typically diagnosed at puberty when primary amenorrhea noted; maintain as females and offer vaginoplasty.

True hermaphroditism: About 70% 46,XX and remainder 46,XY or mosaic; comprises less than 10% of all intersex cases; bilateral ovotestes or ovary and testis on opposite sides; testicular tissue determines virilization degree; gender assignment based on genitalia appearance (~75% assigned male gender); contradictory reproductive structures removed in older patients with assigned gender.

Mixed gonadal dysgenesis: Most 46,XY/45,XO karyotype; testis with Sertoli and Leydig cells, but no germinal elements, on one side and streak gonad on other; hypospadias, partial labioscrotal fusion, and undescended testes most common (incompletely virilized male appearance); usually assigned female gender and undergo gonadectomy (25% of streak gonads develop malignancy); assign as male if testis descended.

Assessment

After obtaining a careful history, a family pedigree should be constructed to identify consanguinity and to document cases of genital ambiguity, infertility, unexpected pubertal changes, or inguinal hernias. Physical findings could support a genetically transmitted intersex condition. The history of an unexplained neonatal death may suggest a family history of CAH. Maternal exposure to endogenous or exogenous androgens should be investigated.

A thorough physical examination is crucial in determining the diagnosis and making the most reasonable gender assignment. A critical physical finding is the presence or absence of a testis in a labioscrotal compartment. Other physical findings include appearance of the labioscrotal folds (hyperpigmentation common in infants with CAH), phallic size and location of urethral opening, and palpation of a uterus on bimanual examination. Evidence of failure to thrive (failure to regain birth weight, progressive weight loss), vomiting, and dehydration in the infant with ambiguous genitalia may signify CAH. **Early consideration of CAH in the infant with ambiguous genitalia is important, given the disease can be life threatening; timely diagnosis and intervention (fluid resuscitation, electrolyte repletion, adrenocorticoid replacement) are paramount to survival.**

Karyotype analysis using activated lymphocytes is an important first step in the laboratory evaluation of infants with ambiguous genitalia. Results with a high degree of accuracy typically can be available in less than 48 hours. To determine mosaicism, repeat studies on multiple tissues may be necessary. If CAH is suspected, biochemical markers might include an elevated **serum 17-hydroxyprogesterone level.** Plasma testosterone levels alone usually are not helpful. Urinary steroids and plasma androgens, measured before and after administration of corticotropin (adrenocorticotropic hormone [ACTH]) and human chorionic gonadotropin (hCG), help to determine whether a block in testosterone synthesis or 5α-reductase deficiency exists.

An ultrasonogram or pelvic magnetic resonance imaging (MRI), urogenital sinus x-ray after contrast injection, and fiberoptic endoscopy may also aid in the evaluation. Laparoscopy usually is not necessary in the newborn because primary emphasis is placed on the external genitalia and the possibilities for adequate sexual function in assigning gender.

Treatment

The major treatment consideration for infants with ambiguous genitalia is the possibility of achieving functionally normal external genitalia by surgical and hormonal means, with judicious emphasis on cosmetic appearance. **Because the presence of ambiguous external genitalia may reinforce doubt about the sexual identity of the infant, reconstructive surgery is performed as early as medically and surgically feasible, usually before 6 months of age.** Feminizing genitoplasty is the most common surgical procedure performed in female pseudohermaphrodites, in true hermaphrodites, and in male pseudohermaphrodites reared as females. The goal of this surgery is to reduce the size of the clitoris while maintaining vascularity and innervation, feminizing the labioscrotal folds, and ultimately creating a vagina. Because of the high incidence of gonadal tumors in individuals with certain forms of gonadal dysgenesis, gonadectomy performed concurrently with the initial repair of the external genitalia is mandatory. **A male with hypospadias often requires multiple procedures to create a phallic urethra. Circumcision is avoided** in these individuals because the foreskin tissue is commonly used for reconstruction.

If steroid production is the underlying etiology of the intersex problem, treatment is provided to prevent further virilization. **Administration of hydrocortisone to individuals with CAH helps to inhibit excessive production of androgens and further virilization.** Hormone substitution therapy in hypogonadal patients is prescribed so that secondary sexual characteristics develop at the expected time of puberty. Oral estrogenic hormone substitution is initiated in females, and repository injections of testosterone are given to males. With the exception of some female pseudohermaphrodites and true hermaphrodites reared as females, disorders that cause ambiguous genitalia usually lead to infertility.

COMPREHENSION QUESTIONS

5.1   A 3650-g term infant has ambiguous genitalia, including an enlarged clitoris or microphallus and one palpable testis in the labioscrotal folds. Sonogram reveals a uterus and ovaries. Which of the following is the most likely explanation for the child's ambiguous genitalia?

A.   Aromatase deficiency

B.   Congenital adrenal hyperplasia

C.   Female pseudohermaphroditism

D.   Male pseudohermaphroditism

E.   True hermaphroditism

5.2   A mother brings in her 1-week-old son who has vomited four times over the last 24 hours. He has no fever or diarrhea. The infant is breast-feeding poorly and is "floppy" per the mother. He has had only one wet diaper in the last 12 hours. Physical examination reveals a lethargic infant who has lost 250 g since birth, with pulse of 110 beats/min, dry oral mucosa, and no skin turgor. You suspect a form of adrenogenital syndrome precipitating salt wasting. Which of the following serum levels should be checked after hemodynamic stabilization and electrolyte measurement?

A.   Cortisol

B.   Pregnenolone

C.   ACTH

D.   17-hydroxyprogesterone

E.   Testosterone

5.3. A mother brings in her 15-year-old daughter because she has never started her periods. She otherwise is healthy and takes no medications. Her past medical history is unremarkable except for inguinal hernia repair as an infant. Family history is unremarkable. She is at the 75th percentile for height and weight, has tanner stage IV breast development, and has no pubic or axillary hair development. Her anogenital examination reveals a short, pocket-like vaginal opening. Which of the following is consistent with her likely diagnosis?

A. 46, XY genotype with male phenotype

B. Bilateral ovaries

C. Normal or elevated testosterone level

D. Delayed puberty

E. Abnormal developmental milestones

5.4. You examine a full-term 3780-g newborn in the nursery and notice that he has unilateral cryptorchidism and a microphallus with hypospadias. You suspect mixed gonadal dysgenesis. Which of the following is most associated with this condition?

A. Normal spermatogenesis

B. Increased risk for germ cell tumor

C. Abnormal gross motor development

D. Umbilical hernia development

E. Normal seminiferous tubules

ANSWERS

5.1 **E.** The gonad in the labioscrotal fold suggests a testis, but a uterus and an ovary on sonography are highly suggestive of a true hermaphrodite. Gender assignment in this case should be based on the possibility of surgical correction of the external genitalia. Assignment of female sex and an attempt to preserve ovarian tissue is appropriate.

5.2 **D.** Male infants with salt-losing CAH develop clinical symptoms similar to pyloric stenosis, intestinal obstruction, heart disease, cow's milk intolerance, and other causes of failure to thrive. Their genitalia appear normal. A serum 17-hydroxyprogesterone level typically is elevated and is the first enzymatic assay considered when CAH is suspected. Without appropriate treatment (hydrocortisone, mineralocorticoid, and sodium supplementation), cardiovascular collapse and death may occur within a few weeks. Many states have neonatal screening programs for CAH, yet infants with salt-losing CAH (21-hydroxylase deficiency) can become very ill and die before the screening results are known.

5.3 **C.** Testicular feminization results from decreased androgen binding to target tissues or androgen insensitivity, the latter being the most common form of male pseudohermaphroditism. Patients have functional testicular tissue, with normal or high testosterone levels. They also have 46,XY karyotypes, yet appear as phenotypically normal females with short or atretic vaginas. Maintaining female gender assignment is appropriate, and vaginoplasty is frequently needed after puberty. Puberty typically is not delayed, and linear growth and developmental milestones are usually normal.

5.4 **B.** A testis typically has immature seminiferous tubules, spermatogenesis is often impaired, and a higher risk for testicular cancer is noted in mixed gonadal dysgenesis. As in other conditions, undescended testes can be associated with inguinal herniation. Although a history of sexual ambiguity in mixed gonadal dysgenesis may impact psychosocial development to some degree, abnormal neuromuscular development is not a typical finding.

CLINICAL PEARLS

▶ The goal of evaluating a neonate with sexual ambiguity is to determine the etiology of the intersex problem, assign gender, and intervene with surgical or other treatment when appropriate and as soon as possible.

▶ Treatment of sexual ambiguity is directed toward achieving cosmetically and functionally normal external genitalia by surgical and hormonal means.

▶ Reconstructive surgery for a patient with ambiguous genitalia is performed as early as medically and surgically feasible, usually before the age of 6 months.

▶ CAH is potentially life threatening in the first several weeks of life, if not considered, evaluated, and treated in a timely manner.

REFERENCES

Ali O, Donohoue PA. Hypofunction of the testes. In: Kliegman RM, Stanton BF, St. Geme JW, Schor NF, Behrman RE, eds. *Nelson Textbook of Pediatrics*. 19th ed. Philadelphia, PA: WB Saunders; 2011:1943-1951.

Diamond DA. Pediatric urology. In: Wein AJ, Kavassi LR, Novick AC, Partin AW, Peters CA, eds. *Campbell's Urology*. 10th ed. Philadelphia, PA: WB Saunders; 2012:3597-3629.

Donohoue PA. Disorders of sex development. In: Kliegman RM, Stanton BF, St. Geme JW, Schor NF, Behrman RE, eds. *Nelson Textbook of Pediatrics*. 19th ed. Philadelphia, PA: WB Saunders; 2011:1959-1968.

Grumbach MM. Disorders of sexual development (DSD). In: Rudolph CD, Rudolph AM, Lister GE, First R, Gershon AA, eds. *Rudolph's Pediatrics*. 22nd ed. New York, NY: McGraw-Hill; 2011: 2063-2074.

Laufer MR, Goldstein DP. Pediatric and adolescent gynecology—Part I. In: Ryan KJ, Berkowitz RS, Barbieri RL, Dunaif A, eds. *Kistner's Gynecology and Women's Health*. 7th ed. St. Louis, MO: Mosby; 1999:233-259.

Lee PA, Houk CP, Ahmed SF, et al. Consensus statement on management of intersex disorders. International Consensus Conference on Intersex. *Pediatrics*. 2006;118:e488.

White PC. Disorders of the adrenal glands. In: Kliegman RM, Stanton BF, St. Geme JW, Schor NF, Behrman RE, eds. *Nelson Textbook of Pediatrics*. 19th ed. Philadelphia, PA: WB Saunders; 2011:1923-1930.

A 6-day-old girl is brought to the emergency room by her mother for a 12-hour history of irritability, decreased oral intake, and fever of 100.4°F (38°C). She was delivered vaginally at 39-weeks gestation to a gravida 2, para 1 woman after an uncomplicated pregnancy with routine prenatal care. The mother denies any past medical history, illness, or infections during pregnancy; her only medication was prenatal vitamin. On examination, the infant has a temperature of 100.2°F (37.9°C), heart rate 145 beats/min, respiratory rate 64 breaths/min, and she is fussy with any movement despite being swaddled. The only findings on physical examination are about 10 small 2-mm, fluid-filled lesions surrounded by an erythematous base on her right shoulder (Figure 6–1). Shortly after her blood, urine, and cerebrospinal fluid (CSF) studies are obtained, she exhibits shaking of the right side of her body that then generalizes. The episode lasts approximately 20 seconds, and afterward she is somnolent. Lumbar puncture results show 850 white blood cells with 90% lymphocytes, 80 red blood cells, and a protein of 200 mg/dL. Computed tomography (CT) of the head is normal. Her complete blood cell count reveals a platelet count of 57,000/mm³ and her ALT is 112 U/L and AST 108 U/L. Her chest x-ray has patchy bilateral ground-glass opacities.

▶ What is the most likely diagnosis?
▶ What is the next step in management?

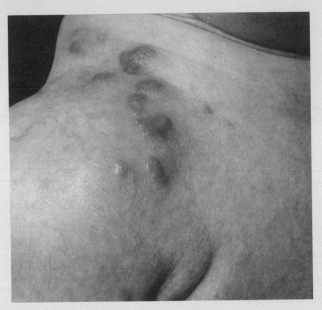

Figure 6–1. Vesicular eruption. (*Reproduced, with permission, from Wolff K, Johnson RA, Saavedra AP. Fitzpatrick's Color Atlas and Synopsis of Clinical Dermatology. 7th ed. New York: McGraw-Hill Education, 2013. Figure 27-40.*)

ANSWERS TO CASE 6:
Neonatal Herpes Simplex Virus Infection

Summary: A 6-day-old previously healthy infant with fever, irritability, decreased oral intake, and **vesicles** on her shoulder has an episode of seizure-like activity. Laboratory studies reveal **lymphocytic meningitis**, thrombocytopenia, **transaminitis**, and **pneumonitis**.

- **Most likely diagnosis:** Neonatal herpes simplex virus (HSV) infection, disseminated.

- **Next step in management:** High-dose intravenous **acyclovir** along with empiric antibiotics is administered until more definitive results are available. Even with early antiviral treatment, mortality is 20% in neonates with disseminated disease.

ANALYSIS

Objectives

1. Recognize the different presentations of neonatal herpes infection including its role as a "TORCH" infection.

2. Know how to diagnose neonatal herpes infection.

3. Know the appropriate management of neonatal herpes infection.

Considerations

A **young infant with fever and irritability is presumed to have a serious bacterial or viral infection.** Bacterial causes in this age include group B *Streptococcus, Listeria,* and gram-negative pathogens such as *Escherichia coli.* The history in this patient of a **fever, a focal seizure,** the finding of **vesicles** on the infant's shoulder, and **the laboratory abnormalities described make HSV the most likely pathogen.** The absence of a maternal history of herpes is not unusual; only 15% to 20% of mothers of HSV-infected infants have a history of herpes and only approximately 25% of these mothers have symptoms at delivery. The risk of maternal passage of HSV to the neonate is 25% to 60% in cases of primary herpes infection because the viral inoculum in the genital tract is high and protective antibody is not present. Conversely, the risk of transmission is less than 2% if the mother is having reactivation of infection at the time of delivery.

Blood, urine, and CSF specimens are obtained for routine bacterial cultures. Investigation for an inborn error of metabolism would be needed if this patient did not have fever, vesicles, or meningoencephalitis. Workup for suspected neonatal HSV infection includes HSV surface cultures obtained from the conjunctiva, nasopharynx, mouth, rectum, and from any vesicular lesion. CSF and blood are tested by polymerase chain reaction (PCR) for HSV DNA. A complete blood count, metabolic panel, and coagulation studies may reveal abnormalities such as cytopenias, transaminitis, and disseminated intravascular coagulation (DIC).

An electroencephalogram (EEG) is indicated because of the seizure, and in HSV infection it is often abnormal early in the disease course while neuroimaging studies may not show abnormalities for several days.

APPROACH TO:
Neonatal Herpes Infection

DEFINITIONS

NEONATE: Infant who is 60 days old or younger.

VESICLE: A fluid-filled elevation in the epidermis that measures less than 1 cm.

PRIMARY HERPES INFECTION: HSV infection in a previously seronegative host. Most primary infections are subclinical, but they can cause localized lesions or severe systemic symptoms.

"TORCH": An acronym to recall several of the intrauterine infections associated with birth anomalies. T = toxoplasmosis, O = other (syphilis, varicella), R = rubella, C = cytomegalovirus, H = herpes simplex virus and HIV.

CLINICAL APPROACH

Approximately 20% to 30% of American women of childbearing age have antibodies to HSV-2, with a higher rate in women of lower socioeconomic groups and those in crowded living conditions. Approximately 75% of neonatal herpes cases are caused by HSV-2, and it is associated with greater morbidity among survivors than HSV-1. Neonatal infection is **most commonly acquired during delivery** but can also be acquired postnatally from an infected caregiver's mouth or hand. **Intrauterine infection** is rare but an affected infant would be expected to be born with **skin vesicles** (or their scars), **chorioretinitis, and microcephaly**.

Other congenital infections have symptoms that overlap with those of HSV but none will also exhibit vesicles. Toxoplasmosis may be characterized by chorioretinitis, seizure, CSF pleocytosis, and thrombocytopenia but the CT scan will show diffuse intracranial calcifications with a predilection for the basal ganglia and obstructive hydrocephalus. Congenital rubella can also present with meningoencephalitis, microcephaly, seizure, and thrombocytopenia but would be characterized by cataracts and a purpuric rash (blue-gray nodules known as "blueberry muffin rash"). Congenital cytomegalovirus (CMV) may exhibit meningoencephalitis, chorioretinitis, microcephaly, seizure, pneumonitis, transaminitis, and thrombocytopenia but CT demonstrates periventricular calcifications and the blueberry muffin rash. Congenital syphilis may have symptoms of chorioretinitis, aseptic meningitis, pneumonitis, transaminitis, thrombocytopenia, and fever; the rash is characteristically maculopapular.

The three presentations of neonatal HSV disease are (1) localized skin, eye, and mouth (SEM) involvement; (2) central nervous system (CNS) disease; or (3) disseminated disease. SEM usually appears at 1 to 2 weeks of life; it requires intravenous acyclovir to prevent progression to one of the other presentations. Lumbar puncture for cell count and HSV PCR must be done at the time of diagnosis to exclude the presence of CNS disease. **CNS disease typically manifests at 2 to 3 weeks of life. Fever occurs in less than half of infants with CNS disease and only 60% of cases will have vesicles.** The infant will be lethargic, irritable, or have seizures. Recognition of the symptoms and laboratory findings is important as 50% of neonates without treatment will die. **Disseminated** disease has multiple signs and symptoms in **1- to 2-week-old neonate:** fever, lethargy, irritability, apnea, a bulging fontanelle, or seizures (focal or generalized). **Skin vesicles** will be present in approximately two-thirds of cases. **Hepatitis, pneumonitis, shock, and DIC** occur in severe cases. An ophthalmologic examination is necessary with any form of HSV infection to detect chorioretinitis.

Viral surface cultures swabbed from conjunctivae, mouth, nasopharynx, and anus in addition to PCR of CSF are the most useful diagnostic tests. Any vesicle fluid should be sent for HSV culture and PCR testing; blood should also be sent for PCR testing. Serologic tests for herpes virus are not helpful in the acute setting because titers rise late in the infection's course. Tzanck preparation of lesions and antigen detection methods applied to the specimens can aid in rapid diagnosis, but the sensitivity is low. Infected individuals often have moderate peripheral leukocytosis, elevated serum transaminase levels, and thrombocytopenia. When the CNS is involved, the CSF frequently contains an elevated number of red cells, lymphocytes, and protein; CSF glucose usually is normal but may be reduced. EEG shows characteristic patterns in acutely affected infants, and brain CT will become abnormal as the disease progresses.

HSV infection most commonly occurs during delivery so **if the woman has an outbreak** of visible lesions or any symptoms consistent with HSV (paresthesia in a dermatomal pattern), then **cesarean delivery is indicated.** HSV surveillance cultures are not recommended in pregnant women because those at greatest risk for infecting their infants do not have a history of prior infection. Suppressive antiviral therapy starting at 36 weeks of gestation can reduce how many symptomatic recurrences the mother has, but it does not completely eliminate viral shedding and does not prevent neonatal infection.

Parenteral acyclovir is the preferred treatment for any neonatal HSV infection. It can stop the viral replication at the site of inoculation (skin, mouth, nares, eyes). Otherwise, HSV can spread in the neonate to the respiratory tract, down neurons, or enter the bloodstream, allowing hematogenous infection of the liver, adrenals, and CNS. Treatment is for 14 days in SEM disease but a minimum of 21 days with CNS or disseminated disease. Ophthalmologic involvement warrants the use of topical ophthalmologic drops in addition to parenteral treatment. About 50% of neonates with HSV infection will have skin recurrences over the subsequent 6 months and require daily suppressive acyclovir.

CASE CORRELATION

- See also Case 3 (Neonatal Hyperbilirubinemia) and Case 4 (Group B Streptococcal Infection). Hyperbilirubinemia can be a sign of sepsis in the newborn, and Group B *Streptococcus* is the most common cause of bacterial infection in the newborn period.

COMPREHENSION QUESTIONS

6.1 A 10-day-old infant presents to clinic with a painful, red vesicular rash in the diaper area. He is mildly fussy but afebrile, and he has good oral intake. Which of the following is the most appropriate management of this infant?

A. Hospitalize the patient, obtain HSV surface and vesicle fluid cultures and CSF for HSV culture and PCR, and initiate intravenous acyclovir.

B. Order an EEG and brain MRI immediately.

C. Perform a Tzanck smear and send the patient home if it is negative.

D. Prescribe an antifungal cream and follow-up by telephone in 24 hours.

E. Schedule an appointment with a pediatric dermatologist.

6.2 A woman presents for her first prenatal visit at 9 weeks of gestation. She reports that she is generally healthy, except that she has an outbreak of genital herpes approximately once per year. To prevent transmission of the virus to her infant, her physician should do which of following?

A. Prescribe her daily acyclovir.

B. Order titers to determine if the infection is HSV-1 or HSV-2.

C. Perform weekly genital viral cultures starting at 36-week gestation.

D. Perform a cesarean delivery if herpetic lesions or prodromal symptoms are present when labor has begun.

E. No change in management is indicated; the risk of infant transmission is low even if she has an outbreak at delivery.

6.3 An 18-day-old male infant is brought to the emergency department by his mother with an 8-hour history of poor feeding and decreased wet diapers. On examination, he is afebrile, cries during venipuncture, urine catheterization, and lumbar puncture but otherwise sleeps through the examination. The remainder of his examination, including the skin, is normal. His CSF shows 78 white blood cells, 80% lymphocytes, 40 red blood cells, protein 130 mg/dL, and no bacteria on Gram stain. The mother has a cold sore at her lower lip. Which of the following would *not* be further part of your management?

A. Consult ophthalmology to assess for chorioretinitis.

B. HSV IgG and IgM titers.

C. Surface swab for HSV culture.

D. Complete blood cell count (CBC), ALT, and AST.

E. CSF for HSV culture and PCR.

6.4   A 38-week gestation male infant was precipitously delivered vaginally in the emergency department. Weight and head circumference are less than 5th percentile, and length at 10th percentile. He has hepatosplenomegaly and a petechial rash. Notable laboratory results include platelets of $22,000/mm^3$ and elevated total and direct bilirubin levels. CT of the head shows bilateral intracranial calcifications with several around the basal ganglia and obstructive hydrocephalus. Ophthalmologic examination reveals chorioretinitis. What is the most likely cause of the patient's findings?

A.   Cytomegalovirus

B.   Rubella virus

C.   Toxoplasmosis gondii

D.   Herpes simplex virus

E.   Treponema pallidum

ANSWERS

6.1   **A.** In contrast to children and adults, neonates with suspected herpes skin lesions require parenteral antiviral therapy to prevent more serious sequelae as well as CSF analysis to define the extent of disease. HSV PCR of the CSF is the standard for diagnosis. Tzanck smears have low sensitivity and EEG may have nonspecific findings. The absence of fever does not indicate that the rash is from a benign etiology.

6.2   **D.** Even though the viral transmission risk in the setting of a recurrent HSV outbreak is low, cesarean section is indicated if lesions are present at the time of delivery because of the severity of neonatal HSV disease. Surveillance cultures are not recommended; negative results a few days prior to delivery do not preclude a later outbreak, and results of analysis of a more recently obtained specimen may not be available. Either type 1 or type 2 HSV can cause neonatal infection and disease. Daily antiviral therapy has not been shown to prevent neonatal infection.

6.3   **B.** Serology is not useful for the diagnosis of neonatal herpes infection. Neonatal herpes infection in any presentation should prompt an ophthalmology examination because topical ophthalmic antiviral therapy will be needed in addition to intravenous acyclovir if chorioretinitis or keratitis is present. A surface swab and CSF for HSV culture along with CSF HSV PCR are key steps in diagnosing neonatal HSV infection. Abnormalities in the CBC, ALT, or AST suggest that he has disseminated disease.

6.4   **C.** The triad of hydrocephalus, intracranial calcifications, and chorioretinitis is a classic presentation for congenital toxoplasmosis. With cytomegalovirus, the intracranial calcifications would be in a periventricular distribution and the typical rash would be the blueberry muffin rash. Rubella would be expected to also have the purpuric rash along with cataracts and no CT findings. Herpes would have either vesicles or scarring. Syphilis infection would not have an abnormal CT.

CLINICAL PEARLS

▶ Most infants with neonatal herpes simplex virus are born to mothers without a prior history of herpes simplex virus infection.

▶ The presenting signs and symptoms of neonatal herpes simplex virus may be nonspecific, without any visible herpetic lesions.

▶ Neonates with suspected herpes simplex virus infection should be hospitalized for testing and parenteral antiviral therapy pending test results.

▶ Neonates with herpes simplex virus skin, eye, and mouth (SEM) disease generally have the best outcomes, whereas the majority of infants with central nervous system disease develop neurologic sequelae. Approximately 30% of infants with systemic infection die despite aggressive antiviral therapy.

REFERENCES

American Academy of Pediatrics. Herpes simplex. In: Pickering LK, Baker CJ, Kimberlin DW, Long SS, eds. *Red Book: 2012 Report of the Committee on Infectious Diseases*. 29th ed. Elk Grove Village, IL: American Academy of Pediatrics; 2012:398-408.

Hong DK, Prober CG. Herpes simplex virus infections. In: Rudolph CD, Rudolph AM, Lister GE, First LR, Gershon AA, eds. *Rudolph's Pediatrics*. 22nd ed. New York, NY: McGraw-Hill; 2011:1149-1152.

Kimberlin DW, Palazzi DL, Whitley RJ. Therapy for perinatal and neonatal infections. In: Rudolph CD, Rudolph AM, Lister GE, First LR, Gershon AA, eds. *Rudolph's Pediatrics*. 22nd ed. New York, NY: McGraw-Hill; 2011:902-904.

Stanberry LR. Herpes simplex virus. In: Kliegman RM, Stanton BF, St. Geme III J, Schor N, Behrman R, eds. *Nelson Textbook of Pediatrics*. 19th ed. Philadelphia, PA: WB Saunders; 2011:1097-1104.

CASE 7

A term 3700-g male infant is born vaginally to a 27-year-old gravida 2 mother following an uncomplicated pregnancy. Shortly after birth, he begins to cough, followed by a choking episode, difficulty handling secretions, and cyanosis. During the resuscitation, placement of an orogastric tube meets resistance at 10 cm. He is transferred to the level II nursery for evaluation and management of respiratory distress.

► What is the most likely diagnosis?
► What is the best test for evaluation?

ANSWERS TO CASE 7:

Esophageal Atresia

Summary: A newborn with cough, choking, cyanosis, and inability to undergo passage of an orogastric tube.

- **Most likely diagnosis:** Esophageal atresia, probably with a tracheoesophageal fistula (TEF).

- **Best test for diagnosis:** A chest and abdomen radiograph will most commonly show the orogastric tube coiled in the esophageal blind pouch with or without air in the stomach.

ANALYSIS

Objectives

1. Become familiar with the presentation of TEF.

2. Understand the anatomic variants of TEF.

3. Understand emergency management of newborns with TEF.

Considerations

In this newborn with choking and coughing, esophageal atresia is suspected when there is failure to pass the orogastric tube. Infants with esophageal atresia cannot handle oral secretions and require constant esophageal pouch drainage to prevent aspiration. They are monitored in the neonatal intensive care unit while awaiting surgical intervention.

APPROACH TO:

Esophageal Atresia

DEFINITIONS

ASSOCIATION: Sporadic occurrence of two or more clinical features occurring together more commonly than would be expected, but without an identifiable cause.

POLYHYDRAMNIOS: Diagnosis of an increased amount of amniotic fluid.

SYNDROME: A constellation of features having a common cause (such as the features of Down syndrome being caused by a trisomy 21).

CLINICAL APPROACH

Esophageal atresia occurs in 1 in 2500 to 3000 live births, usually accompanied by TEF. Prenatal ultrasound findings of polyhydramnios, absence of a fluid-filled stomach, and a distended esophageal pouch are nonspecific findings suggestive of esophageal atresia. Five different TEF anatomic variants occur; the most common (87%) includes proximal atresia (esophageal pouch) with a distal fistula (Figure 7–1).

Infants with TEF usually present in the newborn period with excessive oral secretions and coughing, choking, and cyanosis secondary to aspirated secretions or with initial feeds. Infants with the **"H-type" fistula** (~4% of cases) often present later in life with recurrent aspiration pneumonia or feeding difficulty. Other congenital anomalies occur in approximately 30% to 50% of TEF patients, and a search for them is undertaken. The most common association is the **VACTERL or VATER association** (vertebral abnormality, anal imperforation, cardiac, tracheoesophageal

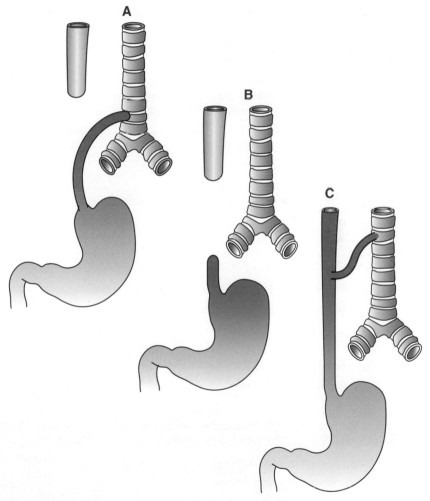

Figure 7–1. Types of esophageal atresia/tracheoesophageal fistula.
A. Proximal esophageal atresia with distal fistula (80%-90%).
B. Esophageal atresia (10%).
C. H-type tracheoesophageal fistula (3%-4%).

fistula, radial, renal and limb anomalies). In addition to esophageal abnormalities, cardiac anomalies are the next most common malformation (~23%) seen with VACTERL or VATER association. Other conditions notable for TEF include CHARGE (coloboma of the eye, heart defects, atresia of the nasal choanae, retardation of growth and/or development, genital and/or urinary abnormalities, and ear abnormalities and deafness) association, DiGeorge syndrome, and trisomy 18, 21, and 13.

Neonates with TEF or esophageal atresia are at risk for respiratory compromise due to aspiration. The esophageal pouch requires constant suctioning while awaiting surgery to ligate the fistula and anastomose the esophagus. Staged surgery is required if anatomic conditions preclude primary anastomosis. Postsurgical complications include leak and stenosis of anastomosis, fistula recurrence, esophageal dysmotility, and chronic gastroesophageal reflux is common.

COMPREHENSION QUESTIONS

7.1   A 2-hour-old term newborn male has coughing, choking, and cyanosis prior to feeding. A nasogastric tube is placed and meets resistance at 10 cm. Prenatal history is significant for polyhydramnios. Which of the following is most likely to be found in this infant?

A.   Congenital cataracts

B.   Gingival hyperplasia

C.   Hepatosplenomegaly

D.   Microcephaly

E.   Fusion of two lower thoracic vertebral bodies

7.2   An infant with a history of recurrent pneumonia is diagnosed with TEF at 8 months of age. Which of the following statements is correct?

A.   The infant most likely has an "H-type" TEF.

B.   The infant most likely has proximal esophageal atresia with distal fistula.

C.   The infant likely has a previously undetected, associated finding of imperforate anus.

D.   The infant is unlikely to have gastroesophageal reflux.

E.   The infant is likely to have cystic fibrosis.

7.3   A 2-year-old girl with a history of esophageal atresia and a ventricular septal defect is hospitalized with *Pneumocystis carinii* pneumonia. Her immunodeficiency is likely a result of which of the following?

A.   Bruton agammaglobulinemia

B.   Chronic granulomatous disease

C.   DiGeorge syndrome

D.   Hyperimmunoglobulin E syndrome

E.   Severe combined immunodeficiency syndrome

7.4   A 2-year-old boy, living with new foster parents for 3 weeks, has become progressively short of breath. When he first arrived at their home, he was active
and playful, but now he is too tired to play. They have few details, but they
know that he had neonatal surgery for a problem with his "esophagus being
connected to his lungs" and that he takes no medications. On examination, he
is afebrile, diaphoretic, tachycardic, and tachypneic. His symptoms can most
likely be attributed to which of the following?

A.   Adjustment disorder

B.   Heart failure secondary to ventricular septal defect

C.   Kawasaki disease

D.   Reactive airway disease

E.   Rheumatic heart disease

ANSWERS

7.1   E. The infant probably has esophageal atresia. VATER or VACTERL association, as described in the case, can have vertebral anomalies such as fused or
bifid vertebral bodies. None of the other findings listed is commonly associated with VATER or VACTERL.

7.2   A. This infant likely has an H-type TEF, found later in infancy with recurrent pneumonias and/or feeding difficulty. Patients with esophageal atresia
and distal fistula present in the first hours of life because of their inability to
swallow oropharyngeal secretions. Infants with imperforate anus also present
as neonates. All patients with TEF are at high risk for gastroesophageal reflux.

7.3   C. DiGeorge syndrome (thymic hypoplasia) results from abnormal third and
fourth pharyngeal pouch formation during fetal development. Neighboring
structures formed during the same fetal growth period are often affected.
Associated conditions include anomalies of the great vessels, esophageal atresia, bifid uvula, congenital heart disease, short philtrum, hypertelorism, anti-
mongoloid slant palpebrae, mandibular hypoplasia, and low-set, notched ears.
DiGeorge syndrome may present in neonates as hypocalcemic seizures because
of parathyroid hypoplasia.

7.4   B. This child likely had undergone TEF repair and has associated congenital
heart disease with heart failure symptoms.

CLINICAL PEARLS

▶ VACTERL or VATER association, vertebral (abnormality), anal (imperforation), tracheoesophageal (fistula), radial, renal, and limb (anomaly), is often seen in patients with tracheoesophageal fistula.

▶ Esophageal atresia is associated with CHARGE (coloboma of the eye, heart defects, atresia of the nasal choanae, retardation of growth and/or development, genital and/or urinary abnormalities, and ear abnormalities and deafness) association, DiGeorge syndrome, and trisomies 13, 18, and 21.

▶ The H-type tracheoesophageal fistula often presents later in infancy as recurrent pneumonitis and can be difficult to diagnose.

REFERENCES

Khan S, Orenstein S. Esophageal atresia and tracheoesophageal fistula. In: Kliegman RM, Stanton BF, St. Geme JW, Schor NF, Behrman RE, eds. *Nelson Textbook of Pediatrics*. 19th ed. Philadelphia, PA: WB Saunders; 2011:1262-1263.

Lal DR. Anatomic disorders of the esophagus. In: Rudolph CD, Rudolph AM, Lister GE, First LR, Gershon AA, eds. *Rudolph's Pediatrics*. 22nd ed. New York, NY: McGraw-Hill; 2011:1400-1403.

McEvoy CF. Developmental disorders of gastrointestinal function. In: McMillan JA, Feigin RD, DeAngelis CD, Jones MD, eds. *Oski's Pediatrics: Principles and Practice*. 4th ed. Philadelphia, PA: Lippincott Williams & Wilkins; 2006:369-370.

A term male is born at 38 weeks of gestation by a scheduled repeat caesarean section prior to the onset of labor. The infant's mother had good prenatal care including vaginal cultures negative for group B *Streptococcus*. At the delivery, the amniotic fluid was clear and was not foul smelling. Apgar scores are 8 at 1 minute and 8 at 5 minutes. Within the first hour of birth, he has tachypnea, nasal flaring, and mild retractions. Chest auscultation reveals good air movement bilaterally; a few rales are noted.

▶ What is the most likely diagnosis?
▶ What is the best management for this condition?

ANSWERS TO CASE 8:

Transient Tachypnea of the Newborn

Summary: A term newborn born by cesarean section has respiratory distress.

- **Most likely diagnosis:** Transient tachypnea of the newborn (TTN).

- **Treatment:** Supportive care including supplemental oxygen, if necessary.

ANALYSIS

Objectives

1. Know the presentation of TTN.
2. Understand the medical care for TTN.

Considerations

This term infant presents soon after birth with mild respiratory distress following an uneventful pregnancy and delivery. Evaluation of this infant begins with auscultation of the lungs and heart.

APPROACH TO:

Transient Tachypnea of the Newborn

DEFINITIONS

TRANSIENT TACHYPNEA OF THE NEWBORN (TTN): Slow absorption of fetal lung fluid with resultant tachypnea. The condition more commonly is associated with cesarean section deliveries.

MECONIUM ASPIRATION SYNDROME: Aspiration of meconium during delivery resulting in respiratory distress. Radiographic findings include hyperinflation with patchy infiltrates. Because meconium may plug small airways, areas of air trapping are often present and may lead to the development of pneumothorax. Commonly associated with persistent pulmonary hypertension of the newborn.

RESPIRATORY DISTRESS SYNDROME: A condition seen in premature infants resulting from surfactant deficiency. Radiographic findings include a characteristic reticulonodular "ground glass" pattern with air bronchograms and decreased aeration.

CONGENITAL DIAPHRAGMATIC HERNIA (CDH): The condition of herniation of abdominal contents through the posterolateral foramen of Bochdalek into the thoracic cavity resulting in pulmonary hypoplasia. The incidence is approximately 1 in 5000 live births. Radiographic findings include bowel gas in the thoracic cavity.

EXTRACORPOREAL MEMBRANE OXYGENATION (ECMO): A system using a modified heart-lung machine utilized in severe pulmonary failure. Cannulation of the carotid artery and jugular vein is required to link the neonate to the system.

CLINICAL APPROACH

Transient tachypnea of the newborn is a self-limited condition usually occurring in a **term infant** after an uneventful cesarean section (more commonly) or precipitous vaginal birth. It is felt to be caused by slow absorption of fetal lung fluid. Infants with TTN develop respiratory distress shortly after birth with tachypnea, mild retractions, nasal flaring, and in more severe cases grunting and cyanosis. Chest radiography reveals **perihilar streaking and fluid in the fissures;** lungs are aerated. Most infants with TTN have resolution of symptoms in 24 to 72 hours and are managed supportively.

For a few infants with TTN, oxygen saturations drop and supplemental oxygen is required. In the rare, more severe case of TTN consideration for ongoing increased pulmonary vascular resistance leading to persistent pulmonary hypertension must be entertained. Infants with TTN do not require antimicrobial therapy; failure of the infant to follow the expected course of mild respiratory distress indicates the need to evaluate the child for more serious pathology.

Infants with **respiratory distress syndrome (RDS)** are usually born prematurely (<34 weeks of gestational age) and deficient in surfactant. Shortly after birth they present with symptoms of respiratory distress including poor oxygenation, grunting, retracting, and poor air movement. Radiographically they have findings including a reticulonodular "ground glass" pattern with air bronchograms and decreased aeration of the lungs. Supportive care includes supplemental oxygen as needed to maintain oxygen saturation of 90% to 95% and intravenous fluids or nasogastric feeding to maintain hydration because the degree of tachypnea usually precludes oral feeding. Exogenous surfactant is available and is administered by the resuscitation team in an effort to ameliorate the effects of surfactant deficiency.

CASE CORRELATION

- See also Cases 2, 4, 6, and 7. The infant born to a diabetic mother (Case 2) has an increased incidence of polycythemia and hypoglycemia, both of which can result in tachypnea. In addition, these infants have a higher incidence of surfactant deficiency at later gestational ages, again resulting in tachypnea. Group B streptococcal infection (Case 4) and neonatal herpes simplex virus infection (Case 6) are common infections in the newborn period; both can cause pneumonia that may present with an increased respiratory rate among other symptoms. The child with tracheoesophageal atresia (Case 7) will have recurrent episodes of aspiration and clinical findings of tachypnea as a result.

COMPREHENSION QUESTIONS

8.1 A term male is born to a 33-year-old woman who had little prenatal care. Immediately after birth he has cyanosis and respiratory distress. Chest auscultation in the delivery room reveals right-sided heart sounds and absent left-sided breath sounds. Which of the following is the most appropriate next step?

    A. Assess the abdomen to evaluate for possible congenital diaphragmatic hernia.

    B. Order a computed tomography of the chest.

    C. Order ultrasonography of the chest.

    D. Perform a needle thoracostomy for possible pneumothorax.

    E. Prepare the infant for extracorporeal membrane oxygenation (ECMO).

8.2 A term male is born via repeat cesarean section to a 30-year-old woman. Immediately after birth he has mild respiratory distress. Chest auscultation in the delivery room reveals clear breath sounds. Which of the following is the most appropriate next step?

    A. Endotracheal intubation with direct suction.

    B. Begin intravenous antibiotic therapy.

    C. Deliver surfactant therapy.

    D. Observe and administer supplemental oxygen as needed.

    E. Bag-mask ventilation.

8.3 A term male is born vaginally to a 22-year-old primigravida woman; the pregnancy was uncomplicated. Just prior to delivery, fetal bradycardia was noted, and at delivery thick meconium is found. The infant has hypotonia and bradycardia. Which of the following is the first step in resuscitation?

    A. Administration of epinephrine through endotracheal tube

    B. Bag-mask ventilation

    C. Endotracheal intubation with direct suction

    D. Oxygen delivered by cannula in close proximity to the nares

    E. Tracheostomy

8.4   A newborn female is delivered by C-section to a 23-year-old mother after 29 weeks of gestation. She has poor respiratory effort at time of delivery with cyanosis, requiring resuscitation and eventually intubated. On examination in the delivery room, the infant continues to have subcostal retractions and is difficult to ventilate. What is the next BEST step in management?

A.   Obtain a chest x-ray.

B.   Administer albuterol.

C.   Administer surfactant.

D.   Closely monitor clinically.

E.   Obtain an echocardiogram (ECHO).

ANSWERS

8.1   **A.** Evaluation of neonates born with respiratory distress and unilateral breath sounds includes an abdominal examination. With asymmetrical breath sounds, pneumothorax and congenital diaphragmatic hernia (CDH) are considered. This infant's scaphoid abdomen and the presence of bowel sounds in the chest suggest CDH; needle thoracostomy is avoided because intestinal perforation may occur. The patient is stabilized and the need for ECMO is ascertained after the infant's initial therapy response is evaluated. Many cases of CDH are diagnosed by prenatal ultrasound. Infants with CDH do not respond to typical steps of neonatal resuscitation, and often have worsening respiratory status upon **bag-mask** ventilation (BMV), ultimately requiring intubation. The diagnosis of CDH can be made by locating on plain imaging the nasogastric feeding tube in the chest where the stomach has been displaced from the abdomen.

8.2   **D.** Because this infant most likely has TTN, the next step is to observe and administer supplemental oxygen, as needed.

8.3   **C.** Endotracheal intubation with direct suctioning of meconium below the vocal cords is performed in a **depressed** infant with thick meconium noted at delivery. Bag-mask ventilation or endotracheal intubation without suction may increase the volume of meconium aspirated. A vigorous infant with a heart rate greater than 100 beats/min, strong respirations, and good muscle tone with meconium-stained need not be suctioned immediately after birth.

8.4   **C.** This infant born prematurely likely has respiratory distress syndrome from surfactant deficiency. Difficulty ventilating arises due to collapsed alveoli. Introduction of surfactant as a treatment in delivery rooms decreases alveoli surface tension thus improving ventilation and has increased premature infants survival. A need for ECHO and chest imaging maybe required if symptoms persist.

CLINICAL PEARLS

▶ Transient tachypnea of the newborn (TTN) is associated with birth by cesarean section in term infants.

▶ TTN is managed with supportive care and does not lead to chronic lung disease.

REFERENCES

Carlo WA, Ambalavanan N. Respiratory distress syndrome (hyaline membrane disease). In: Kliegman RM, Stanton BF, St. Geme JW, Schor NF, Behrman RE, eds. *Nelson Textbook of Pediatrics*. 19th ed. Philadelphia, PA: WB Saunders; 2011:581-590.

Galarza MG, Sosenko IRS. Abnormalities of the lungs. In: Rudolph CD, Rudolph AM, Lister GE, First LR, Gershon AA, eds. *Rudolph's Pediatrics*. 22nd ed. New York, NY: McGraw-Hill; 2011:201-206.

Gross I. Meconium aspiration syndrome. In: McMillan JA, Feigin RD, DeAngelis CD, Jones MD, eds. *Oski's Pediatrics: Principles and Practice*. 4th ed. Philadelphia, PA: Lippincott Williams & Wilkins; 2006:315.

Gross I. Transient tachypnea of the newborn. In: McMillan JA, Feigin RD, DeAngelis CD, Jones MD, eds. *Oski's Pediatrics: Principles and Practice*. 4th ed. Philadelphia, PA: Lippincott Williams & Wilkins; 2006:311.

Hansen TN, Hawgood S. Respiratory distress syndrome. In: Rudolph CD, Rudolph AM, Lister GE, First LR, Gershon AA, eds. *Rudolph's Pediatrics*. 22nd ed. New York, NY: McGraw-Hill; 2011:233-235.

A full-term infant is delivered vaginally after a pregnancy that was uncomplicated. On initial examination it is noted that the baby has cloudiness of both lenses, which obscures the red reflex. The family history is significant for the father having had eye surgery at a young age. The physical examination otherwise is unremarkable.

▶ What is the most likely diagnosis?
▶ What are possible complications of this diagnosis?
▶ What is the next step?

ANSWERS TO CASE 9:
Congenital Cataracts

Summary: A healthy full-term infant with bilateral lens cloudiness and a family history of ophthalmologic condition requiring surgery.

- **Most likely diagnosis:** Congenital cataracts.

- **Possible complications:** Severe visual deprivation accompanied by poor fixation and nystagmus.

- **Next step:** Ophthalmologic evaluation and complete evaluation for possible associated hereditary, chromosomal, metabolic, or infectious causes.

ANALYSIS

Objectives

1. Understand the conditions associated with congenital cataracts.

2. Understand the development of amblyopia.

Considerations

This newborn presents with an isolated eye finding consistent with cataracts and a positive family history of eye disease. It is important to assess the infant for common chromosomal, hereditary, metabolic, and infectious or inflammatory entities associated with congenital cataracts. Because of the varying severity of opacification of the lens, early referral to a pediatric ophthalmologist for treatment and visual rehabilitation is mandatory as unilateral cataracts can cause severe deprivation amblyopia and strabismus.

APPROACH TO:
Congenital Cataracts

DEFINITIONS

CATARACT: Any opacity of the lens. Depending on the size and location, the cataract may be clinically insignificant. Or can significantly affect vision.

APHAKIA: Absence of the lens.

STRABISMUS: Misalignment of the visual axes. Strabismus can result in the loss of vision (amblyopia).

AMBLYOPIA: Decrease or loss of vision caused by underuse of one eye (deprivation amblyopia) or lack of clear image projecting onto the retina (strabismic amblyopia).

CLINICAL APPROACH

Congenital cataracts occur in approximately 2 to 13 of 10,000 births. They are an isolated condition in 60% of cases, part of a syndrome in 20% to 25% of cases, and the remainder is associated with other unrelated major birth defects. Cataracts are more common in low-birth-weight infants, with those that are at or below 2500 g having a three- to fourfold increase incidence in developing infantile cataracts. Many of the cases of isolated congenital cataracts are hereditary in origin, with most being transmitted through autosomal dominance. Developmental cataracts may result from prenatal infections, such as toxoplasmosis, cytomegalovirus, syphilis, rubella, and herpes simplex virus (the TORCH [toxoplasmosis, rubella, cytomegalovirus, and herpes simplex virus] infections), or secondary to metabolic diseases such as **galactosemia**, homocysteinemia, galactokinase deficiency, abetalipoproteinemia, Fabry, Hurlers, Niemann-Pick, and Wilson syndromes. The most common metabolic disorders causing congenital cataracts are hypoglycemia and hypocalcemia; infants born to diabetic mothers or those with hypoparathyroidism are closely evaluated. Intraocular abnormalities including retinopathy of prematurity, retinitis pigmentosa, uveitis, and retinal detachment may lead to the development of cataracts. Chromosomal anomalies associated with cataracts include trisomies 13, 18, and 21; Turner syndrome; and various depletion and duplication syndromes.

Evaluation of infants presenting with congenital cataracts includes full history and physical examination, assessment of TORCH titers, evaluation for galactosemia, and other metabolic disorders, many of which are included in the newborn metabolic screening test, a full ophthalmologic examination by a pediatric ophthalmologist, and ocular ultrasound in cases with completely opaque lenses. Parents should also have full dilated ophthalmologic evaluation including slit lamp examination.

If visual disturbance is significant, surgical removal of lens may be performed as early as 2 to 4 weeks after birth. The infant is then fitted with refraction contact lens; intraocular lens placement is used in older children and has recently been used in children younger than 2 years. If surgery is deemed not necessary, the cataract is monitored for changes and the child is monitored for the development of amblyopia. Infants with unilateral cataracts without surgery may need patching of their good eye to prevent the development of deprivation amblyopia.

The prognosis for congenital cataracts is dependent on multiple factors including the nature of the cataract, age of onset, age at intervention, the underlying disease, and the presence of any other associated ocular abnormalities. Deprivation amblyopia is the most common cause of poor visual recovery following cataract surgery in children.

In addition to deprivation amblyopia (opacity in the visual axis), other forms of amblyopia include strabismic (poorly formed image due to deviated eye), ametropic (high refractive error in both eyes), and anisometropic (unequal vision between the eyes). For all of these lesions, the common cause of pathology for the child is interference with the development of clear images during the critical period of eye development in infancy and early childhood. Amblyopia is usually asymmetric and is diagnosed when an ophthalmologic examination demonstrates reduced acuity otherwise not explained by an organic etiology. Early detection of this condition is key because the recovery of eye function is more likely the younger the child is.

Treatment for amblyopia must first include removal of any opacity and then ensuring well-focused retinal images are being produced in each eye; glasses may be necessary. Strengthening of the "weak" eye in order to stimulate appropriate visual development is accomplished by covering the "good" eye (occlusion therapy) or using atropine eye drops in the "good" eye (penalization therapy) to blur vision in this eye. Close monitoring by a pediatric ophthalmologist will ensure that the treatment maximizes the benefits to the amblyoptic eye while not causing amblyopia to develop in the nonaffected eye. Although it was previously thought that full-time occlusion was the best way to treat amblyopia, recent studies have shown that many children are able to achieve similar results with less patching or through the use of atropine drops. It is also more common now for older children who were previously thought to be "visually mature" to respond to therapy.

CASE CORRELATION

- See also Case 2 (Infant of Diabetic Mother). One of the complications of an infant born to a mother who has diabetes is cataracts. See also Case 6 (Neonatal Herpes Simplex Virus Infection). All the TORCH (toxoplasmosis, rubella, cytomegalovirus, and herpes simplex virus) infection agents may result in neonatal cataracts.

COMPREHENSION QUESTIONS

9.1 A full-term, small for gestational age newborn girl presents with cataracts, petechiae, and a continuous machine-like murmur. Which of the following statements is accurate?

A. This infant needs an audiology evaluation because sensorineural hearing loss is a common association.

B. This infant needs a renal ultrasound because she is likely to have renal abnormalities.

C. Treatment of her condition includes 14 days of intravenous penicillin after evaluation of her cerebrospinal fluid.

D. The infant's condition is likely to have occurred because of a maternal illness during the third trimester.

E. Intravenous antiviral therapy should be initiated and viral cultures should be obtained.

9.2   A healthy 2-week-old girl has yellow discharge from her left eye. Her mother had early prenatal care, the baby was delivered vaginally, and she was discharged at 48 hours of life. Within the first few days of life, the mother noted that the baby had increased tear production in her left eye, which now has yellow discharge. She has red reflexes bilaterally, her pupils are equal and reactive to light, and she has no scleral injection. She has left-sided mucous ocular discharge. The next step is to:

A.   Administer intravenous antibiotic therapy.

B.   Begin a course of oral antimicrobial treatment.

C.   Begin a course of topical antimicrobial treatment and nasolacrimal massage and warm water cleansing.

D.   Incise and drain the area.

E.   Refer the child for an outpatient ophthalmologic evaluation.

9.3   A 4-month-old infant has excessive right-sided tearing. His mother states he becomes irritable in bright light and calms in a darkened room. On examination, he has eye asymmetry, with the right eye appearing to be larger than the left. Which of the following statements is accurate?

A.   Warm compresses and gentle massage are first-line therapy.

B.   In most cases, treatment is nonsurgical.

C.   The infant has the classic features of Down syndrome.

D.   Immediate systemic antibiotic therapy will reduce complications.

E.   Immediate referral to a pediatric ophthalmologist is warranted.

9.4   While examining a term neonate in the newborn nursery, the red reflex is noted to be markedly less bright on one side. The remainder of the newborn examination is normal including all growth parameters. The mother has no history of infections during pregnancy. What of the following is the correct course of action?

A.   Continue routine newborn care and reexamine the baby at the 2 week follow-up appointment.

B.   Consult pediatric ophthalmology for immediate evaluation.

C.   Order an ocular ultrasound.

D.   Obtain laboratory test results including blood for a complete blood count (CBC), comprehensive metabolic panel (CMP), Rubella titers, and karyotype as well as urine for reducing substances.

E.   Provide reassurance to the parents because the condition will resolve over time.

ANSWERS

9.1 **A.** This infant has the classic features of congenital rubella syndrome including low birth weight, heart defect (patent ductus arteriosus), and congenital cataracts. Other clinical findings associated with congenital rubella syndrome include purpura, hepatosplenomegaly, jaundice, retinopathy, glaucoma, pulmonary artery stenosis, meningoencephalitis, thrombocytopenia, and hemolytic anemia. Long-term sequelae of congenital rubella include sensorineural hearing loss, neurodevelopmental abnormalities, growth retardation, endocrine disease (diabetes mellitus, thyroid dysfunction), and hypogammaglobulinemia. Maternal infection may or may not be clinically apparent, and infection during the first month is most likely to result in fetal infection with the involvement of multiple organs.

9.2 **C.** This infant had excessive tear production that later became a mucopurulent discharge but had an otherwise normal ophthalmologic examination. The most likely cause is congenital nasolacrimal duct obstruction (CNLDO) or dacryostenosis. This condition is typically caused by failure of canalization of the cells that form the nasolacrimal duct. Infants with CNLDO are at risk of developing acute infection of the nasolacrimal sac (dacryocystitis) or rarely periorbital cellulitis. Of note, in this case, the conjunctiva is not inflamed and the cornea is not involved. Initial treatment includes topical antibiotic therapy and nasolacrimal duct massage two to three times daily with warm water eyelid cleansing. Most cases of CLDNO resolve spontaneously, usually before 1 year of age.

9.3 **E.** A history of excessive tearing and photophobia, and examination findings of corneal enlargement suggest an immediate need for the evaluation for congenital glaucoma; treatment likely is surgical. Infantile glaucoma occurs in 1 in 100,000 births with a classic triad of tearing, photophobia, and blepharospasm. It may be isolated (primary congenital glaucoma) or occur with various conditions, including congenital rubella, neurofibromatosis type 1, mucopolysaccharidosis I, Lowe oculocerebrorenal syndrome, Sturge-Weber syndrome, Marfan syndrome, and several chromosomal abnormalities. The increased intraocular pressure can lead to expansion of the globe and corneal damage.

9.4 **B.** A positive Bruckner test (also known as "red reflex" test) warrants immediate evaluation by pediatric ophthalmology because the presence of an opacity of the lens or congenital cataracts exists. Leukocoria or a white pupil may indicate the presence of a retinoblastoma. Management of congenital cataracts includes early pediatric ophthalmology involvement for possible cataract extraction usually within the first 4 weeks to 3 months of life. Indications for surgery include opacity greater than 3 mm in diameter, decreased visual response, and onset of strabismus. Babies with unilateral cataracts are at increased risk of developing deprivation amblyopia, and adherence to a postoperative schedule of occlusion therapy with close follow-up with an ophthalmologist is essential to achieve good visual outcome.

CLINICAL PEARLS

▶ Galactosemia is associated with cataracts.

▶ Workup of an infant with congenital cataract includes TORCH titers.

▶ Amblyopia must be diagnosed at an early period so that occlusive or penalization therapy may be instituted on the unaffected eye to maximize improvement to the vision on the affected eye.

REFERENCES

Cazacu AC, Demmler GJ. Rubella (German measles). In: McMillan JA, Feigin RD, DeAngelis CD, Jones MD, eds. *Oski's Pediatrics: Principles and Practice*. 4th ed. Philadelphia, PA: Lippincott Williams & Wilkins; 2006:1272-1275.

Cheng KP, Biglan AW. Ophthalmology. In: Zitelli BJ, McIntire S, Nowalk AJ, eds. *Zitelli and Davis' Atlas of Pediatric Physical Diagnosis*. 6th ed. Philadelphia, PA: Saunders; 2012:756-757.

Mason WH. Rubella. In: Kleigman RM, Stanton BF, St. Geme JW, Schor NF, Behrman RE, eds. *Nelson Textbook of Pediatrics*. 19th ed. Philadelphia, PA: WB Saunders; 2011:1075-1078.

Olitsky SE, Hug D, Plummer LS, Stass-Isern M. Abnormalities of the lens. In: Kleigman RM, Stanton BF, St. Geme JW, Schor NF, Behrman RE, eds. *Nelson Textbook of Pediatrics*. 19th ed. Philadelphia, PA: WB Saunders; 2011:2169-2172.

Olitsky SE, Hug D, Plummer LS, Stass-Isern M. Disorders of eye movement and alignment. In: Kleigman RM, Stanton BF, St. Geme JW, Schor NF, Behrman RE, eds. *Nelson Textbook of Pediatrics*. 19th ed. Philadelphia, PA: WB Saunders; 2011:2157.

Olitsky SE, Hug D, Plummer LS, Stass-Isern M. Disorders of the lacrimal system. In: Kleigman RM, Stanton BF, St. Geme JW, Schor NF, Behrman RE, eds. *Nelson Textbook of Pediatrics*. 19th ed. Philadelphia, PA: WB Saunders; 2011:2165-2166.

Olitsky SE, Hug D, Plummer LS, Stass-Isern M. Disorders of vision. In: Kleigman RM, Stanton BF, St. Geme JW, Schor NF, Behrman RE, eds. *Nelson Textbook of Pediatrics*. 19th ed. Philadelphia, PA: WB Saunders; 2011:2152.

Quinn AG, Levin AV. Amblyopia. In: Rudolph CD, Rudolph AM, Lister GE, First LR, Gershon AA eds. *Rudolph's Pediatrics*. 22nd ed. New York, NY: McGraw-Hill; 2011:2291-2293.

Traboulski EI. Pediatric ophthalmology. In: McMillan JA, Feigin RD, DeAngelis CD, Jones MD, eds. *Oski's Pediatrics: Principles and Practice*. 4th ed. Philadelphia, PA: Lippincott Williams & Wilkins; 2006:801-819.

Walton DS. Visual impairment in children. In: Rudolph CD, Rudolph AM, Lister GE, First LR, Gershon AA eds. *Rudolph's Pediatrics*. 22nd ed. New York, NY: McGraw-Hill; 2011:2289-2290.

A mother brings her 18-month-old girl to your clinic for a well-child visit. She is a new patient without available past medical records, but her mother declares no known health issues. Her diet is varied, but she is a picky eater with frequent tantrums when given anything beyond fried foods and juices. You immediately note the child to be small for her age. Her weight is below the 5th percentile on standardized growth curves (50th percentile for a 12 month old), her length is at the 25th percentile, and her head circumference is at the 50th percentile. Her vital signs and her examination otherwise are normal.

▶ What is the next step in the management of this patient?
▶ What is the most likely diagnosis?
▶ What is the next step in the evaluation?

ANSWERS TO CASE 10:

Failure to Thrive

Summary: An 18-month-old girl has poor weight gain, but no etiology is suggested on examination.

- **Next step:** Gather more information, including birth, past medical, family, social, and developmental histories. A dietary history is especially important.

- **Most likely diagnosis:** Failure to thrive (FTT), most likely nonorganic in etiology.

- **Next step in evaluation:** Limited screening laboratory testing to identify organic causes of FTT, dietary counseling, and frequent office visits to assess weight gain.

ANALYSIS

Objectives

1. Know the historical clues necessary to recognize organic and nonorganic FTT.

2. Understand the appropriate use of the laboratory in an otherwise healthy child with FTT.

3. Appreciate the treatment and follow-up of a child with nonorganic FTT.

4. Understand some of the more common etiologies for FTT.

Considerations

This patient's growth pattern (inadequate weight gain, potentially modest length retardation, head circumference sparing) suggests FTT, most likely nonorganic given that the examination is normal. A nonorganic FTT diagnosis is made after organic etiologies are excluded, and, after adequate nutrition and an adequate environment are assured, growth resumes normally after catch-up growth is demonstrated. Diagnostic and therapeutic maneuvers aimed at organic causes are appropriate when supported by the history (prematurity, maternal infection) or examination (enlarged spleen, significant developmental delay). Although organic and nonorganic FTT can occur simultaneously, attempts to differentiate the two forms are helpful because the evaluation, treatment, and follow-up may be different.

In this case scenario, had the same practitioner followed this patient since birth or had records from the previous health care provider, earlier detection of FTT and its potential etiology might have occurred, thus allowing more rapid intervention. For instance, patients with poor caloric intake usually fail to gain weight, but maintain length and head circumference. As nutrition remains poor, length becomes affected next, and then ultimately head circumference.

APPROACH TO:
Failure to Thrive

DEFINITIONS

FAILURE TO THRIVE (FTT): A physical sign, not a final diagnosis; suspected when a child's growth is below the third or fifth percentile, in a child younger than 6 months who does not gain weight for 2 to 3 months, or in a child whose growth crosses more than two major growth percentiles in a short time frame; usually seen in children younger than 5 years whose physical growth is significantly less than that of their peers.

NONORGANIC (PSYCHOSOCIAL) FTT: Poor growth without a medical etiology; nonorganic FTT often is related to poverty or poor caregiver–child interaction; constitutes one-third to one-half of FTT cases identified in tertiary care settings and nearly all cases in primary care settings.

ORGANIC FTT: Poor growth caused by an underlying medical condition, such as inflammatory bowel disease, renal disease, or congenital heart conditions.

CLINICAL APPROACH

The goals of the history, physical examination, and laboratory testing are to establish whether the child's caregiver is supplying enough calories, and whether the child is consuming enough calories and able to use them for growth. Identification of which factor is the likely source of the problem helps guide management.

Diagnosis

The history and physical examination are the most important tools in an FTT evaluation. Of note, properly defining FTT involves use of adjusted growth curves in select populations; condition-specific curves are available for premature infants and those with select genetic abnormalities (Marfan syndrome, achondroplasia). A dietary history can offer important clues to identify an etiology. The type of milk (breast or bottle) and frequency and quality of feeding, voiding, vomiting, and stooling should be recorded. The milk used (commercial or homemade formula) and the mixing process (to ensure appropriate dilution) should be reviewed (adding too much water to powdered formula results in inadequate nutrition). The amount and type of juices and solid foods should be noted for older children. Significant food aversions might suggest gastric distress of malabsorption. A 2-week food diary (the parent notes all foods offered and taken by the child) and any associated symptoms of sweating, choking, cyanosis, or difficulty sucking can be useful.

Pregnancy and early neonatal histories may reveal maternal infection (toxoplasmosis, cytomegalovirus, rubella, syphilis), maternal depression, drug use, intrauterine growth retardation, prematurity, or other chronic neonatal conditions. When children suspected of having FTT are seen in families whose members are genetically small or with a slow growth history (constitutional delay), affected children are usually normal and do not require an exhaustive evaluation. In contrast, a family history of inheritable disease associated with poor growth (cystic fibrosis) should be evaluated more extensively. Because nonorganic FTT is more commonly associated with poverty, a social history is often useful. The child's living arrangements, including primary and secondary caregivers, housing type, caregiver's financial and employment status, the family's social supports, and unusual stresses (domestic abuse or neglect) should be reviewed. While gathering the history, the clinician can observe for unusual caregiver–child interactions.

All body organ systems potentially harbor a cause for organic FTT (Table 10–1). **The developmental status (possibly delayed in organic and nonorganic FTT) needs evaluation.** Children with nonorganic FTT may demonstrate an occipital bald spot from lying in a bed and failure to attain appropriate developmental milestones resulting from lack of parental stimulation; may be disinterested in their environment; may avoid eye contact, smiling, or vocalization; and may not respond well to maternal attempts of comforting. Children with some types of organic FTT (renal tubular acidosis) and most nonorganic FTT show "catch-up" in developmental milestones with successful therapy. During the examination (especially of younger infants), **the clinician can observe a feeding, which may give clues to maternal-child interaction bonding issues or to physical problems** (cerebral palsy, oral motor or swallowing difficulties, cleft palate).

The history or examination suggestive of organic FTT directs the laboratory and radiologic evaluation. In most cases, results of the newborn state screen are critical. A child with cystic fibrosis in the family requires sweat chloride or genetic testing, especially if this testing is not included on the newborn state screen. A child with a loud, harsh systolic murmur and bounding pulses deserves a chest radiograph, an electrocardiogram (ECG), and perhaps an echocardiogram and cardiology consult. Most FTT children have few or no signs. Thus, laboratory evaluation

Table 10–1 • MAJOR CAUSES OF INADEQUATE WEIGHT GAIN

Inadequate Caloric Intake
- Lack of appetite: depression, chronic disease
- Ingestion difficulties: feeding disorders, neurologic disorders (cerebral palsy), craniofacial anomalies, genetic syndromes, tracheoesophageal fistula
- Unavailability of food: neglect, inappropriate food for age, insufficient volume of food

Altered Growth Potential
- Prenatal insult, chromosomal anomalies, endocrine disorders

Caloric Wasting
- Emesis: intestinal tract disorders, drugs, toxins, CNS pathology
- Malabsorption: GI disease (biliary atresia, celiac disease), inflammatory bowel disease, infections, toxins
- Renal losses: diabetes, renal tubular acidosis

Increased Caloric Requirements
- Increased metabolism: congenital heart disease, chronic respiratory disease, neoplasms, chronic infection, hyperthyroidism
- Defective use of calories: metabolic disorders, renal tubular acidosis

Abbreviations: CNS, central nervous system; GI, gastrointestinal.

is usually limited to a few screening tests: a complete blood count (CBC), lead level (especially for patients in lower socioeconomic classes or in cities with a high lead prevalence), thyroid and liver function tests, urinalysis and culture, and serum electrolyte levels (including calcium, blood urea nitrogen [BUN], and creatinine). A tuberculosis skin test and human immunodeficiency virus testing may also be indicated. Abnormalities in screening tests are pursued more extensively.

Treatment and Follow-up

The treatment and follow-up for organic FTT are disease specific. Patients with nonorganic FTT are managed with improved dietary intake, close follow-up, and attention to psychosocial issues.

Healthy infants in the first year of life require approximately 120 kcal/kg/d of nutrition and about 100 kcal/kg/d thereafter; FTT children require an additional 50% to 100% to ensure adequate catch-up growth. A mealtime routine is important. Families should eat together in a nondistracting environment, with meals lasting between 20 and 30 minutes. Solid foods are offered before liquids; children are not force-fed. Low-calorie drinks, juices, and water are limited; age-appropriate high-calorie foods (whole milk, cheese, dried fruits, peanut butter) are encouraged. Formulas containing more than the standard 20 cal/oz may be necessary for infants, and high-calorie supplementation (PediaSure, Ensure) may be required for older children. Frequent office or home health visits are indicated to ensure weight gain. In some instances, hospitalization of an FTT child is required; some infants often have rapid weight gain, supporting the diagnosis of nonorganic FTT.

Nonorganic FTT treatment requires not only the provision of increased calories, but also attention to contributing psychosocial issues. Referral to community services (Women, Infants, and Children [WIC] Program, Food Stamp Program, and local food banks) may be required. Caregiver help in the form of job training, substance and physical abuse prevention, parenting classes, and psychotherapy may be available through community programs. Older children and their families may benefit from Early Childhood Intervention (ECI) and Head Start programs.

Some children with organic FTT also have nonorganic FTT. For instance, a poorly growing special-needs premature infant is at increased risk for superimposed nonorganic FTT because of psychosocial issues, such as poor bonding with the family during a prolonged hospital stay. In such cases, care for the organic causes is coordinated with attempts to preclude nonorganic FTT.

CASE CORRELATION

- See also Cases 6, 7, and 9. Infants who have had neonatal herpes simplex virus infection (Case 6) often have meningitis as part of their illness; the result often is poor growth and developmental delay. The child with tracheoesophageal atresia (Case 7) will have recurrent episodes of aspiration, pneumonia, and failure to thrive. While the majority of congenital cataracts (Case 9) are isolated findings, many cases are because of congenital infection or inborn errors of metabolism and are also associated with FTT and developmental delay.

COMPREHENSION QUESTIONS

10.1 Parents bring their 6-month-old son to see you. He is symmetrically less than the fifth percentile for height, weight, and head circumference on routine growth curves. He was born at 30 weeks of gestation and weighed 1000 g. He was a planned pregnancy, and his mother's prenatal course was uneventful until an automobile accident initiated the labor. He was ventilated for 3 days in the intensive care unit (ICU), but otherwise did well without ongoing problems. He was discharged at 8 weeks of life. Which of the following is the mostly likely explanation for his small size?

   A. Chromosomal abnormality

   B. Protein-calorie malnutrition

   C. Normal ex-premie infant growth

   D. Intestinal malabsorption

   E. Congenital hypothyroidism

10.2 A 13-month-old child is noted to be at the 25th percentile for weight, the 10th percentile for height, and less than the 5th percentile for head circumference. She was born at term. She was noted to have a small head at birth, be developmentally delayed throughout her life, and have required cataract surgery shortly after birth. She currently takes phenobarbital for seizures. Caloric intake has been deemed appropriate by history, and neither frequent emesis nor excessive stooling is reported. Her examination is remarkable for a small head and liver enlargement on abdominal palpation. Which of the following would most likely explain this child's small size?

   A. Congenital infection

   B. Chromosomal abnormality

   C. Metabolic disorder

   D. Gastrointestinal dysmotility

   E. Increased intracranial pressure

10.3 A 2-year-old boy had been slightly less than the 50th percentile for weight, height, and head circumference, but in the last 6 months he has fallen to slightly less than the 25th percentile for weight. The pregnancy was normal, his development is as expected, and the family reports no psychosocial problems. The mother says that he is now a finicky eater (wants only macaroni and cheese at all meals), but she insists that he eat a variety of foods. The meals are marked by much frustration for everyone. His examination is normal. Which of the following is the best next step in his care?

   A. Sweat chloride testing

   B. Ophthalmologic examination for retinal hemorrhages

   C. Reassurance and counseling for family about normal childhood development

   D. Testing of stool for parasites

   E. Magnetic resonance imaging (MRI) of the brain

10.4   A 10-month-old child is seen in follow-up after a pediatric gastroenterologist visit for poor weight gain. Her current length is at the 10th percentile, head circumference is at the 50th percentile, and weight is less than the 5th percentile. The examination is unremarkable except for small size. She was sent to the gastroenterologist about a month prior by a colleague after her weight was noted to have dropped from the 50th percentile on her 6-month-old visit to less than the 5th percentile on her 9-month-old visit. Perinatal history is unremarkable. Feeding is via breast and bottle with a standard milk-based formula; the quantity of feeds reported seems sufficient and no excessive spit-up is reported. Various table foods are eaten and reportedly tolerated well. The child has had no recent or recurring illness. At the gastroenterology visit, a comprehensive array of laboratory and imaging studies were performed, as outlined in the referral letter, and were unhelpful in diagnosing the cause of the FTT. His recommendations at that time were to begin a 1-month's trial of a 24 cal/oz formula and follow-up with you for a weight check. Which of the following is the best next step in her care?

A.   Commence caloric supplementation with 27 cal/oz formula.

B.   Counsel family regarding diet and schedule follow-up weight check in 6 months.

C.   Commence growth hormone administration.

D.   Refer to nutritionist.

E.   Admit to the hospital for FTT evaluation.

ANSWERS

10.1   **C.** The expected weight versus age must be modified for a preterm infant. Similarly, growth for children with Down or Turner syndrome varies from that for other children. Thus, use of an appropriate growth curve is paramount. For the child in the question, weight gain should follow or exceed that of term infants. For this premature infant, when his parameters are plotted on a "premie growth chart," normal growth is revealed.

10.2   **A.** Developmental delay, intrauterine growth retardation (including microcephaly), cataracts, seizures, hepatosplenomegaly, prolonged neonatal jaundice, and purpura at birth are consistent with congenital cytomegalovirus (CMV) or toxoplasmosis infection. Calcified brain densities of CMV typically are found in a periventricular pattern; in toxoplasmosis, they are found scattered throughout the cortex.

10.3   **C.** Between 18 and 30 months of age, children often become "picky eaters." Their growth rate can plateau, and the period can be distressing for families. Of note, this patient's growth decline has not crossed two major growth percentiles to define FTT. Counseling parents how to provide optimal nutrition, avoid "force-feeding," and avoid providing snacks is usually effective. Close follow-up is required.

10.4 **E.** Without evident abnormality on examination and with a presumed thorough outpatient FTT workup, this infant probably has nonorganic FTT. Of note, the infant is already on a calorie-fortified formula, in addition to breast milk. Although it might be appropriate to solicit advice from a nutritionist, the best response would be to consider admission to the hospital for a multidisciplinary assessment of her FTT. A 2- to 3-day stay to watch intake ('calorie count') and daily weights, while selected services comment on the patient and her family (social services, nutrition, pediatric gastroenterology), might uncover a nonorganic cause for her FTT (parental neglect). Growth hormone administration and further counseling regarding diet without close follow-up are not standard of care.

CLINICAL PEARLS

▶ In the United States, psychosocial failure to thrive is more common than organic failure to thrive; it often is associated with poverty or poor parent-child interaction.

▶ Inexpensive laboratory screening tests, dietary counseling, and close observation of weight changes are appropriate first steps for most healthy-appearing infants with failure to thrive.

▶ Organic failure to thrive can be associated with abnormalities of any organ system. Clues in history, examination, and selected screening laboratory tests may help identify affected organ systems.

▶ Up to one-third of patients with psychosocial failure to thrive have developmental delay, as well as social and emotional problems.

REFERENCES

Bunik M, Treitz M, Fox D. Ambulatory & office pediatrics. In: Hay WW, Levin MJ, Deterding RR, Abzug MJ, eds. *Current Diagnosis & Treatment: Pediatrics*. 22nd ed. New York, NY: McGraw-Hill; 2014:239-247.

Chiesa A, Sirotnak AP. Child abuse & neglect. In: Hay WW, Levin MJ, Deterding RR, Abzug MJ, eds. *Current Diagnosis & Treatment: Pediatrics*. 22nd ed. New York, NY: McGraw-Hill; 2014:240-246.

Kirkland RT. Failure to thrive. In: McMillan JA, Feigin RD, DeAngelis CD, Jones MD, eds. *Oski's Pediatrics: Principles and Practice*. 4th ed. Philadelphia, PA: Lippincott Williams & Wilkins; 2006:900-906.

McLean HS, Price DT. Failure to thrive. In: Kleigman RM, Stanton BF, St. Geme JW, Schor NF, Behrman RE, eds. *Nelson Textbook of Pediatrics*. 19th ed. Philadelphia, PA: WB Saunders; 2011:1147-1149.

Noel RJ. Approach to the infant and child with feeding difficulty. In: Rudolph CD, Rudolph AM, Lister G, First LR, Gershon AA, eds. *Rudolph's Pediatrics*. 22nd ed. New York, NY: McGraw-Hill; 2011:117-123.

Raszka WV. Neonatal toxoplasmosis. In: McMillan JA, Feigin RD, DeAngelis CD, Jones MD, eds. *Oski's Pediatrics: Principles and Practice*. 4th ed. Philadelphia, PA: Lippincott Williams & Wilkins; 2006:530-532.

Shaw JS, Palfrey JS. Health maintenance issues. In: Rudolph CD, Rudolph AM, Lister G, First LR, Gershon AA, eds. *Rudolph's Pediatrics*. 22nd ed. New York, NY: McGraw-Hill; 2011:27-34.

Stagno S. Cytomegalovirus. In: Kleigman RM, Stanton BF, St. Geme JW, Schor NF, Behrman RE, eds. *Nelson Textbook of Pediatrics*. 19th ed. Philadelphia, PA: WB Saunders; 2011:1115-1117.

A 6-month-old child arrives for a well-child examination. His family recently moved to the United States from Turkey. His medical and family histories are unremarkable except that his sole source of nutrition is goat's milk. He appears to be healthy on examination.

- ▶ What hematologic problem is most likely to develop?
- ▶ What nonhematologic concerns are considered in an infant fed on goat's milk?

ANSWERS TO CASE 11:

Megaloblastic Anemia

Summary: This is a 6-month-old child exclusively fed on goat's milk.

- **Likely complication:** Megaloblastic anemia from folate or B_{12} deficiency
- **Other concerns:** Brucellosis if milk is unpasteurized

ANALYSIS

Objectives

1. Appreciate the benefits of breast-feeding.
2. Know the nutritional supplements recommended for breast-feeding mothers.
3. Understand the special needs of infants and toddlers fed on goat's milk and vegan diets.
4. Recognize the clinical syndromes resulting from vitamin excesses and deficiencies.

Considerations

A variety of feeding regimens exist for infants and toddlers—breast-feeding, goat's milk, other types of nonformula milk, and commercial or handmade foods. Health care providers can educate parents about the benefits and potential dangers of various diet choices.

APPROACH TO:

Infant Nutrition

DEFINITIONS

LACTOVEGETARIAN: Diet devoid of animal products but includes milk.

OMNIVORE: Diet includes both animal and vegetable products.

OVOVEGETARIAN: Diet devoid of animal products but includes eggs.

VEGAN: Vegetarian diet devoid of all animal products.

CLINICAL APPROACH

Infant formulas containing goat's milk are not routinely available in the United States, but they are available elsewhere. Goat's milk has lower sodium levels but more potassium, chloride, linoleic acid, and arachidonic acid than does cow's milk. It is low in vitamin D, iron, folate, and vitamin B_{12}; **infants receiving goat's milk as a primary nutrition source should receive folate and vitamin B_{12} supplementation** (to prevent megaloblastic anemia) and iron supplementation (to prevent iron-deficiency anemia). **Goat's milk** should be boiled or pasteurized before ingestion because goats are particularly susceptible to **brucellosis.**

Breast milk is considered the ideal human infant food because it contains optimal nutrition (with the exception of vitamin D and sometimes fluoride); iron levels are low but highly bioavailable and do not require supplementation until 4 to 6 months of age. In addition, it has antimicrobial and immunologic benefits, and the act of breast-feeding promotes bonding between the mother and infant. In developing countries, it is associated with lower infant morbidity and mortality, not only due to a reduction in diarrhea associated by avoidance of contaminated water used in formula preparation but also because it contains **high concentrations of immunoglobulin A (IgA),** which reduces bacterial adherence to the intestinal wall, and macrophages, which inhibit *Escherichia coli* growth. **Disadvantages** include potential **HIV** (and other virus) transmission, occasional **jaundice exacerbation** due to breast-feeding and breast milk jaundice, increased unconjugated bilirubinemia levels (resolved with a 12- to 24-hour breast-feeding interruption), and its association with **low vitamin K** levels, contributing to hemorrhagic disease of the newborn (prevented by vitamin K administration at birth). Iron levels in breast milk are low but highly bioavailable and do not require supplementation until 4 to 6 months of age.

Formula-feeding is substituted for breast-feeding for a variety of reasons. Commercial formula manufacturers strive to provide products similar to human milk. Infant growth rates with cow's milk formula are similar to those in infants receiving breast milk. Improved sterilization procedures and refrigeration in developed and developing countries have reduced to some degree the gastrointestinal (GI) infections noted with formula feedings.

Formulas are available for special-needs infants. Infants with phenylketonuria require formulas low in phenylalanine, and those unable to digest protein require nitrogen in the form of amino acid mixtures.

Vegan diets can supply all necessary nutrients to adults if a variety of vegetables are consumed. Some evidence suggests that high-fiber vegetarian diets lead to faster GI transit time, resulting in reduced serum cholesterol levels, less diverticulitis, and a lower appendicitis incidence. Breast-feeding vegan mothers should receive vitamin B_{12} supplementation to prevent infant development of methylmalonic academia (an amino acid metabolism disorder involving a defect in the conversion of methylmalonyl-coenzyme A ([CoA)] to succinyl-CoA), which presents with failure to thrive, seizure, encephalopathy, stroke, or other neurologic manifestations. Toddlers on a vegan diet should also receive vitamin B_{12} and trace minerals, which may be depleted because of the high fiber content and rapid GI transit time.

Vitamin deficiencies and excesses can result in a variety of clinical syndromes, the majority of which resolve with appropriate nutrition (Table 11–1).

CASE CORRELATION

- See also Case 10 (Failure to Thrive). Poor diet may result in anemia.

Table 11–1 • EFFECTS OF VITAMIN AND MINERAL DEFICIENCY OR EXCESS

	Deficiency	Excess
Vitamin A	Night blindness, xeroph-thalmia, keratomalacia, conjunctivitis, poor growth, impaired resistance to infection, abnormal tooth enamel development	Increased intracranial pressure (ICP), anorexia, carotenemia, hyperostosis (pain and swelling of long bones), alopecia, hepatomegaly, poor growth
Vitamin D	Rickets (with elevated serum phosphatase levels appearing before bone deformities), osteomalacia, infantile tetany	Hypercalcemia, azotemia, poor growth, nausea and vomiting, diarrhea, calcinosis of a variety of tissues including kidney, heart, bronchi, stomach
Vitamin E	Hemolytic anemia in premature infants	Unknown
Ascorbic acid (vitamin C)	Scurvy and poor wound healing	Predisposition to kidney stones
Thiamine (vitamin B_1)	Beriberi (neuritis, edema, cardiac failure), hoarse-ness, anorexia, restlessness, aphonia	Unknown
Riboflavin (vitamin B_2)	Photophobia, cheilosis, glossitis, corneal vascular-ization, poor growth	Unknown
Niacin	Pellagra (dementia, dermatitis, diarrhea)	Nicotinic acid causes flushing, pruritus
Pyridoxine (vitamin B_6)	In infants, irritability, convulsions, anemia; in older patients (on isoniazid [INH]), dermatitis, glos-sitis cheilosis, peripheral neuritis	Sensory neuropathy
Folate	Megaloblastic anemia, glossitis, pharyngeal ulcers, impaired cellular immunity	Usually none, although extremely high levels can cause stomach problems, sleep disturbance, skin reactions, and seizures
Cobalamin (vitamin B_{12})	Pernicious anemia, neurologic deterioration, methylmalonic acidemia	Unknown
Pantothenic acid	Rarely depression, hypo-tension, muscle weakness, abdominal pain	Unknown
Biotin	Dermatitis, seborrhea, anorexia, muscle pain, pallor, alopecia	Unknown
Vitamin K	Hemorrhagic manifestations	Water-soluble forms can cause hyperbilirubinemia

COMPREHENSION QUESTIONS

11.1 A 2-day-old infant has significant nasal and rectal bleeding. The pregnancy was without complications; he was delivered by a midwife at home. His Apgar scores were 9 at 1 minute and 9 at 5 minutes. He has breast-fed well and has not required a health care professional visit since birth. Which of the following vitamin deficiencies might explain his condition?

A. Vitamin A

B. Vitamin B_1

C. Vitamin C

D. Vitamin D

E. Vitamin K

11.2 A 6-month-old infant has been growing poorly. His parents have changed his formula three times without success. His examination is remarkable for a pale, emaciated child with little subcutaneous fat and anterior fontanelle fullness. His laboratory test results are notable for a hemolytic anemia and prolonged bleeding times. Which of the following is the most appropriate next step?

A. Obtain urine for pH and electrolytes.

B. Measure serum factor IX levels.

C. Measure serum immunoglobulins.

D. Obtain a sweat chloride concentration.

E. Perform a hemoglobin electrophoresis.

11.3 An exclusively breast-fed infant with poor routine care is switched at 6 months of age to whole milk and table foods. Screening laboratories at 9 months of age demonstrate the hemoglobin and hematocrit of 8 mg/dL and 25%, respectively. Lead level is less than 2 µg/dL. A follow-up complete blood count (CBC) 2 weeks later shows a hemoglobin of 7.8 mg/dL, hematocrit 25%, the mean corpuscular volume (MCV) 62%, the platelet count to be 750,000/mm³, and a reticulocyte count of 1%. Which of the following is the most appropriate next step in the management of this child?

A. Order a hemoglobin electrophoresis.

B. Obtain a bone marrow aspiration.

C. Initiate iron supplementation.

D. Refer to a pediatric hematologist.

E. Initiate soybean-based formula.

11.4 A 3-week-old boy is admitted for failure to thrive, vomiting, and diarrhea. He appears ill. He initially improves after intravenous fluid resuscitation; when begun on routine infant formula with iron, his symptoms return. It is Saturday and the state health department laboratory is closed. You should switch his feeds to which of the following?

A. Amino acid-based formula (Nutramigen or Pregestimil)

B. Low-phenylalanine formula (Lofenalac or Phenex-1)

C. Low-iron, routine infant formula (Similac with low iron or Enfamil with low iron)

D. Low-isoleucine, low-leucine, low-valine infant formula (Ketonex-1 or MSUD 1)

E. Soy-based formula (Isomil or ProSobee)

ANSWERS

11.1 **E.** Newborn infants have a relative vitamin K deficiency, especially if they are breast-fed; most infants are given vitamin K at birth to prevent deficiency-related bleeding complications.

11.2 **D.** The patient appears to have failure to thrive, with deficiencies of vitamin K (bleeding problems), vitamin A (fontanelle fullness), and vitamin E (hemolytic anemia). Cystic fibrosis (associated with vitamin malabsorption) would explain the condition.

11.3 **C.** The child in the question most likely did not get iron (or vitamin D) supplementation in the first 6 months of life while exclusively breast-feeding, and was switched to whole milk (low in iron) and to table foods (not supplemented with iron as are baby foods) at too young an age. All the laboratory data are consistent with iron-deficiency anemia. He should be started on iron supplementation and then reevaluated; improvement confirms the diagnosis. Failure of the child to respond to the iron therapy would require further evaluation.

11.4 **E.** This patient appears to have galactosemia; uridyl transferase deficiency is the cause, and the condition results in features of jaundice, hepatosplenomegaly, vomiting, hypoglycemia, seizures, lethargy, irritability, poor feeding and failure to thrive, aminoaciduria, liver failure, mental retardation, and an increased risk of *Escherichia coli* sepsis. Children with galactosemia are managed with a lactose-free formula. The low-phenylalanine formulas are for infants with phenylketonuria; low-iron formulas do not have sufficient iron content to fortify infant iron stores and are not routinely recommended; the low-isoleucine, low-leucine, and low-valine infant formulas are useful for patients with maple syrup urine disease (MSUD); and the amino acid-based formulas are excellent for children with malabsorption syndromes.

> ## CLINICAL PEARLS

> ▶ Breast-feeding is associated with lower morbidity and mortality (especially in developing countries) mostly because of a reduction in enteric pathogens and diarrhea associated with contaminated water used in formula preparation.

> ▶ Breast-feeding provides all the nutrients necessary for infant growth with the exception of vitamin D, which should be supplemented in all breast-fed infants.

> ▶ A breast-feeding vegan should supplement her infant's or toddler's diet with trace minerals and also with vitamin B_{12} to prevent methylmalonic acidemia in her infant.

REFERENCES

American Academy of Pediatrics. Committee on Nutrition. Iron fortification of infant formulas. *Pediatrics*. 1999;104:119-123.

American Academy of Pediatrics. Section on breastfeeding. Breastfeeding and the use of human milk. *Pediatrics*. 2012;129:e827-e841.

Baker RD, Greer FR. Diagnosis and prevention of iron deficiency and iron-deficiency anemia in infants and young children (0-3 years of age). *Pediatrics*. 2010;126:1040-1050.

Egan M. Cystic fibrosis. In: Kleigman RM, Stanton BF, St. Geme JW, Schor NF, Behrman RE, eds. *Nelson Textbook of Pediatrics*. 19th ed. Philadelphia, PA: WB Saunders; 2011:1481-1497.

Federico MJ, Kerby GS, Deterding RR, et al. Cystic fibrosis. In: Hay WW, Levin MJ, Sondheimer JM, Deterding RR, eds. *Current Diagnosis & Treatment: Pediatrics*. 20th ed. New York, NY: McGraw-Hill; 2011:501-502.

Finberg L. Feeding the healthy child. In: McMillan JA, Feigin RD, DeAngelis CD, Jones MD, eds. *Oski's Pediatrics: Principles and Practice*. 4th ed. Philadelphia, PA: Lippincott Williams & Wilkins; 2006:109-118.

Greenbaum LA. Rickets and hypervitaminosis D. In: Kleigman RM, Stanton BF, St. Geme JW, Schnor NF, Behrman RE, eds. *Nelson Textbook of Pediatrics*. 19th ed. Philadelphia, PA: WB Saunders; 2011: 200-209.

Greenbaum LA. Vitamin E deficiency. In: Kleigman RM, Stanton BF, St. Geme JW, Schnor NF, Behrman RE, eds. *Nelson Textbook of Pediatrics*. 19th ed. Philadelphia, PA: WB Saunders; 2011: 209-211.

Kirby M. Infant formula and complementary foods. In: Rudolph CD, Rudolph AM, Lister G, First LR, Gershon AA, eds. *Rudolph's Pediatrics*. 22nd ed. New York, NY: McGraw-Hill; 2011:99-105.

Kishnani PS, Chen Y-T. Defects in galactose metabolism. In: Kleigman RM, Stanton BF, St. Geme JW, Schnor NF, Behrman RE, eds. *Nelson Textbook of Pediatrics*. 19th ed. Philadelphia, PA: WB Saunders; 2011:502-503.

Krebs NF, Primak LE, Haemer M. Normal childhood nutrition & its disorders. In: Hay WW, Levin MJ, Sondheimer JM, Deterding RR, eds. *Current Diagnosis & Treatment: Pediatrics*. 20th ed. New York, NY: McGraw-Hill; 2011:277-278.

Lerner NB, Sills R. Iron-deficiency anemia. In: Kleigman RM, Stanton BF, St. Geme JW, Schor NF, Behrman RE, eds. *Nelson Textbook of Pediatrics*. 19th ed. Philadelphia, PA: WB Saunders; 2011: 1655-1658.

Martin PL. Nutritional anemias. In: McMillan JA, Feigin RD, DeAngelis CD, Jones MD, eds. *Oski's Pediatrics: Principles and Practice*. 4th ed. Philadelphia, PA: Lippincott Williams & Wilkins; 2006: 1692-1696.

Orenstein DM. Cystic fibrosis. In: Rudolph CD, Rudolph AM, Lister G, First LR, Gershon AA, eds. *Rudolph's Pediatrics*. 22nd ed. New York, NY: McGraw-Hill; 2011:1977-1986.

Rosenstein BJ. Cystic fibrosis. In: McMillan JA, Feigin RD, DeAngelis CD, Jones MD, eds. *Oski's Pediatrics: Principles and Practice*. 4th ed. Philadelphia, PA: Lippincott Williams & Wilkins; 2006: 1425-1438.

Sachdev HPS, Shah D. Vitamin B complex deficiency and excess. In: Kleigman RM, Stanton BF, St. Geme JW, Schor NF, Behrman RE, eds. *Nelson Textbook of Pediatrics*. 19th ed. Philadelphia, PA: WB Saunders; 2011:191-198.

Shah D, Sachdev HPS. Vitamin C (ascorbic acid). In: Kleigman RM, Stanton BF, St. Geme JW, Schor NF, Behrman RE, eds. *Nelson Textbook of Pediatrics*. 19th ed. Philadelphia, PA: WB Saunders; 2011: 198-200.

Stettler N, Bhatia J, Parish A, Stallings V. The feeding of healthy infants, children, and adolescents. In: Kleigman RM, Stanton BF, St. Geme JW, Schor NF, Behrman RE, eds. *Nelson Textbook of Pediatrics*. 19th ed. Philadelphia, PA: WB Saunders; 2011:160-170.

Suchy FJ. Disorders of carbohydrate metabolism. In: Rudolph CD, Rudolph AM, Lister G, First LR, Gershon AA, eds. *Rudolph's Pediatrics*. 22nd ed. New York, NY: McGraw-Hill; 2011:1503-1504.

Wappner RS. Disorders of carbohydrate metabolism. In: McMillan JA, Feigin RD, DeAngelis CD, Jones MD, eds. *Oski's Pediatrics: Principles and Practice*. 4th ed. Philadelphia, PA: Lippincott Williams & Wilkins; 2006:2181-2192.

Zile M. Vitamin A deficiencies and excess. In: Kleigman RM, Stanton BF, St. Geme JW, Schor NF, Behrman RE, eds. *Nelson Textbook of Pediatrics*. 19th ed. Philadelphia, PA: WB Saunders; 2011: 188-191.

An 8-month-old child has a 24-hour history of increased crying when she moves her right leg. She has a prominent bulge over the mid-right thigh where she had received an immunization the previous day. She has not had fever nor change in appetite, and she seems upset only when the leg is disturbed. The child underwent a failed Kasai procedure for biliary atresia and is awaiting a liver transplant. A radiograph of the leg demonstrates a mid-shaft fracture and poor mineralization.

▶ What is the mechanism for this condition?
▶ What are the best diagnostic tests to diagnose this condition?

ANSWERS TO CASE 12:

Rickets

Summary: An 8-month-old child with a chronic medical condition, including biliary atresia, poor bone mineralization, and a fracture.

- **Mechanism:** Malabsorption of vitamin D (among other fat-soluble vitamins) due to lack of intestinal secretion of bile salts, resulting in rickets.

- **Best diagnostic tests:** Serum 25(OH)D, calcium, phosphorus, and alkaline phosphatase levels. Radiographs demonstrate poor bone mineralization.

ANALYSIS

Objectives

1. Become familiar with the clinical presentation of rickets.

2. Understand the pathophysiology behind nutritional and nonnutritional rickets.

3. Appreciate some of the other causes of childhood fractures.

Considerations

This child has biliary atresia and underwent a failed Kasai procedure. Metabolic aberrations are expected while this child awaits liver transplantation. A review of her medications and compliance in receiving them is warranted. Because of the brittle nature of her bones, her leg was fractured while receiving immunizations.

APPROACH TO:

The Child with Possible Rickets

DEFINITIONS

BILIARY ATRESIA: A congenital condition affecting approximately 1 in 16,000 live births in which the liver's bile ducts become blocked and fibrotic, resulting in reduced bile flow into the bowel.

KASAI PROCEDURE: An operative procedure in which a bowel loop forms a duct to allow bile to drain from a liver with biliary atresia.

RICKETS: Poor mineralization of growing bone or of osteoid tissue.

CRANIOTABES: Thinning of the bones of the skull.

RACHITIC ROSARY: Enlarged costochondral junction along anterior part of chest wall.

GENU VALGUM: "Knock" knees.

GENU VARUM: "Bowed" legs.

CLINICAL APPROACH

Rickets refers to "softening of the bones." Calcium-deficient rickets is due to insufficient intake or metabolism of vitamin D or calcium. Phosphate-deficient rickets is due to renal phosphate wasting.

Calcipenic Rickets

The predominant cause for rickets is vitamin D deficiency. Vitamin D is synthesized in the skin after exposure to ultraviolet (UV) radiation. It then binds to vitamin D–binding protein (DBP), undergoes 25-hydroxylation in the liver, and then further undergoes 1-hydroxylation in the kidney, thereby converting to the metabolically active form. The active form is essential for intestinal calcium absorption.

Stage 1 calcipenic rickets presents with hypocalcemia. Stage 2 presents with normal calcium but low phosphorus and increased alkaline phosphatase because of increased parathyroid hormone (PTH) secretion. Stage 3 presents with low calcium because PTH compensation reaches its limit.

Populations at risk for vitamin D deficiency include children who are exclusively breast-fed, born to vitamin D–deficient mothers, are dark skinned, are born prematurely, have limited sun exposure (especially during winter season), partake of vegetarian or vegan diets, use of anticonvulsant or antiretroviral medications, are obese, have conditions associated with malabsorption (celiac disease, inflammatory bowel disease [IBD], cystic fibrosis, gut resection), and have liver or kidney disease. Vitamin D deficiency is uncommon in formula-fed infants but can occur if the mother was vitamin D deficient during pregnancy and the quantity formula intake or vitamin D content of the formula is insufficient to compensate.

Symptoms of severe hypocalcemia include seizures, tetany (neuromuscular excitability leading to muscle contractions), poor feeding, vomiting, apneic spells, stridor, wheezing, hypotonia, lethargy, hyperreflexia, and arrhythmias.

Symptoms of rickets include bone pain, motor delays, muscle weakness, failure to thrive, delayed closure of fontanelles, craniotabes, frontal bossing, dental abnormalities, widening of wrists and ankles, genu valgum, genu varus, and the "rachitic rosary." Infants can also demonstrate increased respiratory distress (due to softening of the ribs) and increased susceptibility to respiratory infections. Deformities of the forearms are more common in infants, whereas angular bowing of the legs is more common in toddlers.

The changes of rickets are best visualized at the growth plate of rapidly growing bones; the best sites to examine to find clinical evidence are the distal ulna and the metaphyses of the knees. On radiographs, it is typical to see widened distal ends of long bones with cupping and fraying, osteopenia, and deformities of the long bone shafts. In severe rickets, pathological fractures and Looser zones (pseudofractures, fissures, or radiolucent lines) can be present.

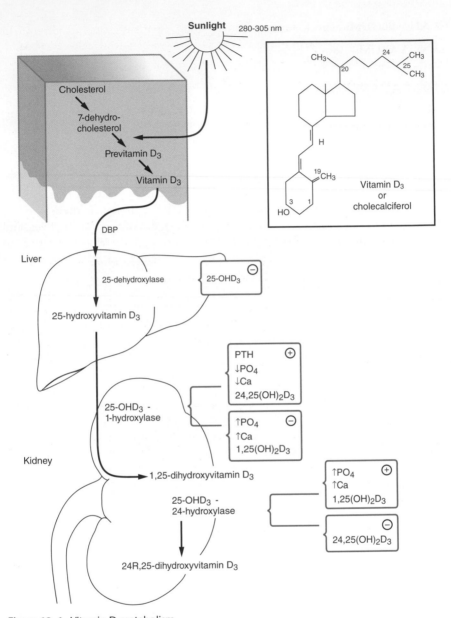

Figure 12–1. Vitamin D metabolism.

Categories of Calcipenic Rickets

1. **Nutritional rickets:** Inadequate intake of vitamin D and/or calcium (Figure 12–1)

2. **Vitamin D–dependent rickets type I:** Defective conversion of 25(OH)D to 1,25(OH)$_2$D, which leads to early onset of skeletal disease, enamel hypoplasia, and severe hypocalcemia

3. **Hereditary vitamin D resistant rickets**: End-organ resistance to vitamin D secondary to a mutation in the vitamin D (autosomal recessive disorder)

4. **Defects in vitamin D metabolism** (liver or kidney disease), **defections in absorption of calcium or vitamin D**, and **biochemical abnormalities in calcium or phosphorus metabolism** (Table 12–1)

Phosphopenic Rickets

Renal phosphate wasting causes phosphopenic rickets; low serum phosphorus combined with normal PTH concentrations is the most defining symptom. Causes may include renal tubular disorders (Fanconi syndrome), X-linked hypophosphatemic rickets, tumor-induced osteomalacia, and hereditary hypophosphatemic rickets with hypercalciuria.

X-linked hypophosphatemic rickets is the most common cause of isolated renal phosphate loss and is caused by mutations in the PHEX gene. This congenital condition becomes clinically apparent when the child begins to walk. In affected children phosphate reabsorption is defective, and conversion of 25(OH) D to 1,25$(OH)_2$D in the proximal tubules of the kidneys is abnormally affected. Children at the age of walking present with smooth lower-extremity bowing (as compared to angular bowing of calcium-deficient rickets), a waddling gait, genu varum, genu valgum, short stature, craniostenosis, and spontaneous dental abscesses.

Premature Infants

This population (<37 gestational weeks) is at risk for bone disease because substantial mineralization occurs between 32 and 36 weeks of gestation; 80% of calcium and phosphorus is acquired through placental transfer during the third trimester.

Parenteral nutrition vitamin D supplementation is weight based. Therefore, infants receiving parenteral nutrition alone do not receive 400 IU/d vitamin D supplementation until reaching a weight of 2.5 kg. Infants taking preterm infant formula also may receive inadequate vitamin D supplementation, depending on weight and enteral intake. Vitamin D supplementation in this population is dependent on weight and is adjusted accordingly.

Diagnosis of Vitamin D–Deficient Rickets

The level of **25(OH)D** is the best indicator of vitamin D status and stores.

1. **Vitamin D sufficiency:** >20 ng/mL

2. **Vitamin D insufficiency:** 15-20 ng/mL

3. **Vitamin D deficiency:** <15 ng/mL

Alkaline phosphatase is also a good screening tool; if the result is greater than 95th percentile for age, 25(OH)D, calcium, phosphorus, and PTH levels should be checked.

Table 12–1 • COMMON CAUSES OF ABNORMAL METABOLISM OF CALCIUM AND PHOSPHORUS

	Serum Calcium	Phosphorus	Serum Alkaline Phosphatase	Urine Amino Acids	Comments
Calcium deficiency with secondary hyperparathyroidism [vitamin D deficiency or low 25(OH)D without stimulation of 1,25(OH)$_2$D production]					
Lack of vitamin D (lack of exposure to sunlight; dietary deficiency vitamin D, congenital)	N or ↓	↓	↑	↑	Unusual except in dark-skinned infants without vitamin D supplementation, or in exclusively breast-fed infants without exposure to sunlight
Malabsorption of vitamin D	N or ↓	↓	↑	↑	Such as in celiac disease, cystic fibrosis, or steatorrhea
Hepatic disease	N or ↓	↓	↑	↑	See discussion of case
Anticonvulsive drugs	N or ↓	↓	↑	↑	Usually phenobarbital and phenytoin; patients have reduced 25(OH)D levels, possibly because of increased cytochrome P450 activity; treatment is with vitamin D$_2$ and adequate dietary calcium
Renal osteodystrophy	N or ↓	↓	↑	Variable	Hypophosphaturia results in hypocalcemia that then stimulates parathyroid secretion and enhanced bone turnover. In addition, diminished conversion of 25(OH)D to 1,25(OH)$_2$D occurs as renal damage progresses
Vitamin D–dependent type I	↓	N or ↓	↑	↑	Autosomal recessive; believed to be reduced activity of 25(OH)D$_1$ α-hydroxylase; responds to massive doses of vitamin D$_2$ or low-dose 1,25(OH)$_2$D
Phosphate deficiency without secondary hyperparathyroidism					
Genetic primary hypophosphatemia	N	↓	↑	N	X-linked dominant; most common form of nonnutritional rickets (see text)
Fanconi syndrome	N	↓	↑	↑	Includes cystinosis, tyrosinosis, Lowe syndrome, and acquired forms. Cystinosis and tyrosinosis are autosomal recessive, Lowe syndrome is X-linked recessive

Renal tubular acidosis, type II (proximal)	N	↓	↑	N	Bicarbonaturia, hyperkaluria, hypercalciuria, hypophosphatemia, and phosphaturia are common. Rickets may result from leaching of bone calcium bicarbonate in an attempt to buffer retained hydrogen ions seen in this condition
Oncogenic hypophosphatemia	N	↓	↑	Usually N	Caused by tumor section of a phosphate-regulating gene product (PEX), which results in phosphaturia and impaired conversion of 25(OH)D to 1,25(OH)$_2$D. The tumors are often hard to detect but are found in the small bones of the hands and feet, abdominal sheath, nasal antrum, and pharynx. Resolution occurs after tumor removal
Phosphate deficiency or malabsorption	N	↓	↑	N	Caused by parenteral hyperalimentation or low-phosphate intake
End-organ resistance to 1,25(OH)$_2$D$_3$					
Vitamin D–dependent type II	↓	↓ or N	↑	↑	Autosomal recessive; very high serum levels of 1,25(OH)$_2$D; may result from 1,25(OH)$_2$D receptor–binding disorder

N = normal

Treatment

Treatment for vitamin D deficiency consists of the following supplementation:

Infants who are younger than 1 month: 1000 IU daily

Infants 1 to 12 months old: 1000-2000 IU daily

Children who are older than 12 months: 2000 IU daily

Treatment continues for average of 3 months or until there is chemical or radiographic evidence of healing. Concurrent calcium supplementation is also recommended.

Supplementation

In November 2008, the American Academy of Pediatrics (AAP) recommended an increase for vitamin D supplementation. **All infants younger than 12 months should receive 400 IU daily beginning within the first few days after birth. Healthy children 1 to 18 years of age should receive 600 IU daily.** Formula-fed infants and older children who consume at least 33 oz of formula or fortified beverages daily meet the current AAP standards. However, many children fail to consume the recommended levels and should also receive supplementation. Vitamin D fortification is found in many foods, especially milk, dairy products, orange juice, bread, and cereals. To optimize an infant's vitamin D status, pregnant mothers should maintain sufficient vitamin D intake throughout pregnancy; 600 IU per day is recommended.

Limited sunlight exposure and outdoor activities should be encouraged in older infants and children, while maintaining an emphasis on sun safety. Direct sunlight exposure generally is not recommended in infants younger than 6 months.

CASE CORRELATION

- See also Case 10 (Failure to Thrive). Poor diet may result in nutritional rickets.

COMPREHENSION QUESTIONS

12.1 An 18-month-old infant is seen in the pediatrician's office as a new patient for a well-child visit having moved from Minnesota to Texas. A comparison of new to previous growth parameters suggest he has dropped to less than fifth percentile for height, weight, and head circumference. Physical examination findings are significant for lower-extremity bowing, wrist enlargement, frontal bossing, and some hypotonia. The mother is concerned because he does not pull to stand nor walking. She reports that he was exclusively breast-fed until he was 9 to 10 months old, currently drinks about 24 oz of whole milk daily, and has never taken medications or dietary supplements. The mother also has a question about whether he needs allergy testing given his history of frequent upper respiratory infections. Which of the following laboratory findings would be expected?

A. Low calcium, normal phosphorus, elevated alkaline phosphatase, elevated parathyroid hormone (PTH)

B. Low calcium, low phosphorus, low alkaline phosphatase, elevated PTH

C. Low calcium, low phosphorus, elevated alkaline phosphatase, elevated PTH

D. Low calcium, high phosphorus, elevated alkaline phosphatase, elevated PTH

E. Low calcium, low phosphorus, low alkaline phosphatase, low PTH

12.2 Which of the following would be the most likely radiographic finding in a child who has been diagnosed with calcium-deficient rickets?

A. Widening of the ribs

B. Shortening of the radius and ulna

C. Vertebral fissures and fractures

D. Prominence of the costochondral junctions

E. Increased densities in the long bone shafts

12.3 A 12-month-old patient is seen in the clinic. His mother reports that she exclusively breast-fed the child until he was 6 months of age. He still breast-feeds approximately four to five times daily but the mother reports he also drinks 2 to 3 oz of water daily, 8 to 10 oz of juice daily, and has been doing well eating table foods. What dosing of vitamin D would be the most appropriate for this child?

A. 200 IU daily

B. 400 IU daily

C. 600 IU daily

D. 800 IU daily

E. 1000 IU daily

12.4 Which of the following is a potentially distinguishing feature of osteogenesis imperfecta versus rickets?

A. Poor muscle tone

B. Easily fractured long bones

C. Increased susceptibility to respiratory infections

D. Small stature

E. Blue sclera

ANSWERS

12.1 **C.** Rickets secondary to vitamin D deficiency frequently presents with low to normal serum calcium (depending on the duration of the disease), elevated serum PTH (to compensate for the calcium deficiency), elevated serum alkaline phosphatase, and low serum phosphorous. PTH mobilizes calcium from the bone and subsequently increases renal phosphate loss.

12.2 **D.** Common bony abnormalities associated with calcium-deficient rickets include delayed closure of fontanelles, craniotabes, frontal bossing, dental hypoplasia, rachitic rosary, widening of the wrists and ankles, softening of the ribs (which may demonstrate fractures), bowing of the tibia or fibula, cupping or fraying at the distal ends of long bones, and deformities of the long bone shafts such as pseudofractures, pathologic fractures, fissures, or radiolucent lines.

12.3 **C.** All infants younger than 12 months should receive 400 IU daily beginning within the first few days after birth. Healthy children 1 to 18 years of age should receive 600 IU daily. Children with liver disease, kidney disease, or malabsorption (ie, secondary to cystic fibrosis, celiac disease, inflammatory bowel disease [IBD], etc.) as well as premature infants need even higher doses to account for the limitations in vitamin D metabolism or absorption brought on by these health issues.

12.4 **E.** Osteogenesis imperfecta is a congenital bone disorder that is caused by defective connective tissue formation secondary to collagen deficiency. Diagnosis is confirmed via collagen or DNA testing. Inheritance can be either autosomal dominant or autosomal recessive (depending on the type). There are eight different types of osteogenesis imperfecta with varying degrees of disability, but many of the features bare similarities to rickets. A few exceptions to this, however, are bluish sclera, triangular facies, and degrees of hearing loss.

CLINICAL PEARLS

▶ Nutritional rickets (inadequate dietary vitamin D or sunlight exposure) is rare in healthy children in industrialized countries. Medical conditions (liver or renal failure) or abnormalities in calcium and phosphorus metabolism usually are responsible.

▶ Primary hypophosphatemia (X-linked dominant) is the most common cause of nonnutritional rickets; proximal kidney tubule defects in phosphate reabsorption and conversion of 25(OH) D to 1,25(OH)$_2$D are seen. Findings include low normal serum calcium, moderately low serum phosphate, elevated serum alkaline phosphatase, and low serum 1,25(OH)$_2$D levels, hyperphosphaturia, and no evidence of hyperparathyroidism.

REFERENCES

Abrams S. Dietary guidelines for calcium and vitamin D: a new era. *Pediatrics*. 2011;127:566-568.

Beary J, Chines A. Osteogenesis imperfecta: clinical features and diagnosis. In: Rose BD ed. *UpToDate*. http://www.uptodate.com/home/index.html. Accessed May 25, 2014.

Brewer ED. Pan-proximal tubular dysfunction (Fanconi syndrome). In: McMillan JA, Feigin RD, DeAngelis CD, Jones MD, eds. *Oski's Pediatrics: Principles and Practice*. 4th ed. Philadelphia, PA: Lippincott Williams & Wilkins; 2006:1892-1897.

Chesney RW. Metabolic bone disease. In: Kleigman RM, Stanton BF, St. Geme JW, Schor NF, Behrman RE, eds. *Nelson Textbook of Pediatrics*. 19th ed. Philadelphia, PA: WB Saunders; 2011:2446-2447.

Chiang ML. Disorders of renal phosphate transport. In: McMillan JA, Feigin RD, DeAngelis CD, Jones MD, eds. *Oski's Pediatrics: Principles and Practice*. 4th ed. Philadelphia, PA: Lippincott Williams & Wilkins; 2006:1898-1901.

Egan M. Cystic fibrosis. In: Kleigman RM, Stanton BF, St. Geme JW, Schor NF, Behrman RE, eds. *Nelson Textbook of Pediatrics*. 19th ed. Philadelphia, PA: WB Saunders; 2011:1481-1497.

Federico MJ, Kerby GS, Deterding RR, et al. Cystic fibrosis. In: Hay WW, Levin MJ, Sondheimer JM, Deterding RR. *Current Diagnosis & Treatment: Pediatrics*. 20th ed. New York, NY: McGraw-Hill; 2011:501-502.

Geary DF. Chronic kidney disease. In: Rudolph CD, Rudolph AM, Lister G, First LR, Gershon AA, eds. *Rudolph's Pediatrics*. 22nd ed. New York, NY: McGraw-Hill; 2011:1749-1755.

Greenbaum LA. Rickets and hypervitaminosis D. In: Kleigman RM, Stanton BF, St. Geme JW, Schor NF, Behrman RE, eds. *Nelson Textbook of Pediatrics*. 19th ed. Philadelphia, PA: WB Saunders; 2011: 200-209.

Hill LL, Chiang ML. Renal tubular acidosis. In: McMillan JA, Feigin RD, DeAngelis CD, Jones MD, eds. *Oski's Pediatrics: Principles and Practice*. 4th ed. Philadelphia, PA: Lippincott Williams & Wilkins; 2006:1886-1892.

Joiner T, Foster C, Shope T. The many face of vitamin deficiency rickets. *Pediatr Rev*. 2000;21:296-302.

Kohaut EC. Chronic renal failure. In: McMillan JA, Feigin RD, DeAngelis CD, Jones MD, eds. *Oski's Pediatrics: Principles and Practice*. 4th ed. Philadelphia, PA: Lippincott Williams & Wilkins; 2006: 1841-1844.

Lauer B, Spector N. Vitamins. *Pediatr Rev*. 2012;33:339-352.

Linglart A, Biosse-Duplan M, Briot K, et al. Therapeutic management of hypophosphatemic rickets from infancy to adulthood. *Endocrine Connections*. 2014;3:R13-R30.

Lum GM. Chronic renal failure. In: Hay WW, Levin MJ, Sondheimer JM, Deterding RR, eds. *Current Diagnosis & Treatment: Pediatrics*. 20th ed. New York, NY: McGraw-Hill; 2011:686-688.

Madhusmita M. Vitamin D insufficiency and deficiency in children and adolescents. In: Rose BD, ed. *UpToDate*. http://www.uptodate.com/home/index.html. Accessed May 25, 2014.

Orenstein DM. Cystic fibrosis. In: Rudolph CD, Rudolph AM, Lister G, First LR, Gershon AA, eds. *Rudolph's Pediatrics*. 22nd ed. New York, NY: McGraw-Hill; 2011:1977-1986.

Porter CC, Avner ED. Toxic nephropathies-renal failure. In: Kleigman RM, Stanton BF, St. Geme JW, Schor NF, Behrman RE, eds. *Nelson Textbook of Pediatrics*. 19th ed. Philadelphia, PA: WB Saunders; 2011:1816-1818.

Root AW. Rickets and osteomalacia. In: Rudolph CD, Rudolph AM, Lister G, First LR, Gershon AA, eds. *Rudolph's Pediatrics*. 22nd ed. New York, NY: McGraw-Hill; 2011:2097-2101.

Rosenstein BJ. Cystic fibrosis. In: McMillan JA, Feigin RD, DeAngelis CD, Jones MD, eds. *Oski's Pediatrics: Principles and Practice*. 4th ed. Philadelphia, PA: Lippincott Williams & Wilkins; 2006: 1425-1438.

Sokol RJ, Narkewicz MR. Biliary atresia. In: Hay WW, Levin MJ, Sondheimer JM, Deterding RR. *Current Diagnosis & Treatment: Pediatrics*. 20th ed. New York, NY: McGraw-Hill; 2011:639-640.

Taylor S, Hollis B, Wagner C. Vitamin D needs of preterm infants. *NeoReviews*. 2009;10:e590-e599.

Thomas C. Etiology and treatment of calcipenic rickets in children. In: Rose BD, ed. *UpToDate*. http://www.uptodate.com/home/index.html. Accessed May 25, 2014.

Thomas C. Overview of rickets in children. In: Rose BD, ed. *UpToDate*. http://www.uptodate.com/home/index.html. Accessed May 25, 2014.

Zeitler PS, Travers SH, Nadeau K, et al. Disorders of calcium & phosphorus metabolism. In: Hay WW, Levin MJ, Sondheimer JM, Deterding RR, eds. *Current Diagnosis & Treatment: Pediatrics*. 20th ed. New York, NY: McGraw-Hill; 2011:959-963.

Zhou P, Markowitz M. Hypocalcemia in infants and children. *Pediatr Rev*. 2009;30:190-192.

A 10-year-old child presents to the emergency department with the complaint of right thigh pain. This child is one of your well-known sickle cell disease (SCD) patients, having been followed by your practice since birth. His previous history includes two previous hospitalizations, once at 6 months for fever and another at 12 months for a swollen, painful left wrist. On examination, he is afebrile, but his heart rate is 130 beats/min. You notice tenderness to palpation over the right femur with an otherwise benign physical examination.

▶ What is the most likely diagnosis?
▶ What is the next step in the care of this patient?
▶ What long-term strategies might be employed to prevent recurrence?

ANSWERS TO CASE 13:

Sickle Cell Disease with Vaso-Occlusive Crisis

Summary: An otherwise healthy 10-year-old boy with known SCD is found to have pain localized to his right thigh and tachycardia.

- **Most likely diagnosis:** Vaso-occlusive pain crisis.

- **Next step:** Admit to the hospital to administer intravenous fluids (IVF) and to provide pain management, possibly with narcotics.

- **Long-term strategy:** Administration of hydroxyurea will increase the concentration of fetal hemoglobin, thus reducing the frequency of sickle cell crisis episodes.

ANALYSIS

Objectives

- Learn the common complications and treatment strategies for a child with SCD.

- Become familiar with the goals of routine well-child (or health supervision) session for a patient with SCD.

Considerations

Vaso-occlusive crisis is the most commonly experienced complication for children with SCD. Risk factors for development of this condition include increasing age and high baseline hemoglobin level. Episodes can be triggered by infection, stress, cold temperatures, or high altitude, but often no trigger can be identified for an episode. The site of pain may vary from child to child, but the most common sites are the extremities or back. For many children experiencing recurrent vaso-occlusive crises, the pain tends to occur in similar locations with repeat episodes. The severity of these episodes varies; some successfully treated outpatient. When oral medications are insufficient to control the pain, hospital admission for IVF and intravenous (IV) narcotic medication are required.

APPROACH TO:

The Child with Sickle Cell Disease

DEFINITIONS

SICKLE CELL DISEASE (SCD): A group of disorders affecting at least one of the β-globulin genes, resulting in some degree of sickling of the red blood cells (RBCs).

VASO-OCCLUSIVE CRISIS: An episode of severe pain caused by increased sickling of RBCs, which leads to bone marrow ischemia and infarction.

DACTYLITIS: A form of vaso-occlusive crisis that involves painful swelling of hands and/or feet.

ACUTE CHEST SYNDROME (ACS): A new pulmonary infiltrate on chest x-ray (CXR) in addition to one of the following signs: fever, chest pain, shortness of breath, tachypnea, or low oxygen saturations.

APLASTIC CRISIS: Infection with parvovirus B19 (most commonly), which leads to temporary cessation of RBC formation. Reduced lifespan of RBCs in SCD coupled with reduced production may result in profound anemia.

CLINICAL APPROACH

Vaso-occlusive crises are the most common complication among children with SCD. Pain is the most common presenting symptom, but patients may also have erythema, edema, or joint effusions near the site of the pain. No specific laboratory work is diagnostic of the crisis, but affected patients may have decreased hemoglobin or increased white blood cells (WBCs). Children whose pain is inadequately controlled with home medication regimens must be evaluated. Additional pain medications, such as morphine or hydromorphone, along with hydration, may be attempted in the outpatient setting. If more than one or two doses of these additional pain medications are required, inpatient hospitalization is required. Additional inpatient strategies include IVF (often given at higher than maintenance rates) and IV narcotics with doses and frequencies titrated to control the patient's pain. RBC transfused typically are not used for simple vaso-occlusive crises, because they have not been found to be effective. Prevention of recurrent episodes of vaso-occlusive crises is attempted by avoidance of known triggers, as well as administration of hydroxyurea. This medication increases the concentration of fetal hemoglobin, thus decreasing sickling.

A patient with SCD with fever (with or without vaso-occlusive crisis) can have a medical emergency. Any SCD child presenting with a fever greater than 38.5°C is evaluated emergently, because SCD causes functional asplenia and predisposes patients to invasive encapsulated organisms (typically pneumococcal disease). In such situations complete blood count (CBC) and blood cultures are warranted, and if the screening results are concerning for infection without obvious source, empiric antibiotics are typically initiated (usually with ceftriaxone).

A variety of other complications occur with SCD. Children with SCD who have significant respiratory symptoms, such as severe cough, shortness of breath, or chest pain may be exhibiting symptoms of acute chest syndrome. Criteria for diagnosis include new pulmonary infiltrate on chest radiograph in addition to one of the following: fever, dyspnea, tachypnea, chest pain, or decreased oxygen saturations. Because of potentially fatal complications of acute chest syndrome, immediate treatment is warranted and includes empiric antibiotics, supplemental oxygen, pain medications, and IVF. Close inpatient observation for respiratory failure is warranted.

Parents of the child with SCD are taught to palpate the abdomen of their younger children to observe for splenic enlargement. A child who has abdominal pain, distension, or acute enlargement of the spleen likely has acute splenic sequestration and requires hospitalization, possibly in the intensive care unit, to observe for cardiovascular collapse. Blood transfusions, perhaps even emergently, may be required and could potentially be lifesaving. As the child ages, the spleen usually auto-infarcts. Although lack of a functional spleen eliminates the complication of splenic sequestration, it also increases the odds of an infection with an encapsulated organism.

About 10% of children with SCD have acute strokes, with peak incident between 4 and 8 years of age. Symptoms might include paresis, aphasia, seizures, cranial nerve palsy, headache, or coma; all such children are admitted to the hospital. Emergency neuroimaging is warranted, repeated neurologic examinations are conducted, and partial or simple transfusions are performed to reduce the percentage of sickled cells. Physical therapy and rehabilitation are provided as the patient recovers. Chronic transfusions are instituted to reduce the risk of recurrence. As part of the routine well-child care of a patient with SCD, transcranial Doppler (TCD) ultrasonography is often recommended to identify those with increased flow velocity in the large cerebral blood vessels, and thus are at high-risk for developing a first stroke. Routine chronic transfusion among these high-risk children has resulted in reduced risk of first stroke.

A child with SCD who presents with a significant increase in pallor, fatigue, or lethargy may be exhibiting signs of aplastic crisis, most often caused by infection with parvovirus B19. These children will have a hemoglobin level below their normal baseline and a low reticulocyte count. They require hospitalization to observe for evidence of cardiovascular collapse, and blood transfusions may be required.

A boy with SCD who has a priapism episode persisting for more than 3 to 4 hours must be evaluated by a urologist. Intravenous fluid hydration and pain control are provided; ice is not to be used. The urologist may be required to aspirate and irrigate the corpora cavernosa to achieve detumescence. Failure of three or four aspirations in the outpatient setting requires more extensive inpatient management, including exchange blood transfusions, further pain control, and additional surgical intervention.

Children with SCD require multiple evaluations by both primary care providers and hematologists per year, especially when young, and should receive screening for the various known complications of the disease. Goals of a health supervision visit for all children, including those with sickle cell and other diseases, incorporate evaluating a child's physical, developmental, psychosocial, and educational status to identify problems early. Prompt intervention can then be instituted. Anticipatory guidance aims to foster good health habits, prevent illness, and assist in family communication. For the child with a diagnosis such as SCD, another important part improving the overall good health of the patient is to ensure he or she is linked to a comprehensive SCD program.

Routine care for children with SCD includes initiation of prophylactic penicillin as early as possible, the pneumococcal PCV13 series at 2, 4, 6, and 12 to 15 months, and the pneumococcal and meningococcal vaccines starting at 2 years of age. Frequent CBCs are performed, and renal, liver, and lung function are monitored annually beginning at 1 year of age. Parents must also take an active role in the child's health care supervision, and his or her education is an important part of the well-child checks. Routine spleen palpation should be performed at home and enlargement should prompt an urgent evaluation. Parents should also check temperatures with any illness and bring the child to the primary care physician (PCP) or emergency department (ED) with a temperature of 38.5°C or higher.

COMPREHENSION QUESTIONS

13.1 Appropriate advice for a mother of a 2-week-old child identified on newborn state screen to have sickle cell disease (SCD) includes which of the following?

 A. Initiation of iron therapy

 B. Emergent genetic testing of both parents for hemoglobinopathy status

 C. Initiation of hydroxyurea therapy

 D. Purchase of an apnea monitor

 E. Enrollment in a comprehensive sickle cell program

13.2 A 14-year-old boy with known SCD has been admitted for vaso-occlusive crisis. He has been receiving IV fluids and IV narcotics for the last 2 days. He seemed to be getting better, but the nurse has just called and stated his temperature is now 101.8°F. On examination, you find his respiratory rate to be 32 breaths/min, and his oxygen saturation is 90%. What is the next step in management?

 A. Order spiral CT.

 B. Initiate antibiotics and provide supplemental oxygen via nasal cannula.

 C. Obtain STAT hemoglobin level.

 D. Initiate incentive spirometry.

 E. Administer another dose of narcotics.

13.3 Evaluation of a 9-year-old girl with known SCD reveals right-sided weakness and slurring of speech without any associated pain. Her vital signs are within normal limits for her age. Which of the following screening tests might have helped to prevent this complication of SCD?

 A. Annual CT of head

 B. Annual MRI of head

 C. Biannual check of hemoglobin level

 D. Annual transcranial Doppler ultrasound

 E. Annual neurologic assessments during well-child checks

13.4 Which of the following statements about routine procedures for a patient with SCD is accurate?

A. All children with SCD have baseline and then periodic complete blood count (CBC) and reticulocyte measurement screenings beginning at about 2 months of age.

B. To reduce the risk of sepsis, polysaccharide pneumococcal 23 vaccines are administered at 2, 4, and 6 months of age.

C. To identify new infiltrates, chest radiographs are obtained at all routine visits beginning at about 12 months of age.

D. Yearly gallbladder ultrasounds are indicated beginning in adolescence to identify the presence of stones.

E. Human papilloma virus vaccines are contraindicated in the SCD population.

ANSWERS

13.1 **E.** This child must be enrolled in a comprehensive SCD program to ensure the best possible outcome. At 2 weeks of age, the child has no reason to be iron deficient, and combined with future blood transfusions that may be required, iron therapy could result in iron overload. The newborn state screen has shown the child to have SCD and that both parents have at least a single sickle cell gene; further testing of the family may be warranted, but not as an emergency. Hydroxyurea is used to increase the levels of fetal hemoglobin; this child in the first months of life already has significant quantities of that hemoglobin present. SCD is not an indication for an apnea monitor.

13.2 **B.** This patient has been admitted for vaso-occlusive crisis and is at high risk of developing acute chest syndrome (ACS). Given that he currently has a fever, tachypnea, and decreased oxygen saturation, he meets ACS criteria. Prompt initiation of antibiotics and supplemental oxygen is imperative in preventing deadly complications of ACS. Although pulmonary embolism is in the differential for this patient and an acute drop in hemoglobin might cause tachypnea, initiation of antibiotics should be your first step in management. Incentive spirometry is an important part of the prevention of ACS, but antibiotics are more important in its treatment. Although increased pain may result in tachypnea, it would not usually cause a decrease in the patient's oxygen saturation.

13.3 **D.** Transcranial Doppler ultrasound should initially be performed at 2 years of age. If normal, it should be repeated annually until the patient is 16 years old. If two ultrasounds are abnormal, transfusion therapy typically is initiated and continued indefinitely to help prevent stroke. CT and MRI without any signs of stroke are not indicated. A change in hemoglobin level does not indicate potential stroke in a patient with SCD, but may be concerning for infection or aplastic crisis. Although neurological examinations are an important part of any physical examination, changes in the examination would indicate an already evolving process, rather than help to predict the potential for future disease.

13.4 **A.** Patients with SCD require baseline and periodic blood counts as described. The 23-valent polysaccharide pneumococcal vaccine is initiated at 2 years of age, whereas the 13-valent conjugate pneumococcal vaccine is administered at the younger ages outlined. Chest radiographs typically are obtained at approximately 2 years of age and periodically thereafter for screening purposes, for recent acute chest syndrome, or if the child has chronic cardiac or pulmonary disease. Ultrasounds of the gallbladder are reserved for patients with symptoms referable to that area.

CLINICAL PEARLS

▶ Children with SCD who have fever (risk of sepsis), pallor (aplastic crisis), abdominal pain or distension (splenic sequestration), pain crisis, evidence of lower respiratory disease (acute chest syndrome) priapism, new neurologic findings (stroke), or dehydration must be evaluated urgently.

▶ Additions to routine care required for all children include initiation of penicillin and folate therapies, as well as administration of meningococcal and polysaccharide vaccines at earlier than typical ages.

▶ A variety of screening tests, such as routine CBC and reticulocyte measurements, begin at 2 months of age or at diagnosis.

REFERENCES

Ambruso DR, Hays T, Goldenberg NA. Sickle cell disease. In: Hay WW, Levin MJ, Sondheimer JM, Deterding RR. *Current Diagnosis & Treatment: Pediatrics.* 20th ed. New York, NY: McGraw-Hill; 2011:846-848.

Debaun, MR, Frei-Jones M, Vichinsky E. Sickle cell disease. In: Kleigman RM, Stanton BF, St. Geme JW, Schor NF, Behrman RE, eds. *Nelson Textbook of Pediatrics.* 19th ed. Philadelphia, PA: WB Saunders, 2011;1663-1670.

National Institutes of Health. National Heart, Lung, and Blood Institute. The management of sickle cell disease. NIH Publication No. 02-2117. June 2002. http://www.nhlbi.nih.gov/health/prof/blood/sickle/sc_mngt.pdf. Accessed April 12, 2014.

McCavit TL. Sickle cell disease. *Pediatr Rev.* 2012;33:195-206. http://pedsinreview.aappublications.org/content/33/5/195.short. Accessed July 24, 2015.

Lane PA, Buchanan GR, Hutter JJ, et al. Sickle cell disease in children and adolescents: diagnosis, guidelines for comprehensive care, and care paths and protocols for management of acute and chronic complications. Sickle Cell Disease Care Consortium. http://www.dshs.state.tx.us/WorkArea/DownloadAsset.aspx?id=8589985663. Accessed April 12, 2014.

Martin PL. Sickle cell disease and trait. In: McMillan JA, Feigin RD, DeAngelis CD, Jones MD, eds. *Oski's Pediatrics: Principles and Practice.* 4th ed. Philadelphia, PA: Lippincott Williams & Wilkins; 2006:1696-1698.

Quinn CT. Hemoglobinopathies. In: Rudolph CD, Rudolph AM, Lister G, First LR, Gershon AA, eds. *Rudolph's Pediatrics.* 22nd ed. New York, NY: McGraw-Hill; 2011:1556-1561.

A 4-year-old boy has a 2-day history of runny nose, productive cough, and wheezing. Subjective fever and decreased appetite also were noted today. He has no known cardiorespiratory disease, and his immunizations are current. His two younger siblings are recovering from "chest colds." On examination, he is febrile to 103.2°F (39.6°C), with a respiratory rate of 22 breaths/min. His examination is remarkable for congested nares, clear rhinorrhea, coarse breaths sounds in all lung fields, and bibasilar end-expiratory wheezes.

▶ What is the most likely diagnosis?
▶ What is the next step in evaluation?

ANSWERS TO CASE 14:

Pneumonia

Summary: A toddler presents with cough, fever, and an abnormal chest examination.

- **Most likely diagnosis:** Pneumonia.

- **Next step in evaluation:** A chest x-ray (CXR) often is indicated to ascertain if radiographic changes support clinical findings. In addition to chest radiography, pulse oximetry and selected laboratory tests (complete blood count [CBC], blood culture, and nasal swab for respiratory viral polymerase chain reaction [PCR]) may help elucidate the etiology and extent of infection, as well as direct possible antimicrobial therapy.

ANALYSIS

Objectives

1. Describe the etiologies of pneumonia and their age predilections.

2. Describe various clinical and radiographic findings in pneumonia.

3. Describe the evaluation and treatment of pneumonia.

Considerations

The most important initial goal in managing this patient is to ensure adequacy of the **ABC's** (maintaining the **A**irway, controlling the **B**reathing, and ensuring adequate **C**irculation). A patient with pneumonia may present with varying degrees of respiratory compromise. Oxygen may be required, and in severe cases respiratory failure may be imminent, necessitating intubation and mechanical ventilation. The patient with pneumonia and sepsis also may have evidence of circulatory failure (septic shock) and require vigorous fluid resuscitation. After the basics of resuscitation have been achieved, further evaluation and management can be initiated.

APPROACH TO:

The Child with Pneumonia

DEFINITIONS

RALES: Wet or "crackly" inspiratory breath sounds due to alveolar fluid or debris; usually heard in pneumonia or congestive heart failure (CHF).

PLEURAL RUB: Inspiratory and expiratory "rubbing" or scratching breath sounds heard when inflamed visceral and parietal pleurae come together.

STACCATO COUGH: Coughing spells with quiet intervals, often heard in pertussis and chlamydial pneumonia.

PLEURAL EFFUSION: Fluid accumulation in the pleural space; may be associated with chest pain or dyspnea; can be transudate or exudate depending on results of fluid analysis for protein and lactate dehydrogenase; origins include cardiovascular (congestive heart failure), infectious (mycobacterial pneumonia), and malignant (lymphoma).

EMPYEMA: Purulent infection in the pleural space; may be associated with chest pain, dyspnea, or fever; usually seen in conjunction with bacterial pneumonia or pulmonary abscess.

PULSE OXIMETRY: Noninvasive estimation of arterial oxyhemoglobin concentration (SPO_2) using select wavelengths of light.

CLINICAL APPROACH

Pneumonia or lower respiratory tract infection (LRTI) is a diagnosis made clinically and radiographically. The typical pediatric patient with pneumonia may have traditional findings (fever, cough, tachypnea, toxicity) or very few signs, depending on the organism involved and the patient's age and health status.

Pathophysiology

LRTI typically begins with organism acquisition via inhalation of infected droplets or contact with a contaminated surface. Depending on the organism, spread to distal airways occurs over varying intervals. Bacterial infection typically progresses rapidly over a few days; viral pneumonia may develop more gradually. With infection progression, an inflammatory cascade ensues with airways affected by humoral and cellular mediators. The resulting milieu adversely affects ventilation-perfusion, and respiratory symptoms develop.

Clinical and Radiologic Findings

The pneumonia process may produce few findings or may present with increased work of breathing manifested as nasal flaring, accessory muscle use, or tachypnea, the latter being a relatively sensitive indicator of pneumonia. Associated symptoms may include malaise, headache, abdominal pain, nausea, or emesis. Toxicity can develop, especially in bacterial pneumonia. Fever is not a constant finding. Subtle temperature instability may be noted in neonatal pneumonia. Clinically, pneumonia can be associated with decreased or abnormal breathing (rales, wheezing). Chest examination may be equivocal, especially in the neonate. Hypoxia can be seen. Pneumonia complications (pleural effusion) may be identified by finding localized decreased breath sounds or rubs.

Radiographic findings in LRTI may be limited, nonexistent, or lag the clinical symptoms, especially in the dehydrated patient. Findings may include single or multilobar consolidation (pneumococcal or staphylococcal pneumonia), air trapping with a flattened diaphragm (viral pneumonia with bronchospasm), or perihilar lymphadenopathy (mycobacterial pneumonia). Alternatively, an interstitial pattern may predominate (mycoplasmal pneumonia). Finally, pleural effusion and abscess formation are more consistent with bacterial infection.

Causative Organisms: Viral, Bacterial, and Fungal

LRTI occurs more frequently in the fall and winter and with greater frequency in younger patients, especially those in group environments (large households, day care facilities, elementary schools). When all age groups are considered, approximately 60% of pediatric pneumonias are bacterial in origin, with pneumococcus topping the list. Viruses (respiratory syncytial virus [RSV], adenovirus, influenza, parainfluenza, enteric cytopathic human orphan [ECHO] virus, Coxsackie virus) run a close second.

Identifying an organism in pediatric pneumonia may prove difficult; causative organisms are identified in only 40% to 80% of cases. Routine culturing of the nasopharynx (poor sensitivity or specificity) or sputum (difficulty obtaining specimens in young patients) usually is not performed. Thus, diagnosis and treatment usually are directed by a patient's symptoms, physical and radiographic findings, and age.

In the first few days of life, *Enterobacteriaceae* and group B *Streptococcus* (GBS) are the primary bacterial etiologies; other possibilities include *Staphylococcus aureus*, *Streptococcus pneumoniae* (pneumococcus), and *Listeria monocytogenes*. In the newborn with pneumonia, broad-spectrum antimicrobials (ampicillin with either gentamicin or cefotaxime) are customarily prescribed. **During the first few months of life, *Chlamydia trachomatis* is a possibility, particularly in the infant with staccato cough and tachypnea, with or without conjunctivitis or known maternal chlamydia history.** These infants also may have **eosinophilia, and bilateral infiltrates with hyperinflation on chest radiograph;** treatment is erythromycin. **Viral etiologies include herpes simplex virus (HSV), enterovirus, influenza, and RSV;** of these, HSV is the most concerning and prevalent viral pneumonia in the first few days of life. Intravenous acyclovir is an important consideration if HSV is suspected.

Beyond the newborn period and **through approximately 5 years of age, viral pneumonia is common; adenovirus, rhinovirus, RSV, influenza, and parainfluenza are possibilities. Bacterial etiologies include pneumococcus and nontypeable *Haemophilus influenzae*.** Patients with nasal and chest congestion with increased work of breathing, wheezing, and hypoxemia regularly present to the emergency room during the winter months and are admitted for observation, hydration, oxygen, and bronchodilator therapies. The diagnosis of a viral process may be made clinically or with CXR findings (perihilar interstitial infiltrates). Nucleic acid PCR amplification of secretions from a nasal swab or wash often is performed to confirm a viral etiology. A mixed viral and bacterial pneumonia can be present in approximately 20% of patients. Antibacterial coverage should be considered if the clinical scenario, examination, or radiographic findings suggest bacterial infection.

The pediatric patient older than approximately 5 years of age with LRTI typically has *Mycoplasma*. However, most of the viral and bacterial etiologies previously listed are possible, except GBS and *Listeria*. Antibiotics in this age group are directed toward *Mycoplasma* and typical bacteria (pneumococcus). Treatment options include penicillins (amoxicillin, ampicillin), cephalosporins (ceftriaxone, cefuroxime), or macrolides (azithromycin). Vancomycin or clindamycin should be added if community-acquired methicillin-resistant *Staphylococcus aureus* is suspected.

Pneumonia in the intubated intensive care patient with central lines may be related to *Pseudomonas aeruginosa* or fungal species (*Candida*). *Pseudomonas* and *Aspergillus* are possibilities in the patient with chronic lung disease (cystic fibrosis). Varicella-zoster virus should be considered in the patient with typical skin findings and pneumonia; cytomegalovirus (CMV) if concomitant retinitis is present; *Legionella pneumophila* if the patient has been exposed to stagnant water; and *Aspergillus* if a patient has refractory asthma or a classic "fungal ball" on chest radiograph. Travel to the southwestern United States may expose patients to *Coccidioides immitis*, infected sheep or cattle to *Coxiella burnetti*, and spelunking or working on a farm east of the Rocky Mountains to *Histoplasma capsulatum*.

Causative Organisms: Mycobacterial

One important subset of LRTI is tuberculosis (TB). *Mycobacterium tuberculosis* has become more problematic over the past decade; multidrug resistance is increasingly seen. Patients may present with symptoms ranging from a traditional cough, bloody sputum, fever, and weight loss to subtle or nonspecific symptoms. A positive purified protein derivative (PPD), also known as a positive tuberculin skin test (TST), is defined by induration diameter in the context of a patient's exposure history, radiographic findings, and immune status. For instance, 5-mm induration may be considered a "positive PPD" at 48 to 72 hours in a patient with confirmed exposure, abnormal chest radiograph, or immunodeficiency. This same measurement in an otherwise healthy child without exposures would not be considered positive. Possible sources for acid-fast bacilli for stain and culture (depending on the age of the patient) include sputum samples, first-morning gastric aspirates, cerebrospinal fluid, bronchial washes or biopsy obtained through bronchoscopy, and empyema fluid analysis or pleural biopsy if surgical intervention is required. Standard antituberculous therapy, while awaiting culture and sensitivities, includes isoniazid, rifampin, and pyrazinamide. For possible drug-resistant organisms, ethambutol can be added temporarily as long as visual acuity can be followed. The typical antibiotic course consists of an initial phase of approximately 2 months' duration on three or four medications, followed by a continuation phase of 4 to 7 months on isoniazid and rifampin. Therapy for 9 to 12 months is recommended for CNS or disseminated TB. Ultimately, total therapy duration is dependent upon the extent of imaging abnormalities, resistance patterns, and results of follow-up sputum samples in the age-appropriate patient. Directly observed therapy should be routinely advised.

A recent TB testing modality, the interferon gamma release assay (IGRA), was FDA approved in stages between 2005 and 2008. These include the Quantiferon Gold In-Tube (QFT-GIT) test and the T-SPOT.TB (T-Spot) test. Both screen whole blood for *M. tuberculosis* proteins not found in Bacillus Calmette–Guérin (BCG) (thus excludes false-positive TST in BCG patients), but may cross react with proteins in nontuberculous mycobacteria (*Mycobacterium kansasii*, *Mycobacterium bovis*) and cause false-positives. White blood cells infected with *M. tuberculosis* release interferon gamma (IFN-g) when infected blood is incubated with the synthetic peptides in QFT-GIT (quantifies amount IFN-g released). In contrast, T-Spot measures the number of "spots" or cells with IFN-g release. Sensitivity and specificity for both are around 90% in children. Results are usually known within 2 to 3 days.

An IGRA can be used in place of the TST, and preferentially should be considered in pregnant patients, patients having received BCG, and serial assessment of those infected and treated. In children older than 5 years and patients who may not return for interpretation, QFT-GIT is the recommended modality. TST or IGRA can be used in children older than 5 years and in patient contact evaluation. Performing both a TST and IGRA is not recommended in routine screening, except in select situations (initial negative or indeterminate independent testing but high clinical suspicion, independent testing delivers indeterminate results). IGRA results are reported as positive, negative, or indeterminate (QFT-GIT) or borderline (T-spot), with indeterminate or borderline results warranting retesting; if results continue elusive, another modality such as TST should be considered. After noting a positive TST or IGRA, a thorough physical examination and CXR should be performed.

CASE CORRELATION

- See also Cases 4, 6, 7, 8, 10, and 13. Group B streptococcal infection (Case 4) and neonatal herpes simplex virus infection (Case 6) are common infections in the newborn period; both can present as pneumonia. The child with tracheoesophageal atresia (Case 7) will have recurrent episodes of aspiration resulting in pneumonia. In the first hours of life transient tachypnea of the newborn (Case 8) may result in increased respiratory rate and streakiness on the radiograph; the condition typically self-resolves in the first 2 days of life but occasionally may be confused with neonatal pneumonia. Depending on the cause of the pneumonia (ie, tuberculosis) failure to thrive (Case 10) may result. The child with sickle cell disease (Case 13) is prone to acute chest syndrome, a life-threatening condition of new pulmonary infiltrate on chest radiograph in addition to one of the following: fever, dyspnea, tachypnea, chest pain, or decreased oxygen saturations.

COMPREHENSION QUESTIONS

14.1 A 6-week-old boy, born by vaginal delivery after an uncomplicated term gestation, has experienced cough and "fast breathing" for 2 days. His mother relates that he has a 1-week history of nasal congestion and watery eye discharge, but no fever or change in appetite. He has a temperature of 99.4°F (37.4°C) and a respiratory rate of 44 breaths/min. He has nasal congestion, clear rhinorrhea, erythematous conjunctivae bilaterally, and watery, right eye discharge. His lungs demonstrate scattered crackles without wheezes. Which of the following is the most likely pathogen?

A. *Chlamydia trachomatis*

B. *Listeria monocytogenes*

C. Respiratory syncytial virus

D. Rhinovirus

E. *Streptococcus pneumoniae*

14.2 A 2-year-old girl has increased work of breathing. Her father notes she has had cough and subjective fever over the past 3 days. She has been complaining that her "belly hurts" and has experienced one episode of posttussive emesis, but no diarrhea. Her immunizations are current, and she is otherwise healthy. Her temperature is 102°F (38.9°C). She is somnolent but easily aroused. Respirations are 28 breaths/min, and her examination is remarkable for decreased breath sounds at the left base posteriorly with prominent crackles. Which of the following acute interventions is the next best step in your evaluation?

A. Blood culture

B. Chest radiography

C. Pulse oximetry

D. Sputum culture

E. Viral nasal swab

14.3 You are evaluating a previously healthy 8-year-old boy with subjective fever, sore throat, and cough over the past week. There has been no rhinorrhea, emesis, or diarrhea, and his appetite is unchanged. According to your clinic records, his immunizations are current and his weight was at the 25th percentile on his examination 6 months ago. Today, he is noted at the 10th percentile for weight. He is afebrile, with clear nares and posterior oropharynx, and a normal respiratory effort. He has bilateral cervical and right supraclavicular lymphadenopathy. Chest auscultation is notable for diminished breath sounds at the left base. Beyond obtaining a chest radiograph, which of the following is the best next step in your evaluation?

A. Rapid strep throat swab

B. Viral nasal swab

C. Purified protein derivative (PPD) placement

D. Lymph node biopsy

E. *Bordetella pertussis* direct fluorescent antibody testing

14.4 A 12-year-old boy presents to your clinic complaining of 1 week of fever, cough, and chest pain. He recently went on a boy scouts trip to Arizona, where he camped outside for 2 weeks, and excitedly describes how he became trapped in a "haboob" (massive dust storm) for an hour with his troop mates. His mother mentions that one of the other boys in his troop developed an unidentified, painful rash on his shins shortly after returning from the trip. The patient has a temperature of 101°F (38.3°C), but otherwise stable vital signs, and his physical examination reveals bibasilar rales. Which of the following is the most likely pathogen?

A. *Mycobaterium tuberculae*

B. *Coccidioides immitis*

C. *Myocoplasma pneumoniae*

D. *Staphylococcus aureus*

E. Influenza

ANSWERS

14.1 **A.** Cough and increased respiratory effort in an afebrile infant with eye discharge are consistent with *Chlamydia*. Transmission typically occurs during vaginal delivery. Approximately 25% of infants born to mothers with *Chlamydia* develop conjunctivitis; about half of these develop pneumonia. Most infants present with respiratory infection in the second month of life, but symptoms can be seen as early as the second week. Inner eyelid swabs are sent for polymerase chain reaction (PCR), and oral erythromycin or sulfisoxazole (latter only in infants >2 months) is given for 2 weeks for either conjunctivitis or pneumonia.

14.2 **C.** Tachypnea and lethargy are prominent in this patient with clinical pneumonia. Pulse oximetry should urgently be performed to ascertain whether oxygen is required. Sputum culturing is reasonable for an older patient who can produce sputum, but an adequate and diagnostically useful specimen can only be obtained from a 2-year-old by endotracheal aspirate or bronchoscopy. In this otherwise healthy toddler for whom concerns for atypical pneumonia are high, invasive maneuvers are not indicated. Viruses (respiratory syncytial virus [RSV] and adenovirus) are prominent at this age; one might consider performing a nasal swab viral PCR. Abdominal pain, as noted in this question, can be seen as a presenting symptom in pneumonia, probably because of irritation of the diaphragm by pulmonary infection.

14.3 **C.** The scenario is typical for pediatric tuberculosis. Neck and perihilar or mediastinal lymphadenopathy and pulmonary or extrapulmonary manifestations can occur, with miliary disease and meningitis more common in infants and younger children. Fever, weight loss, and lower respiratory tract signs and symptoms (possible left pleural effusion in this patient) are archetypal TB findings. A PPD should be placed or IGRA drawn, and consideration given to hospitalizing this patient in negative pressure isolation for further evaluation beyond initial screening (pleurocentesis, bronchoalveolar lavage, gastric aspirates) and possible antituberculous treatment.

14.4 **B.** Coccidioides spores often are found in the soil in the southwestern Unites States. Coccidioidomycosis typically results from inhalation of spores during dust-generating events. Symptoms may include constitutional (fatigue, weight loss), isolated cutaneous (erythema nodosum), and LRTI, akin to community-acquired pneumonia (cough, pleuritic chest pain). The incubation period ranges from 1 to 4 weeks. Treatment for symptomatic infection is with systemic antifungal (fluconazole, itraconazole).

CLINICAL PEARLS

▶ The etiology of pneumonia varies according to the patient's age. Neonates have the greatest risk of group B *Streptococcus*, toddlers are more likely to have respiratory syncytial virus, and adolescents usually contract *Mycoplasma*.

▶ Historical clues, including travel history and exposures, may help define an atypical pathogen in LRTI.

▶ Efforts in tuberculosis management should be directed toward isolating an organism and obtaining sensitivities, thus allowing selection of the optimal antituberculous regimen.

REFERENCES

American Academy of Pediatrics. Coccidioidomycosis. In: Pickering LK, ed. *2012 Red Book: Report of the Committee on Infectious Diseases*. 29th ed. Elk Grove Village, IL: American Academy of Pediatrics; 2012:289-291.

American Academy of Pediatrics. Tuberculosis. In: Pickering LK, ed. *2012 Red Book: Report of the Committee on Infectious Diseases*. 29th ed. Elk Grove Village, IL: American Academy of Pediatrics; 2012:736-759.

Kennedy WA. Disorders of the lungs and pleura. In: Osborn LM, DeWitt TG, First LR, Zenel JA, eds. *Pediatrics*. 1st ed. Philadelphia, PA: Elsevier-Mosby; 2005:803-818.

Moscona A, Murrell MT, Horga M, Burroughs M. Respiratory infections. In: Katz SL, Hotez PJ, Gerson AA, eds. *Krugman's Infectious Diseases of Children*. 11th ed. Philadelphia, PA: Mosby; 2005: 493-524.

Roosevelt GE. Acute inflammatory upper airway obstruction. In: Kliegman RM, Stanton BF, St. Geme JW, Schor NF, Behrman RE, eds. *Nelson Textbook of Pediatrics*. 19th ed. Philadelphia, PA: WB Saunders; 2011:1445-1449.

Sandora TJ, Sectish TC. Pneumonia. In: Kliegman RM, Stanton BF, St. Geme JW, Schor NF, Behrman RE, eds. *Nelson Textbook of Pediatrics*. 19th ed. Philadelphia, PA: WB Saunders; 2011:1474-1479.

The University of Texas Health Science Center at Tyler Heartland National TB Center. *Tuberculosis at a Glance: A Reference for Practitioners on Basic Tuberculosis Information*. www.heartlandntbc.org/assets/products/tb_at_a_glance.pdf. Accessed September 20, 2014.

A mother brings her 2-year-old son to your clinic for a 3-day history of his having about one tablespoon of bright red blood in his diaper with each stool and spots of red blood when she wipes him after his stooling. He has not had any abdominal pain but for the past week, has sometimes cried with stooling and now cries when she wipes him. The mother denies fever, vomiting, and diarrhea. She reports he previously had two soft bowel movements per day but over the past month, he has been having only one bowel movement per day. The stool has become hard and bulky. The mother and the child's father are his only caregivers, and she notes that the change occurred after she started trying to get him to stool in the toilet. He acts afraid of the toilet and avoids it. Instead, he goes behind the sofa and she will hear him grunt and see his face turn red. He is eating his regular diet of grilled cheese sandwiches with 20 oz of milk and 20 oz of a fruit-flavored beverage each day. On examination, his heart rate is 112 beats/min, temperature is 98.4°F (36.9°C), and he is playing on the examination table with his toy cars. His height and weight are in the 90th percentile for his age. On palpation of his abdomen, he has no tenderness, guarding, nor hepatosplenomegaly. On inspection of the rectal area, you find a 7-mm linear split in the posterior midline traversing from the anocutaneous junction to the dentate line. A fecal occult blood test (FOBT) is positive.

► What is the most likely diagnosis?
► What is the best management for this condition?

ANSWERS TO CASE 15:
Rectal Bleeding

Summary: A 2-year-old boy presents with rectal bleeding and painful defecation following a period of constipation and stool-withholding behavior. His examination is normal except for a fissure in the perianal region.

- **Most likely diagnosis:** Anal fissure, one of the most common causes of rectal bleeding in children of all ages.

- **Best management:** Begin dietary changes and a stool softener to ameliorate constipation. Parents should minimize foods known to be constipating (such as dairy products), increase water intake, and avoid bulking agents (such as fiber). Oral polyethylene glycol (PEG) 3350 is the most commonly used stool softener for children because it is an odorless, flavorless powder that can be dissolved in any liquid. Suppositories should be avoided because they will further traumatize the fissured skin. Application of petrolatum and gentle wiping should be performed after each stool until the skin no longer bleeds.

ANALYSIS

Objectives

1. Know the differential diagnosis for rectal bleeding at various ages.

2. Know how to manage rectal bleeding.

3. Be familiar with methods of investigating the cause of bleeding.

Considerations

Anal fissures are one of the most common causes of rectal bleeding in infants, toddlers, children, and adolescents. It is a benign diagnosis that usually results from constipation; large or dried hard stool can cause splitting of the skin. A cycle can then ensue in which the child avoids stooling due to the pain at the fissure site during defecation, which leads to accumulation of bulkier stool. Anal fissures can also occur with Crohn disease. Even though the diagnosis of an anal fissure is made by physical examination, certain details are often found in the child's history that will suggest the diagnosis. Behaviors in which the child is either resisting stooling (such as infants extending their legs), finding encopresis in an older child, or noting the patient may be struggling to stool (grunting or taking long periods in the bathroom to stool). The constipation and these accompanying behaviors may precede the bleeding by weeks to months and usually are provoked by a change in either the child's diet (such as beginning more solid foods) or when the child no longer has a designated time to spend for stooling (such as school entry). The bleeding that occurs with a fissure will be small in volume, may be associated with pain during or following defecation and with wiping the perianal area.

APPROACH TO:
Rectal Bleeding

DEFINITIONS

FECAL OCCULT BLOOD TEST (FOBT): A small amount of stool is placed on a test strip and mixed with a reagent containing guaiacum (usually called guaiac). If the reagent combines with hemoglobin, a blue color appears.

HEMATOCHEZIA: Blood in the stool that is red or maroon colored; may sometimes be referred to as bright red blood per rectum (BRBPR).

LOWER GASTROINTESTINAL (GI) TRACT BLEEDING: Bleeding within any part of the intestine that is distal to the ligament of Treitz, which encompasses the small bowel beginning with the jejunum and extends to the rectum.

MECKEL DIVERTICULUM: A 3- to 6-cm pouch off the ileum and is a remnant of the omphalomesenteric duct. It is often lined with an endothelium that can secrete acid similar to gastric mucosa, causing ulceration of the adjacent ileal mucosa. It causes half of the lower GI bleeds in children aged 2 years or older. It can have a chronic presentation with only occult blood detected in the stool by FOBT, or it can present with acute large volume hematochezia and a child in shock.

CLINICAL APPROACH

Lower GI tract bleeding most often presents with **hematochezia**. Distinguishing whether the cause of the bleeding is serious or benign begins with the history. The patient should be asked to **quantify the amount** of blood as well as **its distribution**, such as if the stool is mixed with blood streaks, is brick colored, if the toilet water was stained red, or if there was blood with wiping. If the patient's stooling is still supervised, then the parent should also provide the history. Information should also be obtained about the baseline and recent **stooling pattern**, such as frequency, size, texture, time needed to stool, ease of stooling, and the presence of encopresis. **Accompanying symptoms** of fever, weight loss, pain, and diarrhea would suggest inflammatory bowel disease in a school-age child or adolescent, especially if a positive family history of autoimmune-mediated disease is found. Fever, myalgias, vomiting, diarrhea, and recent antibiotics or contact with a potential contaminated food or water source can identify infectious enteritis or colitis. **Painless rectal bleeding** with a history of normal stooling **and no associated symptoms could be caused by a juvenile polyp or a Meckel diverticulum.** Juvenile polyps are benign and will cause bleeding when dislodged by the passage of stool.

Physical examination begins with the **vital signs and the patient's general appearance**. Tachycardia and diaphoresis may be present before hematochezia appears. Hypotension or lethargy is a late and ominous finding, indicating the patient is in shock. Signs of pain may be seen when there is bowel ischemia, such as with intussusception or volvulus. The conjunctiva and oral mucosa **may not reflect any pallor** with acute bleeding. Hepatosplenomegaly, petechiae, or purpura would indicate a coagulopathy is the underlying cause of the rectal bleeding. Palpation may elicit abdominal pain in areas where inflammation is present, or if constipation is present, hard stool may be palpable. As part of the abdominal examination, the perirectal skin is inspected. Findings might include a fissure, skin tag, fistula, or hemorrhoid. Rectal examination is useful because hard or impacted stool and benign polyps can be identified. In addition, stool can be obtained for FOBT; some red-pigmented food products, such as beets, gelatin, or beverages can pass unchanged through the GI tract and mimic blood.

Management of the rectal bleeding is determined by the patient's examination. If any vital sign is abnormal, if the child is ill appearing or is exhibiting pain, then stabilization and transfer to an emergency room are the first steps in management. Similarly, a large volume bleed or increasing bleeding may warrant urgent evaluation to identify the cause and have ongoing monitoring of hemoglobin or hematocrit. In such situations intravascular volume is initially restored with isotonic saline, then packed red blood cells may be needed. Laboratory evaluation for contributing coagulopathic conditions should be performed, which includes measurement of platelets, prothrombin time (PT), activated partial thromboplastin time (APTT), liver enzymes, and creatinine. Blood urea nitrogen (BUN) levels may be elevated due to urea being produced from hemoglobin breakdown in the GI tract. Stool studies, erythrocyte sedimentation rate (ESR), and C-reactive protein should be sent if a history of fever or diarrhea is found. A single-view supine, frontal view radiograph of the abdomen (KUB) may show an obstructive pattern which could signal intussusception or volvulus and urgent surgical consultation is indicated. The KUB can be normal in these conditions, so air-contrast enema or ultrasound should follow if these life-threatening causes are still suspected. When the child is well appearing, the blood loss is a small quantity, and the expected course of the underlying cause of GI bleeding is benign, no laboratory investigation or imaging may be necessary. However, if the bleeding continues to recur or worsens, a Meckel radionuclide scan may be indicated. If the scan is normal and a Meckel diverticulum is still suspected, diagnostic laparoscopy will follow because the scan has a high false-negative rate. Consultation with a pediatric gastroenterologist and colonoscopy are usually part of the management of lower GI bleeding when inflammatory bowel disease is the suspected cause or if the source of the bleeding cannot be identified, but colonoscopy is performed after the patient has been stabilized.

CASE CORRELATION

- See also Case 28 (Bacterial Enteritis) and Case 53 (Inflammatory Bowel Disease).

COMPREHENSION QUESTIONS

15.1 A 5-year-old boy is brought to clinic by his mother for evaluation of blood in his stool. Yesterday, the boy told her mother that he saw "red stuff" on his stool and when the mother visualized the stool, it appeared to have "threads of blood" over the surface. The child denies any blood with wiping. Which of the following would indicate that an anal fissure is NOT the cause of the rectal bleeding?

A. The boy has a 1-month history of encopresis.

B. The child's height and weight are at the 75th percentile for his age.

C. The boy's conjunctiva, gingiva, and nail beds are pale.

D. The child affirms that it has been painful to wipe after stooling.

E. The mother reports that since starting kindergarten, her son prefers to eat the school lunch, consisting of pizza and chocolate milk, rather than a homemade sandwich with water.

15.2 A 2-year-old girl presents to the emergency room with her second episode of bloody stool. The mother has brought in the diaper which is filled with about one-fourth cup of brick-colored stool. The first episode of hematochezia occurred 6 months ago but the stools returned to normal within 2 days. The mother denies constipation, diarrhea, and fever. On physical examination, the child is awake and alert, her heart rate is 150 beats/min, she has no tenderness on palpation of the abdomen, and rectal examination is normal except her fecal occult blood test (FOBT) is positive. What would be the next best steps in management?

A. Prescribe a stool softener and have the child follow-up with her pediatrician the next day.

B. Reassure the mother that the cause of bleeding is a benign polyp and no treatment is needed.

C. Inquire more about the amount of ibuprofen the girl has been taking and prescribe omeprazole.

D. Administer a normal saline bolus and order a Meckel scan.

E. Ask the mother about any family history of Crohn disease or ulcerative colitis, and send an erythrocyte sedimentation rate (ESR).

15.3 A 14-year-old girl reports she has intermittent periods of blood in her stools that lasts 2 days. Once the bleeding stops, it does not recur for about 2 weeks. She denies fever, abdominal pain, and diarrhea. She affirms that she has constipation. On physical examination, you see an anal fissure. You counsel her on how to take PEG 3350 and how to apply petrolatum to the site of the fissure. What else should you discuss with her in order to prevent a recurrence of the fissure?

A. She should use a suppository if she feels constipated again.

B. She should increase her dietary fiber intake.

C. She needs to return to the clinic for further evaluation if the fissure recurs despite resolution of the constipation.

D. She should decrease the number of times she goes to defecate.

E. She should apply triple antibiotic ointment to the fissure.

15.4 A 15-month-old boy is brought to the emergency room by his mother for increasing bloody diarrhea over the past 2 days. She reports he was febrile 3 days ago with several episodes of emesis that had resolved by yesterday. In the past 24 hours he has had more than 10 episodes of diarrhea, with the most recent appearing to consist of only blood with no identifiable stool mixed with it. On physical examination, he is somnolent. Which of the following is NOT part of his immediate management?

A. A bolus of isotonic (normal) saline

B. Measurement of prothrombin time (PT) and activated partial thromboplastin time (APTT)

C. Ultrasound of the abdomen

D. A colonoscopy

E. A complete blood cell count (CBC)

ANSWERS

15.1 **C.** Bleeding from an anal fissure is not chronic and the amount of hematochezia is small. A hemoglobin that is low enough to cause pallor of the mucosal membranes is not produced from an anal fissure.

15.2 **D.** The child is tachycardic and the amount of GI bleeding is significant. She requires her intravascular volume to be restored. Given her age, the most likely cause of her painless rectal bleeding is Meckel diverticulum.

15.3 **C.** A suppository, increased fiber, and stool withholding will worsen the stool bulk and are likely to cause a fissure. The etiology for her fissure formation is not infectious. If she no longer has constipation but the fissure recurs, then Crohn disease may be the cause and she should have further evaluation.

15.4 **D.** Given the child's somnolence, immediate intravascular volume is needed. Isotonic saline should be given until volume is restored and then based on the hemoglobin and clotting studies, he may need red blood cells or plasma. His clinical presentation could represent intussusception and if seen on ultrasound, surgical consultation is needed. Colonoscopy would not be indicated until the patient is stabilized.

CLINICAL PEARLS

▶ Anal fissures are the most common cause of hematochezia in infants, children, and adolescents.

▶ Tachycardia is the first indication that the rate or volume of bleeding is significant and warrants stabilization with isotonic saline and transfer to a hospital.

▶ If the patient is lethargic or ill appearing and has abdominal pain, emergent laboratory and radiographic evaluation is indicated.

▶ Lower GI bleeding with a benign etiology identified on physical examination does not require any laboratory or radiographic studies.

REFERENCES

Densmore JC, Lal DR. Intussusception. In: Rudolph CD, Rudolph AM, Lister GE, First LR, Gershon AA, eds. *Rudolph's Pediatrics*. 22nd ed. New York, NY: McGraw-Hill; 2011:1428-1429.

Klinker DB, Gourlay DM. Omphalo-mesenteric duct remnants. In: Rudolph CD, Rudolph AM, Lister GE, First LR, Gershon AA, eds. *Rudolph's Pediatrics*. 22nd ed. New York, NY: McGraw-Hill; 2011:1425-1427.

Noel RJ. Upper and lower gastrointestinal bleeding. In: Rudolph CD, Rudolph AM, Lister GE, First LR, Gershon AA, eds. *Rudolph's Pediatrics*. 22nd ed. New York, NY: McGraw-Hill; 2011:1389-1391.

Stafford SJ, Klein MD. Anal fissure. In: Kliegman RM, Stanton BF, St. Geme III J, Schor N, Behrman R, eds. *Nelson Textbook of Pediatrics*. 19th ed. Philadelphia, PA: WB Saunders; 2011:1359.

A 4-year-old child is seen by the pediatrician for ear pain. His mother reports he was in his usual state of good health until about 5 days ago when he developed an upper respiratory infection (URI) consisting of clear nasal discharge and cough. He had been having normal activity and intake until about 48 hours prior when he developed a temperature of 102.1°F (38.9°C) and complaints that his left ear hurts. She denies nausea, vomiting, diarrhea, headache, or change in urine output. She reports that he did not sleep well the previous evening, awakening several times complaining of ear pain, but remains somewhat interested in his toys earlier in the day.

▶ What is the most likely diagnosis?
▶ What is the best therapy?

ANSWERS TO CASE 16:

Acute Otitis Media

Summary: A preschool child presents with ear pain and fever.

- **Most likely diagnosis:** Acute otitis media (AOM)
- **Best therapy:** Oral antibiotics

ANALYSIS

Objectives

1. Be familiar with the epidemiology of otitis media (OM) in children.
2. Understand the treatment of this condition.
3. Learn the consequences of severe infection.

Considerations

OM is high on the differential diagnosis for this child with URI and ear pain. The diagnosis can be confirmed by pneumatic otoscopy and treatment started. A "telephone diagnosis" should be avoided. Figure 16–1 illustrates the anatomy of the middle ear.

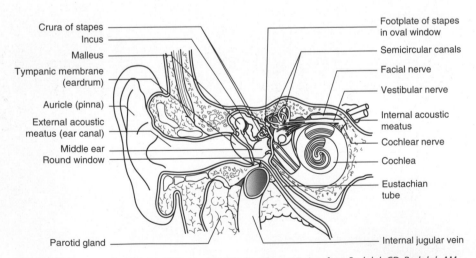

Figure 16–1. Anatomy of the middle ear. (*Modified, with permission, from Rudolph CD, Rudolph AM, Hostetter MK, et al. Rudolph's pediatrics, 21st ed. New York: McGraw-Hill Education, 2003:1240.*)

APPROACH TO:
Acute Otitis Media

DEFINITIONS

ACUTE OTITIS MEDIA (AOM): A condition of otalgia (ear pain), fever, and other symptoms along with findings of a red, opaque, poorly moving, bulging tympanic membrane (TM).

MYRINGOTOMY AND PLACEMENT OF PRESSURE EQUALIZATION (PE) TUBES: A surgical procedure involving TM incision and placement of PE tubes (tiny plastic or metal tubes anchored into the TM) to ventilate the middle ear and help prevent reaccumulation of middle ear fluid.

OTITIS MEDIA WITH EFFUSION: A condition in which fluid collects behind the TM but without signs and symptoms of AOM. Sometimes also called serous OM.

PNEUMATIC OTOSCOPY: The process of obtaining a tight ear canal seal with a speculum and then applying slight positive and negative pressure with a rubber bulb to verify TM mobility.

TYMPANOMETRY: An examination that measures the transfer of acoustic energy at varying levels of ear canal pressures, which will reflect TM mobility.

TYMPANOCENTESIS: A minor surgical procedure in which a small incision is made into the TM to drain pus and fluid from the middle ear space. This procedure is rarely done in the primary care office, but rather is done by the specialist.

CLINICAL APPROACH

Otitis media is a common childhood diagnosis. **Common bacterial pathogens include** *Streptococcus pneumoniae,* **nontypeable** *Haemophilus influenzae,* **and** *Moraxella catarrhalis.* Other organisms, *Staphylococcus aureus, Escherichia coli, Klebsiella pneumoniae,* and *Pseudomonas aeruginosa,* are seen in neonates and patients with immune deficiencies. Viruses can cause AOM, and in many cases the etiology is unknown. Acute OM is diagnosed in a child with fever (usually $<104°F$ [$40°C$]), ear pain (often nocturnal, awakening child from sleep), and generalized malaise. Systemic symptoms may include anorexia, nausea, vomiting, diarrhea, and headache. The cornerstone of diagnosis is the physical examination findings on pneumatic otoscopy of a **red, bulging TM with middle ear effusion and decreased mobility by either pneumatic otoscopy and/or tympanometry.** The TM may be opaque with pus behind it, the middle ear landmarks may be obscured, and, if the TM has ruptured, pus may be seen in the ear canal. Normal landmarks are shown in Figure 16–2.

In some situations and in a child older than 6 months with mild symptoms (ie, mild otalgia for <48 hours, temperature $<39°C$), a "watchful waiting" period of a few days may be indicated because many AOM cases self-resolve. Numerous studies have shown that only about one-third of children with evidence of AOM initially observed for a period of time had persistent or worsening symptoms that

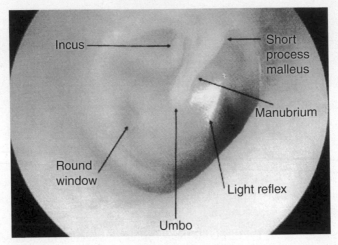

Figure 16–2. The tympanic membrane. (*Redrawn, with permission, from Rudolph CD, Rudolph AM, Hostetter MK, et al. Rudolph's pediatrics, 21st ed. New York: McGraw-Hill Education, 2003:1240.*)

required rescue antibiotics. Ensuring close medical follow-up is paramount if the choice is made to withhold antibiotics and to observe children with mild AOM.

Should antibiotics be deemed necessary and depending on a community's bacterial resistance patterns, amoxicillin at doses up to 80 to 90 mg/kg/d for 7 to 10 days is often the initial treatment. If the child has received amoxicillin in the previous 30 days, has a history of recurrent AOM unresponsive to amoxicillin, or has concurrent purulent conjunctivitis, an antibiotic with β-lactamase coverage is warranted. In the child begun on amoxicillin who demonstrates clinical failure after 3 treatment days, a change to amoxicillin-clavulanate, cefuroxime axetil, cefdinir, azithromycin, ceftriaxone, or tympanocentesis is considered. Adjuvant therapies (analgesics or antipyretics) are often indicated, but other measures (antihistamines, decongestants, and corticosteroids) are ineffective.

After an AOM episode, middle ear fluid can persist for up to several months. If hearing is normal, middle ear effusion often is treated with observation; some practitioners treat with antibiotics. **When the fluid does not resolve or recurrent episodes of AOM occur (defined as ≥3 in the previous 6 months or ≥4 in the previous year with 1 in the previous 6 months), especially if hearing loss is noted, myringotomy with PE tubes is often implemented.**

Rare but serious AOM **complications** include **mastoiditis, temporal bone osteomyelitis, facial nerve paralysis,** epidural and subdural abscess formation, meningitis, lateral sinus thrombosis, and otitic hydrocephalus (evidence of increased intracranial pressure with OM). An AOM patient whose clinical course is unusual or prolonged should be evaluated for one of these conditions.

> **CASE CORRELATION**
>
> - See also Case 10 (Failure to Thrive). A thorough exploration for a patient with chronic or recurrent OM and with failure to thrive is warranted. An anatomic abnormality or immune deficiency may be a contributing factor.

COMPREHENSION QUESTIONS

16.1 A 1-year-old boy presents with fever, ear pain, and purulent discharge from both eyes. On examination, bilateral erythematous, bulging tympanic membranes (TMs), and purulent conjunctivitis are noted. Based on his symptoms and examination, amoxicillin-clavulanate is prescribed. The mother asks what she could do to prevent future ear infections. Which of the following is NOT one of the current recommendations to reduce the incidence of otitis media?

   A. Pneumococcal vaccine

   B. Influenza vaccine

   C. Xylitol

   D. Eliminating exposure to tobacco smoke

   E. Breast-feeding

16.2 Three days after beginning oral amoxicillin therapy for otitis media (OM), a 4-year-old boy has continued fever, ear pain, and swelling with redness behind his ear. His ear lobe is pushed superiorly and laterally. He seems to be doing well otherwise. Which of the following is the most appropriate course of action?

   A. Change to oral amoxicillin-clavulanate

   B. Myringotomy and parenteral antibiotics

   C. Nuclear scan of the head

   D. Topical steroids

   E. Tympanocentesis

16.3 A 5-year-old girl developed high fever, ear pain, and vomiting a week ago. She was diagnosed with OM and started on amoxicillin-clavulanate. On the third day of this medication she continued with findings of OM, fever, and pain. She received ceftriaxone intramuscularly and switched to oral cefuroxime. Now, 48 hours later, she has fever, pain, and no improvement in her OM; otherwise she is doing well. Which of the following is the most logical next step in her management?

   A. Addition of intranasal topical steroids to the oral cefuroxime

   B. Adenoidectomy

   C. High-dose oral amoxicillin

   D. Oral trimethoprim-sulfamethoxazole

   E. Tympanocentesis and culture of middle ear fluid

16.4 A 1-month-old boy has a fever to 102.7°F (39.3°C), is irritable, has diarrhea, and has not been eating well. On examination he has an immobile red TM that has pus behind it. Which of the following is the most appropriate course of action?

A. Admission to the hospital with complete sepsis evaluation

B. Intramuscular ceftriaxone and close outpatient follow-up

C. Oral amoxicillin-clavulanate

D. Oral cefuroxime

E. High-dose oral amoxicillin

ANSWERS

16.1 **C.** Although some research shows xylitol use can reduce AOM, compliance issues make it an ineffective therapy. With the pneumococcal vaccine, a 2009 Cochrane review showed the overall incidence of AOM has reduced by 6% to 7%. Because as many as two-thirds of children who have influenza have AOM, studies have demonstrated the influenza vaccine has a 30% to 55% efficacy of preventing AOM during respiratory season. Breast-feeding for at least 4 to 6 months reduces episodes of AOM and recurrent AOM. In addition to other benefits, elimination of passive tobacco smoke exposure has been linked to a reduction of AOM in infancy.

16.2 **B.** The child has mastoiditis, a clinical diagnosis that can require computed tomography scan confirmation. Treatment includes myringotomy, fluid culture, and parenteral antibiotics. Surgical drainage of the mastoid air cells may be needed if improvement is not seen in 24 to 48 hours.

16.3 **E.** After failing several antibiotic regimens, tympanocentesis and culture of the middle ear fluid are indicated.

16.4 **A.** Very young children with OM (especially if irritable or lethargic) are at higher risk for bacteremia or other serious infection. Hospitalization and parenteral antibiotics often are needed.

CLINICAL PEARLS

▶ The most common bacterial pathogens causing otitis media (OM) are *Streptococcus pneumoniae*, nontypeable *Haemophilus influenzae*, and *Moraxella catarrhalis*.

▶ Examination findings of OM include a red, bulging tympanic membrane that does not move well with pneumatic otoscopy, an opaque tympanic membrane with pus behind it, obscured middle-ear landmarks, and, if the tympanic membrane has ruptured, pus in the ear canal.

▶ Initial treatment of OM often includes amoxicillin (depending on local bacterial resistance patterns). If a clinical failure is seen on day 3, a change to amoxicillin-clavulanate, cefuroxime axetil, ceftriaxone, or a tympanocentesis is indicated.

▶ Administration of the pneumococcal and influenza vaccines, tobacco smoke avoidance, and increase in breast-feeding are linked to a reduction in the incidence of AOM.

▶ Complications are rare but include mastoiditis, temporal bone osteomyelitis, facial nerve palsy, epidural and subdural abscess formation, meningitis, lateral sinus thrombosis, and otitic hydrocephalus.

REFERENCES

Haddad J. External otitis (otitis externa). In: Kleigman RM, Stanton BF, St. Geme JW, Schor NF, Behrman RE, eds. *Nelson Textbook of Pediatrics*. 19th ed. Philadelphia, PA: WB Saunders; 2011:2196-2199.

Kerschner JE. Otitis media. In: Kleigman RM, Stanton BF, St. Geme JW, Schor NF, Behrman RE, eds. *Nelson Textbook of Pediatrics*. 19th ed. Philadelphia, PA: WB Saunders; 2011:2199-2213.

Klein JO. Otitis media. In: Rudolph CD, Rudolph AM, Lister G, First LR, Gershon AA, eds. *Rudolph's Pediatrics*. 22nd ed. New York, NY: McGraw-Hill; 2011:973-979.

Kline MW. Otitis externa. In: McMillan JA, Feigin RD, DeAngelis CD, Jones MD, eds. *Oski's Pediatrics: Principles and Practice*. 4th ed. Philadelphia, PA: Lippincott Williams & Wilkins; 2006:1496-1497.

Kline MW. Mastoiditis. In: McMillan JA, Feigin RD, DeAngelis CD, Jones MD, eds. *Oski's Pediatrics: Principles and Practice*. 4th ed. Philadelphia, PA: Lippincott Williams & Wilkins; 2006:1501-1502.

Lieberthal AS, Carroll AE, Chonmaitree T, et al. Diagnosis and management of acute otitis media. *Pediatrics*. 2013;131:e964-e999.

Rudolph C. Otitis externa. In: Rudolph CD, Rudolph AM, Lister G, First LR, Gershon AA, eds. *Rudolph's Pediatrics*. 22nd ed. New York, NY: McGraw-Hill; 2011:979.

Schwarzwald H, Kline MW. Otitis media. In: McMillan JA, Feigin RD, DeAngelis CD, Jones MD, eds. *Oski's Pediatrics: Principles and Practice*. 4th ed. Philadelphia, PA: Lippincott Williams & Wilkins; 2006:1497-1500.

Yoon PJ, Kelley PE, Friedman NR. Acute otitis media. In: Hay WW, Levin MJ, Sondheimer JM, Deterding RR. *Current Diagnosis & Treatment: Pediatrics*. 20th ed. New York, NY: McGraw-Hill; 2011:453-464.

Yoon PJ, Kelley PE, Friedman NR. Mastoiditis. In: Hay WW, Levin MJ, Sondheimer JM, Deterding RR. *Current Diagnosis & Treatment: Pediatrics*. 20th ed. New York, NY: McGraw-Hill; 2011:464-465.

Yoon PJ, Kelley PE, Friedman NR. Otitis externa. In: Hay WW, Levin MJ, Sondheimer JM, Deterding RR. *Current Diagnosis & Treatment: Pediatrics*. 20th ed. New York, NY: McGraw-Hill; 2011:452-453.

A 12-month-old boy whom you have followed since birth arrives for a well-child visit. The mother is concerned that the baby's manner of crawling, where he drags his legs rather than using a four-limbed movement, is abnormal. She says that the child only recently began crawling and he does not pull to a stand. You noted at his 6-month visit that he was not yet rolling over or sitting; previous visits were unremarkable as was the mother's pregnancy and vaginal delivery. On examination today, you note that he positions his legs in a "scissoring" posture (ie, legs extended and crossed) when held by the axillae.

► What is the initial step in the evaluation of this child?
► What is the most likely diagnosis?
► What is the next step in the evaluation?

ANSWERS TO CASE 17:

Cerebral Palsy

Summary: A 12-month-old boy crawls using primarily his upper extremities and holds his legs in a "scissoring" posture when suspended.

- **Initial step:** Gather detailed history, focusing on the age at which developmental milestones were achieved; obtain thorough pregnancy, birth, social, and family histories; and perform a detailed neurologic examination.

- **Most likely diagnosis:** Cerebral palsy (CP).

- **Next step:** Vision and hearing testing, consider a brain magnetic resonance imaging (MRI) scan, and arrange for therapy with a developmental specialist.

ANALYSIS

Objectives

1. Know the definition of CP.

2. Recognize the classifications of CP.

3. Know the basic therapeutic approach to CP.

Considerations

The described spasticity of the baby's lower extremities is abnormal and is suggestive of CP. He has gross motor delay. A complete developmental and neurologic assessment is crucial for initiating therapies that will help him achieve maximal functional outcome. Although often of low yield, an attempt should be made to identify the etiology of the child's CP. Knowing the etiology can aid in developing a treatment plan, subsequent family planning (especially if the etiology is inherited), and assuaging parental guilt for this child's condition.

APPROACH TO:

Cerebral Palsy

DEFINITIONS

CEREBRAL PALSY (CP): A disorder of nonprogressive movement and posture that results from an insult to or anomaly of the developing central nervous system (CNS). This definition recognizes the central origin of the dysfunction, thus distinguishing it from neuropathies and myopathies.

DEVELOPMENTAL DELAY: Failure of a child to reach developmental milestones of gross motor, fine motor, language, or social-adaptive skills at anticipated ages.

NEUROLOGIC DEFICIT: Abnormal functioning or lack of function of a part of the nervous system.

CLINICAL APPROACH

With a prevalence of 3 to 4 cases per 1000 live births, **CP is the most common child-hood movement disorder. Approximately one-third of CP patients also have seizures, and approximately 60% of affected children are mentally retarded.** Deafness, visual impairments, swallowing difficulty with concomitant aspiration, limb and sensory impairments, and behavioral disturbances are common comorbidities.

Most children with CP have no identifiable risk factors, and low Apgar scores are not a risk for CP. Current research indicates that CP **is most likely because of antenatal insults,** and subsequent difficulties during the pregnancy, delivery, and perinatal period are thought to reflect these already-present insults. Only 10% of cases of CP have a positive family history and may then be caused by a **chromosomal or metabolic** disorder. Acquired conditions that carry a risk for CP are **infection (cytomegalovirus, group B *Streptococcus*, herpes simplex virus), intraventricular hemorrhage, especially if it extends into the white matter and causes cystic periventricular leukomalacia (PVL), acute bilirubin encephalopathy (kernicterus), stroke, and brain trauma.** Cerebral palsy, or "static" encephalopathy, is because of a one-time CNS insult. In contrast, progressive encephalopathies destroy brain function with time. The term *static* is misleading, however, because the manifestations of CP may change with age. Contractures and postural deformities may become more severe with time or may improve with therapy. Also, a child's changing developmental stages early in life can alter the expression of his or her neurologic deficits.

Immaturity of the CNS at birth makes diagnosis of CP nearly impossible in a neonate and difficult in infants younger than 6 months because primitive reflexes may persist until that age. If a CNS insult is suspected, head imaging (by ultrasound or MRI) can be helpful in recognizing CP early. Possible imaging findings include periventricular leukomalacia, atrophy, or focal infarctions. Beyond infancy, CP is suspected when a child fails to meet anticipated developmental milestones.

Examples of concerning findings are as follows:

- A stepping response after the age of 3 months

- A Moro reflex beyond 6 months

- An asymmetrical tonic neck reflex beyond 6 months

Cerebral palsy can be classified in terms of physiologic, topographic, or functional categories. Physiologic descriptors identify the major motor abnormality and are divided into pyramidal (spastic) and extrapyramidal (nonspastic) categories. Extrapyramidal types can be subdivided further into choreoathetoid, ataxic, dystonic, or rigid types.

The topographic classification categorizes CP types according to limb involvement. **Hemiplegia** refers to involvement of a single lateral side of the body, with greater impairment of the upper extremities than the lower extremities. **Diplegia** describes a four-limb involvement, with greater impairment of the lower extremities. **Spastic quadriplegia** is a four-limb involvement with significant impairment of all extremities, although the upper limbs may be less impaired than the lower limbs. (The term *paraplegia* is reserved for spinal and lower motor neuron disorders.)

The functional classification of CP relies on the "motor quotient" to place patients into minimal, mild, moderate, and severe (profound) categories. The motor quotient is derived by dividing the child's "motor age" (ie, motor skills developmental age) with the chronologic age. A motor quotient of 75 to 100 represents minimal impairment, 55 to 70 is mild impairment, 40 to 55 is moderate impairment, and lesser quotients indicate severe impairment. These categories help clinicians identify children with less obvious impairments so that early treatment can be provided.

The evaluation of CP is based on the history and physical examination. The yield of diagnostic findings with brain imaging and metabolic or genetic testing is low but can be helpful in managing the patient, in future family planning, and in reassuring the parents. Identification of comorbid conditions includes cognitive testing for mental retardation and electroencephalography (EEG) for seizures.

Treatment goals include maximizing motor function and preventing secondary handicaps. During the preschool years, the child's communication ability is important. Maintaining optimal vision and auditory function is a priority. School performance and peer acceptance become important issues for older children. Physical therapy for motor deficits may be supplemented with pharmacologic and surgical interventions. Occupational therapy improves positioning and allows for better interaction with the environment and eases care as the child grows. The family's psychological and social needs should not be overlooked.

CASE CORRELATION

- See also Cases 2, 3, 4, 6, 9, and 10. Some patients with cerebral palsy (CP) may have failure to thrive (Case 10). Among myriad causes of CP are birth asphyxia and prematurity, more common in an infant of a diabetic mother (Case 2), severe neonatal hyperbilirubinemia (Case 3), neonatal infections such as group B streptococcal infection (Case 4) and neonatal herpes simplex virus infection (Case 6), and infants having sustained a TORCH (toxoplasmosis, cytomegalovirus, syphilis, rubella, and herpes simplex virus) infection may result in neonatal cataracts (Case 9).

COMPREHENSION QUESTIONS

17.1 You are performing a routine 2-week well-child visit. The mother had routine prenatal care with no complications. During delivery, prolapse of the cord necessitated an emergent Cesarean section. The Apgar scores were 3, 7, and 9. The remainder of the hospital course was routine. The mother reports that her niece has cerebral palsy (CP). She asks about the risk for her baby having CP and you inform her that:

A. Having a family history of CP makes it likely that her child will also have it.

B. The low Apgar score is a risk for her child to develop CP.

C. Your examination today will determine if her infant has CP.

D. Most children with CP do not have a genetic risk, and at each well-child visit, you will continue to perform a careful developmental assessment.

E. You will refer her infant to a pediatric neurologist to do further workup.

17.2 A 4-year-old child with CP comes to your clinic for the first time for a routine visit. He walks with the help of leg braces and a walker, and his speech is slurred and limited to short phrases. He has never been hospitalized, and he does not have swallowing problems. He began walking at the age of 2.5 years, and he is unable to take off his clothes and use the toilet without help. On examination, you find that the boy has only minimally increased tone in the upper extremities but good fine motor coordination; he has significantly increased tone and deep tendon reflexes in the lower extremities. How would you categorize this child's CP?

A. Mild, diplegic

B. Mild, hemiplegic

C. Moderate, diplegic

D. Moderate, quadriplegic

E. Severe, diplegic

17.3 A female is born via spontaneous vaginal delivery at 28 weeks of gestation because of preterm labor. Which of the following would be a risk factor for CP?

A. Hypoglycemia

B. Apnea of prematurity

C. Intraventricular hemorrhage

D. Blood transfusion

E. Mechanical ventilation

17.4 You are seeing a 4-year-old boy with moderate diplegic CP for his well-child visit. He is nonverbal. How will your management of his visit differ from that of a child without CP?

A. You would not need to perform a hearing test because he is unable to respond.

B. You will ask which therapies he receives, who provides them, the frequency and goals.

C. You would not administer any vaccines.

D. You would ask his parents about any behavior that would suggest a seizure.

E. You would not perform a developmental assessment.

ANSWERS

17.1 **D.** Most children with CP do not have identifiable risk factors. Even in the presence of a risk factor, many children do not develop CP. The Apgar score at 1 minute reflects the neonatal environment immediately prior to birth; it does not predict an infant's neurologic outcome. CP cannot be ruled out on the basis of a normal neonatal physical examination. It is difficult to diagnose in children younger than 6 months. Assessing a child's development at each checkup is important for detecting abnormalities. If there is abnormal development or an abnormal examination finding, then referral to a neurologist may be appropriate.

17.2 **C.** In diplegia all four extremities are affected, with greater impairment of the lower extremities. Because most children walk by the age of 14 months, this child's motor quotient is 14 months/30 months = 0.47, which classifies him as moderately impaired.

17.3 **C.** Intraventricular hemorrhage can later result in periventricular leukomalacia, which has been associated with an increased chance of CP.

17.4 **B.** Optimal treatment for CP is multidisciplinary, and it is important to insure the child is receiving the services that are needed for ongoing treatment of his condition. Even though the office-based hearing evaluation cannot be done for him because it requires verbal participation, his hearing still needs to be assessed; a hearing test that does not require the patient to give a verbal response should be ordered. He should receive the recommended vaccines for his age. Asking about behavior that suggests a seizure is part of the review of systems for all children. Although his development is delayed, it is still important to assess in order to identify the age level that he is at for each area of development.

CLINICAL PEARLS

▶ Cerebral palsy is a disorder of movement or posture resulting from an insult to, or an anomaly of, the central nervous system before it has matured.

▶ Most children with cerebral palsy have no identifiable risk factors for the disorder.

▶ Optimal treatment plans for cerebral palsy use a multidisciplinary approach.

REFERENCES

Johnston MV. Cerebral palsy. In: Kliegman RM, Stanton BF, St. Geme III JW, Schor NF, Behrman RE, eds. *Nelson Textbook of Pediatrics*. 19th ed. Philadelphia, PA: Elsevier WB Saunders; 2011: 2061-2065.

Rust RS, Urion DK. Cerebral palsy and static encephalopathies. In: Rudolph CD, Rudolph AM, Lister GE, First LR, Gershon AA, eds. *Rudolph's Pediatrics*. 22nd ed. New York, NY: McGraw-Hill; 2011: 2178-2181.

A 2½-year-old boy comes to your clinic for the first time with complaints of fever and increasing "wet" cough for 8 days. His mother reports that he has been diagnosed with asthma and has an albuterol inhaler to use for wheezing or cough. Since 6 months of age, he has had several similar episodes of "wet" cough and fever, which were diagnosed as bronchitis or pneumonia, and he would improve when treated with antibiotics and albuterol. However, over the past year, these episodes have become more frequent and the cough occurs almost daily now. Sometimes the mother sees him expectorate the sputum, which is thick and purulent. He has daily nasal congestion for which she uses saline and bulb suction in his nares. She is able to obtain some thick yellow discharge but the symptoms mainly improve when he is treated with antibiotics. He is not in daycare and has no tobacco exposure. She is concerned that his frequent illnesses are causing him to be "small for his age." The mother notes his stools are malodorous, and since starting him on potty-training she has observed that his stools float and sometimes appear to have drops of oil on them. Your examination reveals a moderately ill-appearing child whose height and weight are at the third percentile for age. His temperature is 101°F (38.3°C) and respiratory rate is 32 breaths/min. He is breathing with his mouth open. Over the upper lung fields, he has crackles and rhonchi and also a few expiratory wheezes over all lung fields. He has no heart murmur; S1 and S2 are normal. His fingers show clubbing. You obtain a chest radiograph that shows linear opacities in a parallel tram-track configuration in the upper lobes with some ring-shaped opacities; the radiologist interprets the findings as bronchiectasis.

▶ What is the most likely diagnosis?
▶ What is the next step in evaluation?

ANSWERS TO CASE 18:

Cystic Fibrosis

Summary: A 2½-year-old boy has recurrent sinopulmonary infections and bronchiectasis. He exhibits failure to thrive due to the recurrent illness and steatorrhea.

- **Most likely diagnosis:** Cystic fibrosis (CF).

- **Next step in evaluation:** Obtain a sweat chloride test.

ANALYSIS

Objectives

1. Know the historical clues and physical signs to distinguish CF from more common conditions.

2. Know how to accurately diagnose CF.

3. Have a basic understanding of the complications of CF and its treatment.

Considerations

Several causes for bronchiectasis exist, with asthma and infection being the most common. However, the child's poor growth and clubbing suggest a more diffuse pulmonary disease or that other organ systems are involved. Bronchiectasis typically improves with antibiotics. Rhinosinusitis caused by viral respiratory pathogens should improve within 10 days; otherwise a bacterial etiology is assumed and treatment with antibiotics is indicated. Recurrent bacterial sinusitis is not typical for a child this age unless an underlying disorder is found.

APPROACH TO:

Cystic Fibrosis

DEFINITIONS

BRONCHIECTASIS: Condition in which a bronchus or bronchi remains dilated after an infection or obstruction.

CLUBBING: Increase in the angle between the nail and nail base of 180° or greater, and softening of the nail base to palpation. Although the condition can be familial, clubbing is uncommon in children, usually indicating chronic pulmonary, hepatic, cardiac, or gastrointestinal disease.

CYSTIC FIBROSIS (CF): The major cause of chronic debilitating pulmonary disease and pancreatic exocrine deficiency in the first three decades of life. It is characterized by the triad of chronic obstructive pulmonary disease, pancreatic exocrine deficiency, and abnormally high sweat electrolyte concentrations. Characteristic pancreatic changes give the disease its name.

CLINICAL APPROACH

Cystic fibrosis afflicts all ethnicities with the highest prevalence in Caucasians. CF shows autosomal recessive inheritance; it is caused by an abnormal CFTR (cystic fibrosis **transmembrane conductance regulator) protein.** The most common mutation causing the abnormal protein is known as **delta 508.** The altered CFTR protein allows excess loss of sodium and chloride. The loss from the eccrine glands of the skin causes a **hyponatremic, hypochloremic alkalosis.**

With excess loss of sodium chloride from the respiratory tract, mucus thickens and obstructs airways, leading to **bronchiectasis** in most CF patients by the age of 18 months. These children will have symptoms of **cough and wheezing that mimic asthma and bronchiolitis.** Bacteria then proliferate in the inspissated mucus and damaged respiratory cilia, resulting in **pneumonia. Pseudomonas** is a particular threat and is rarely found in other conditions outside CF. Lung function is lost with the destruction from recurrent inflammation, obstruction, and infection. The upper respiratory tract is also involved and the finding of **pansinusitis,** which is rarely seen in healthy children, often signals an underlying disorder such as CF.

The other site where CF commonly manifests is the gastrointestinal tract, particularly the pancreas. Exocrine function is usually lost, resulting in **frequent passage of oily, malodorous, and floating stools** which can eventually **lead to malnutrition and failure to thrive.** The resulting fat-soluble vitamin deficiencies may manifest as peripheral neuropathy and hemolytic anemia (vitamin E), night blindness (vitamin A), or mucosal bleeding (vitamin K). In 20% of neonates with CF, **meconium ileus** occurs in the first 1 to 2 days of life. In this condition, meconium becomes inspissated in the ileum and the infant will not pass stool; abdominal distention and emesis follow. Intestinal perforation can occur without prompt intervention and treatment.

The **diagnosis of CF requires two positive sweat tests in conjunction with any of the characteristic respiratory, gastrointestinal, or genitourinary symptoms.** Table 18–1 lists the common indications for sweat chloride testing. A positive sweat test is defined by a sweat chloride content of 60 mEq/L or greater. However, false-negative results can occur so **DNA testing** is then employed **to detect the presence of mutations known to cause CF.** If two mutations are detected, then CF is confirmed. Routine screening for CF is performed on all newborns in the United States. The test detects a pancreatic enzyme, immunoreactive trypsinogen (IRT), which is elevated in infants with CF. Infants with positive results on the newborn screen undergo sweat chloride testing for definitive diagnosis.

Long-term management of CF patients is best coordinated by experienced pediatric **pulmonary specialists.** Bronchodilators, inhaled corticosteroids, antibiotics, and inhaled recombinant human DNAse are used to minimize airway reactivity, infections, and secretions. Optimal nutrition is dependent on pancreatic enzyme replacement and vitamin supplements. The prognosis varies depending on disease severity, and most patients reach adolescence or adulthood. Mean survival for persons with CF is 35 years; respiratory disease accounts for the majority of deaths.

Table 18–1 • INDICATIONS FOR SWEAT TESTING
Gastrointestinal
Chronic diarrhea
Steatorrhea
Meconium ileus or plug syndrome
Rectal prolapsed
Cirrhosis or portal hypertension
Prolonged neonatal jaundice
Pancreatitis
Deficiency of fat-soluble vitamins (especially A, E, K)
Respiratory Tract
Upper
• Nasal polyps
• Pansinusitis on radiographs
• Lower
• Chronic cough
• Recurrent "wheezing" bronchiolitis
• Recurrent or intractable asthma
• Obstructive pulmonary disease
• Staphylococcal pneumonia
• *Pseudomonas aeruginosa* (especially mucoid) from throat, sputum, or bronchoscopy cultures
Other
Digital clubbing
Family history of cystic fibrosis
Failure to thrive
Hyponatremic, hypochloremic alkalosis
Severe dehydration or heat prostration incompatible with history
"Tastes salty"
Male infertility

Reproduced, with permission, from Rudolph CD, Rudolph AM, Hostetter MK, Lister G, Siegel NJ, eds. Rudolph's Pediatrics. *21st ed. New York, NY: McGraw-Hill; 2003:1973.*

CASE CORRELATION

- See also Case 10 and Case 20 (Asthma). Patients with CF often have nutritional deficiencies as well as pneumonia (Case 14) and recurrent sinusitis and otitis media (Case 16).

COMPREHENSION QUESTIONS

18.1 An 18-month-old girl is seen in the clinic for cough and fever. Her weight is in the third percentile. The mother reports she is concerned her daughter is around "toxic mold" because she has had five to six prior episodes of bronchitis since they moved to a new apartment at 6 months of age. She states that albuterol and an antibiotic are always given for treatment, and symptoms resolve in 2 weeks. A chest radiograph is obtained. What finding on the radiograph would prompt you to perform a sweat chloride test?

A. An enlarged cardiac silhouette

B. Absent thymus

C. Bronchiectasis

D. Dextrocardia

E. Hilar lymphadenopathy

18.2 A 7-year-old girl is admitted to the hospital in respiratory distress due to pneumonia. This is her third admission in the past 6 months. At this time you are suspecting cystic fibrosis (CF) and order a sputum culture. Which organism would be most consistent with a diagnosis of cystic fibrosis?

A. *Streptococcus pneumoniae*

B. *Mycobacterium tuberculosis*

C. *Pseudomonas aeruginosa*

D. *Bacillus cereus*

E. *Haemophilus influenzae*

18.3 A 10-year-old Caucasian boy has a history of recurrent sinusitis and multiple episodes of pneumonia. You suspect CF and order a sweat chloride test. The sweat electrolyte test result is within the normal range. What is your next step in management?

A. Perform DNA testing for CFTR (cystic fibrosis transmembrane conductance regulator) gene mutations.

B. Perform a pH probe test for gastroesophageal reflux.

C. Referral to pulmonologist.

D. Reassure parents that he does not have CF.

E. Place him on a high-calorie, high-protein diet.

18.4 A 3-month-old infant is admitted to the hospital with her third episode of lobar pneumonia and wheezing. Findings that would increase your suspicions for CF and prompt sweat chloride testing include all of the following EXCEPT:

    A. Hyponatremia, hypochloremia, and metabolic alkalosis

    B. Failure to thrive

    C. Lymphocytosis

    D. Digital clubbing

    E. Oily appearing stools

ANSWERS

18.1 **C.** Bronchiectasis occurs as a sequela to impaired mucus clearance combined with inflammation and injury to the bronchial walls. CF is the most common noninfectious and chronic cause of this finding; sweat chloride testing is a standard for diagnosis. The other findings are not characteristics of CF.

18.2 **C.** The presence of *P aeruginosa* on a sputum sample strongly suggests the diagnosis of CF. Patients with CF have a high prevalence of colonization with *P aeruginosa*, *Staphylococcus aureus*, and *Burkholderia cepacia*. The innate defenses of the airway epithelium cells of CF patients may be compromised, making them unable to fight these organisms.

18.3 **A.** The child has recurrent upper and lower respiratory tract infections suggesting CF. The sweat chloride test can yield falsely low values, so the next step would be to perform DNA testing to identify any of the common CFTR mutations. Negative sweat chloride test results do not exclude CF.

18.4 **C.** Infants with CF will lose excess amounts of sodium chloride in their sweat resulting in a hyponatremic, hypochloremic metabolic alkalosis. Malabsorption of fats and protein due to pancreatic exocrine insufficiency usually presents as steatorrhea and is a major cause of morbidity for patients with CF, resulting in failure to thrive. Lymphocytosis can occur with viral infections or pertussis but is not a hallmark of CF.

CLINICAL PEARLS

▶ Cystic fibrosis (CF) involves a defect in chloride channels leading to excess loss of sodium chloride and water with resultant accumulation of thick mucus in the lumina of the respiratory, digestive, and genitourinary tracts.

▶ Extrapulmonary signs and symptoms, such as digital clubbing, recurrent sinusitis, failure to thrive, fat malabsorption, and a history of meconium ileus are clues to the diagnosis of CF.

▶ A negative sweat chloride test result does not exclude CF.

▶ CF is diagnosed by two positive sweat chloride tests or if DNA testing detects two gene mutations known to cause CF.

REFERENCES

Egan M. Cystic fibrosis. In: Kliegman RM, Stanton BF, St. Geme III J, Schor N, Behrman R, eds. *Nelson Textbook of Pediatrics*. 19th ed. Philadelphia, PA: WB Saunders; 2011:1481-1497.

Orenstein DM. Cystic fibrosis. In: Rudolph CD, Rudolph AM, Lister GE, First LR, Gershon AA, eds. *Rudolph's Pediatrics*. 22nd ed. New York, NY: McGraw-Hill; 2011:1977-1986.

A mother brings her previously healthy 6-year-old son to your clinic because he has been limping and complaining of left leg and knee pain for 1 week. He has experienced no recent trauma, and his past medical history is unremarkable. His physical examination reveals a temperature of 100°F (37.8°C) orally with no lower extremity swelling, misalignment, or weakness. He has tenderness over the right knee, hepatosplenomegaly, and petechiae on his cheeks and chest.

▶ What is the most likely diagnosis?
▶ What is the next step in the evaluation?

ANSWERS TO CASE 19:

Acute Lymphoblastic Leukemia

Summary: A 6-year-old boy has a 1-week history of leg pain and limping. He has a low-grade fever, hepatosplenomegaly, and petechiae on his face and chest.

- **Most likely diagnosis:** Acute lymphoblastic leukemia (ALL)

- **Next step in the evaluation:** Complete blood count with platelets and differential

ANALYSIS

Objectives

1. Describe the clinical manifestations of ALL.

2. Describe the laboratory and radiologic tests used in diagnosing ALL.

3. Know the treatment plan for a child with newly diagnosed ALL.

4. Understand the long-term survival and follow-up issues for children with ALL.

Considerations

This patient has several manifestations of ALL, including leg and joint pain, fever, petechiae, and hepatosplenomegaly. Most of the signs and symptoms of ALL result from either replacement of normal bone marrow components with clonal proliferation of a single lymphoblast that has undergone malignant transformation, or from infiltrates of extramedullary sites by these malignant lymphoid cells. Rapid diagnosis and referral to a pediatric cancer center can increase survival.

APPROACH TO:

Acute Lymphoblastic Leukemia

DEFINITIONS

EXTRAMEDULLARY: Areas of the body outside the bone marrow.

LYMPHOBLAST: A large, primitive, undifferentiated precursor cell not normally seen in the peripheral circulation.

GRANULOCYTOPENIA: A reduction in total circulating leukocytes.

PANCYTOPENIA: A reduction in circulating erythrocytes, leukocytes, and platelets.

THROMBOCYTOPENIA: A reduction in circulating platelets.

CLINICAL APPROACH

Leukemia is the most common childhood cancer, with an incidence of 2.8 cases per 100,000 children, accounting for **approximately 40% of all pediatric malignancies.** **Acute lymphoblastic leukemia** affects the **lymphoid cell line** and comprises approximately 75% of leukemia cases in children. Acute myeloblastic leukemia (AML) affects the myeloid cell line (granulocytes, monocytes, and can affect erythrocytes or megakaryocytes) and comprises approximately 20% of childhood leukemia. The clinical manifestations of AML and ALL are similar. In the United States, childhood **ALL has a peak incidence at age 2 to 4 years** and occurs more frequently in **boys.** Children with certain chromosomal abnormalities, such as Down syndrome and Fanconi anemia, have an increased risk of ALL.

ALL is often called the "great imitator" because of its nonspecific symptoms, including anorexia, irritability, lethargy, pallor, bleeding, petechiae, leg and joint pain, lymphadenopathy, and fever. A physical examination includes the child's general appearance and energy level, vital signs (note if antipyretics taken), bleeding, bruising, petechiae, pallor, pain upon palpating bones or joints, and hepatosplenomegaly. Differential diagnoses include idiopathic thrombocytopenic purpura (ITP), aplastic anemia, mononucleosis, juvenile idiopathic arthritis, and leukemoid reaction:

- Idiopathic thrombocytopenic purpura is a common cause of bruising and petechiae because of low platelet levels. However, anemia, leukocyte disturbances, and hepatosplenomegaly are absent.

- Aplastic anemia causes pancytopenia and fever. Lymphadenopathy, arthralgias, bone pain, and hepatosplenomegaly are unusual findings.

- Children with infectious mononucleosis (ie, Epstein-Barr virus [EBV]) or other acute viral illnesses may present with fever, malaise, adenopathy, splenomegaly, and lymphocytosis. Atypical lymphocytes resembling leukemic lymphoblasts are characteristic of these viral illnesses.

- Leukemoid reactions may be observed in bacterial sepsis, pertussis, acute hemolysis, granulomatous disease, and vasculitis. The leukemoid reaction resolves as the underlying disease is treated.

Children with ALL who present with fever, arthralgias, arthritis, or a limp frequently are diagnosed initially with juvenile idiopathic arthritis (JIA). Anemia, leukocytosis, and mild splenomegaly may also be seen in JIA, causing even more confusion. **A bone marrow examination may be required to differentiate ALL from other diagnoses.**

Infiltration of the marrow by other types of malignant cells (neuroblastoma, rhabdomyosarcoma, Ewing sarcoma, and retinoblastoma) occasionally produces pancytopenia. These tumor cells usually are found in clumps in the normal marrow but occasionally replace the marrow completely.

Almost half of the children with newly diagnosed leukemia have total leukocyte counts less than 10,000/mm³. Leukemic blasts may not be seen in the peripheral blood smear. Therefore, the diagnosis of leukemia is established by **examination of bone marrow,** most commonly aspirated from the posterior iliac crest. **A normal**

marrow contains less than 5% blasts; a minimum of 25% blasts confirms the diagnosis. Approximately two-thirds of children with ALL have leukemic cell karyotypic abnormalities, including changes in chromosome number (ie, hypodiploidy or hyperdiploidy) or chromosome structure (translocation, deletions, inversions).

Pediatric ALL patients are classified as standard or high risk at the time of diagnosis. A variety of markers can help gauge prognosis. Children 1 to 9 years of age, with white blood cell (WBC) counts less than 500,000, without adverse cytogenetic features are considered standard risk. Meanwhile, children older than 10 years or those with higher WBC counts are considered higher risk and have an overall worse prognosis. Infants also have a worse prognosis and up to 60% of infants with ALL have the t(4;11) translocation which is correlated with a poor outcome. Another translocation with a poor outcome is the t(9;22) (Philadelphia chromosome) in patients with pre-B ALL.

In general, **girls have a better prognosis. African American and Hispanic populations** historically have **lower remission and higher relapse rates,** although newer studies suggest this might be due to factors other than race. The karyotypes of leukemic cells have diagnostic, prognostic, and therapeutic significance. Patients with hyperdiploidy generally have a more favorable prognosis; those with hypodiploidy and pseudodiploidy do less well.

Workup includes a **lumbar puncture** to examine the central nervous system (CNS) for early leukemic involvement; a **higher number of blasts in the cerebrospinal fluid are associated with a worse prognosis.** A **chest radiograph** is performed to detect a **mediastinal mass.**

Combination chemotherapy is the principal therapy. The therapy involves several phases: remission induction, CNS therapy, consolidation and intensification, and maintenance. Induction therapy, a combination of prednisone, vincristine, and asparaginase, produces remission within 4 weeks in approximately 98% of children with non–high-risk ALL. Intrathecal therapy (± craniospinal irradiation) has decreased the incidence of CNS leukemia as a primary site of relapse from 50% to approximately 3% to 6%. Consolidation treatment, aimed at further reducing residual leukemia, delivers multiple chemotherapies in a relatively short period of time. Maintenance therapy with methotrexate and 6-mercaptopurine, vincristine, and prednisone is given for 2 to 3 years to prevent relapse; therapy is discontinued for children who remain in complete remission for 2 to 3 years.

The 5-year survival rate for childhood ALL has steadily improved over the last 40 years and now is greater than 80%. Treatment response is key for determining the overall outcome. Patients with greater than 25% blasts after induction chemotherapy or greater than 5% blasts after consolidation chemotherapy have a high risk of relapse. Therefore, allogeneic hematopoietic stem cell transplantation is recommended after the first complete remission in this patient population.

Late effects to be considered include neuropsychological deficits, seizures, and endocrine disturbances (ie, growth hormone deficiency) related to CNS prophylaxis; spermatogenesis dysfunction related to cyclophosphamide; delayed sexual maturation in boys who received irradiation of gonadal tissue due to leukemic invasion of the testes; leukoencephalopathy and neurodevelopmental problems (especially in post–CNS radiation patients); and secondary malignancies.

CASE CORRELATION

- See also Case 10 (Failure to Thrive). Any chronic condition (such as malignancy) may result in failure to thrive. The hematologic finding of sickle cell disease (Case 13) typically is isolated to the red blood cell while that of leukemia affects all cell lines. Both may present with pallor and bone pain.

COMPREHENSION QUESTIONS

19.1 A mother brings her 3-year-old son with Down syndrome to the clinic because his gums have been bleeding for 1 week. She reports that he has been less energetic than usual. Examination reveals that the child has an oral temperature of 100°F (37.8°C), pallor, splenomegaly, gingival bleeding, and bruises on the lower extremities. Which of the following is most likely?

   A. Aplastic anemia

   B. Idiopathic thrombocytopenic purpura (ITP)

   C. Leukemia

   D. Leukemoid reaction

   E. Megaloblastic anemia

19.2 A father brings to the clinic his 6-year-old son who currently is undergoing induction chemotherapy for ALL. The school will not allow the child to register until his immunizations are up-to-date. Which of the following is the best course of action?

   A. Call the school nurse or principal to inform him or her that this child should not receive immunizations while he is taking chemotherapy.

   B. Update all immunizations except for measles, mumps, and rubella (MMR) and varicella.

   C. Update all immunizations except for oral polio vaccine.

   D. Update all immunizations.

   E. Call the school nurse or principal to inform him or her that this child will never receive immunizations because of the alteration in his immune system.

19.3 A mother brings to the clinic her 4-year-old son who began complaining of right knee pain 2 weeks ago, is limping slightly, is fatigued, and has had a fever to 100.4°F (38°C). Which of the following laboratory tests is most important?

A. Antinuclear antibodies

B. Complete blood count (CBC) with differential and platelets

C. Epstein-Barr virus titer

D. Rheumatoid factor

E. Sedimentation rate

19.4 Two weeks after a viral syndrome, a 2 year old develops bruising and generalized petechiae that is more prominent over the legs. He has neither hepatosplenomegaly nor lymph node enlargement. Laboratory testing reveals a normal hemoglobin, hematocrit, and white blood cell count and differential. The platelet count is 15,000/mm^3. Which of the following is the most likely diagnosis?

A. Acute lymphoblastic leukemia

B. Aplastic anemia

C. Immune thrombocytopenic purpura

D. Thrombotic thrombocytopenic purpura

E. von Willebrand disease

ANSWERS

19.1 **C.** A high susceptibility to leukemia is associated with certain heritable diseases (Klinefelter syndrome, Bloom syndrome, Fanconi syndrome, ataxia telangiectasia, neurofibromatosis) and chromosomal disorders such as Down syndrome. Children with Down syndrome have a 10- to 15-fold increased risk for developing leukemia and should have routine screening performed at well-child checks. Siblings of an acute lymphoblastic leukemia (ALL) patient have a two- to fourfold increased risk for ALL, and the monozygotic twin of a child who develops ALL in the first year of life has a more than 70% chance of also developing ALL. A few cases of ALL are associated with p53 gene aberrations. Overall, these genetic links account for a small number of total ALL cases.

19.2 **A.** Live virus vaccines are contraindicated for the child with ALL (and all members of the household) during chemotherapy and for at least 6 months after completion of treatment. Although the viruses in the vaccine are attenuated, immunosuppression from treatment can be profound and viral disease can result. Immunizations without live virus (diphtheria, tetanus, inactivated poliovirus vaccine, hepatitis A and B) are not absolutely contraindicated in this case, but the immunosuppression with chemotherapy often inhibits antibody responses.

19.3 **B.** This child has symptoms consistent with both juvenile idiopathic arthritis (JIA) and leukemia. The CBC with differential and platelets is the best initial screening test. The leukocyte and platelet counts are normal to increased in JIA, and no blast cells are present. Frequently, blast cells are found on the peripheral smear with ALL. The child in the question ultimately may require a bone marrow aspiration.

19.4 **C.** Immune (or idiopathic) thrombocytopenic purpura (ITP) is common in children. In most cases, a preceding viral infection can be documented. The platelet count frequently is less than $20,000/mm^3$, but other laboratory test results are normal, including the bone marrow aspiration (which may show an increase in megakaryocytes). Treatment consists of observation or possibly intravenous immunoglobulin (IVIG), intravenous anti-D (in Rh-positive patients), immunosuppressives, or steroids. The history must be reviewed for other possible causes of thrombocytopenia, including recent MMR vaccination, drug ingestion, and human immunodeficiency virus.

CLINICAL PEARLS

▶ Leukemias are the most common childhood cancers, and acute lymphoblastic leukemia (ALL) represents approximately 75% of all leukemia cases in children.

▶ Acute lymphoblastic leukemia has a peak incidence at the age of 2 to 4 years, and boys are affected more frequently.

▶ Acute lymphoblastic leukemia is often called the "great imitator" because of its nonspecific symptoms of anorexia, irritability, lethargy, pallor, bleeding, petechiae, leg and joint pain, and fever.

▶ Combination chemotherapy is the principal therapy for childhood ALL. Induction therapy produces remission within 4 weeks in approximately 98% of children with average-risk ALL.

REFERENCES

Campana D, Pui CH. Childhood leukemia. In: Abeloff MD, Armitage JD, Niederhuber JE, Kastan MB, McKenna WG, eds. *Abeloff's Clinical Oncology.* 4th ed. Philadelphia, PA: Churchill Livingston Elsevier; 2008:2139-2160.

Mahoney DH. Acute lymphoblastic leukemia. In: McMillan JA, Feigin RD, DeAngelis CD, Jones MD, eds. *Oski's Pediatrics: Principles and Practice.* 4th ed. Philadelphia, PA: Lippincott Williams & Wilkins; 2006:1750-1758.

Maloney K, Foreman NK, et al. Neoplastic disease. In: Hay WW, Levin MJ, Sondheimer JM, Deterding RR, eds. *Current Diagnosis & Treatment Pediatrics.* 20th ed. New York, NY: McGraw-Hill; 2011:882-885.

Nachman JB. Acute lymphoblastic leukemia. In: Rudolph CD, Rudolph AM, Lister GE, First LR, Gershon AA, eds. *Rudolph's Pediatrics.* 22nd ed. New York, NY: McGraw-Hill; 2011:1620-1625.

Neunert CE, Yee DL. Immune thrombocytopenic purpura (ITP). In: Rudolph CD, Rudolph AM, Lister GE, First LR, Gershon AA, eds. *Rudolph's Pediatrics*. 22nd ed. New York, NY: McGraw-Hill; 2011:1582-1583.

Rytting M, Choroszy M, Petropoulous D, Chan K. Acute leukemia. In: Chan K, Raney R, eds. *MD Anderson Cancer Care Series Pediatric Oncology*. New York, NY: Springer; 2005:1-17.

Tubergen DT, Bleyer A, Ritchey AK. The leukemias. In: Kliegman RM, Stanton BF, St. Geme JW, Schor NF, and Behrman RE, eds. *Nelson Textbook of Pediatrics*. 19th ed. Philadelphia, PA: Elsevier; 2011:1732-1737.

Wallace CA, Cabral DA, Sundel RP. Juvenile idiopathic arthritis. In: Rudolph CD, Rudolph AM, Lister GE, First LR, Gershon AA, eds. *Rudolph's Pediatrics*. 22nd ed. New York, NY: McGraw-Hill; 2011:800-806.

A 10-year-old boy in respiratory distress arrives to the emergency department (ED) with his mother. She reports he developed nasal congestion and sore throat 24 hours prior, then a cough a few hours previously. Over the past 2 hours, he has complained of chest pain and has been breathing rapidly. His mother administered a unit dose of albuterol via the nebulizer and then a second dose 5 minutes later. He showed no improvement. She reports he has had two similar episodes in the past year. Your examination reveals an afebrile man with a respiratory rate of 40 breaths/minute, oxygen saturation of 88% by pulse oximetry, and a heart rate of 130 beats/min. You note that his radial pulse becomes weak in amplitude with inspiration. His blood pressure is normal, but his capillary refill is sluggish at 4 to 6 seconds. He appears drowsy and is using accessory chest muscles to breathe. You hear faint inspiratory wheezes and no breath sounds during expiration.

▶ What is the most likely diagnosis?
▶ How would you manage this patient?
▶ What other medical history should you obtain?

ANSWERS TO CASE 20:
Asthma Exacerbation

Summary: A 10-year-old boy presents with tachypnea, pulsus paradoxus, use of accessory muscles of breathing, inspiratory wheezing, absent expiratory breath sounds, delayed capillary refill, and drowsiness.

- **Most likely diagnosis:** Asthma exacerbation.

- **Management:** Treating this patient's respiratory distress is of immediate concern. Initial management includes administration of oxygen, an inhaled short-acting β-agonist (SABA), and a systemic dose of prednisone. Intravenous administration of fluids and medications is indicated for a patient with this degree of distress.

- **Next step in evaluation:** After initial stabilization, information on his asthma medications, triggers, frequency and severity of previous exacerbations, especially how many have needed hospitalization or intensive care unit admission, should be obtained.

ANALYSIS

Objectives

1. Know how to diagnose asthma.

2. Know the acute management of an asthma exacerbation.

3. Know how to classify asthma severity and give the management of each level (Table 20–1).

Considerations

This child's history of ED visits for respiratory difficulty and his acute symptoms point to asthma as the most likely diagnosis. Less likely conditions include anaphylaxis, cystic fibrosis, foreign-body aspiration, and congestive heart failure. The National Institutes of Health, National Heart, Lung, and Blood Institute (NHLBI) asthma guidelines suggest this child's exacerbation is severe and requires immediate, intensive treatment. **His drowsiness is of particular concern, indicating impending respiratory failure;** his respiratory and circulatory status must be assessed frequently. The **paucity of wheezes** results from **severe airway obstruction** and reduced air movement; **wheezing is likely to increase when therapy allows more air movement.**

Table 20-1 • Classification of asthma severity and its treatment in school-age children

Components of Severity	Classification of Asthma Severity (5-11 years of age)			
	Intermittent	Persistent		
		Mild	Moderate	Severe
Daytime symptoms	≤2 d/wk	>2 d/wk (but not daily)	Daily	Throughout the day
Nighttime awakenings	≤2×/month	3-4×/mo	>1×/wk (but not nightly)	Nightly
Short-acting β₂-agonist use for symptom control (excludes using it for prevention of EIB)	≤2 d/wk	>2 d/wk (but not daily)	Daily	Several times per day
Interference with activity	None	Minor limitation	Some limitation	Extremely limited
Lung function	Normal FEV1 between exacerbations FEV1 >80% predicted FEV1/FVC >85%	FEV1 >80% of predicted FEV1/FVC >80%	FEV1 = 60%-80% of predicted FEV1/FVC = 75%-80%	FEV1 <60% of predicted FEV1/FVC <75%
Number of exacerbations requiring systemic steroids	0-1/y	≥2/y		
Therapy	Short-acting β-agonist (SABA) prn	Add low-dose inha ed corticosteroid (ICS)	Low-dose ICS + montelu-kast or medium-dose ICS	Refer to pulmonologist Medium-dose ICS + long-acting β-agonist

APPROACH TO:
Asthma Exacerbation

DEFINITIONS

ASTHMA: The diagnosis when: (1) episodic symptoms of airflow obstruction are present; (2) airflow obstruction is at least partially reversible; and (3) alternative diagnoses are excluded.

ASTHMA EXACERBATION: Characterized by the triad of acute, progressively worsening bronchoconstriction, airway inflammation, and mucus plugging.

PULSUS PARADOXUS: A fall in systolic blood pressure that varies more widely than normal between inspiration and expiration, and the amplitude of the pulse will decrease or disappear when airway obstruction is severe. A variance of greater than 10 mm Hg between inspiration and expiration suggests severe obstructive airway disease, pericardial tamponade, or constrictive pericarditis.

SPIROMETRY: A test of pulmonary function that can generally be performed in children aged 5 years or older. For patients with asthma, this test demonstrates airflow obstruction and reversibility, and can be used to determine an individual's response to treatment. The most common measure demonstrating airflow obstruction is forced expiratory volume in 1 second (FEV1).

CLINICAL APPROACH

The prevalence of asthma in children in the United States is 6 million with almost 140,000 requiring hospitalization in a year. The **median age at onset is 4 years,** but 20% of children develop symptoms within the first year of life. **Atopy and a family history** of asthma are strong risk factors for its development, as is respiratory infection early in life; between 40% and 50% of children with **respiratory syncytial virus (RSV) bronchiolitis** later develop asthma. More than half of children with asthma have symptom resolution by young adulthood. Heavy exposure to pollution, allergens, or cigarette smoke makes resolution less likely.

    Airway inflammation in asthma is because of mast cell activation. An immediate immunoglobulin (Ig) E response to environmental triggers occurs within 15 to 30 minutes and includes vasodilation, increased vascular permeability, smooth-muscle constriction, and mucus secretion. Symptoms result from these changes and may include **wheezing, cough (especially if worse at night), difficulty breathing, or chest tightness.** These symptoms will be **triggered by dust mites, animal dander, cigarette smoke, pollution, weather changes, pollen, upper respiratory infections, or exercise** (particularly when performed in a cold environment). Two to four hours after this acute response, a **late-phase reaction (LPR)** begins. The LPR is **characterized by infiltration of inflammatory cells into the airway parenchyma;** it is responsible for the chronic inflammation seen in asthma. Airway hyperresponsiveness and the accompanying symptoms may persist for weeks after the LPR.

Physical examination findings that suggest asthma are wheezing, hyperexpansion of the thorax or a prolonged phase of forced exhalation. The presence of other atopic diseases such as allergic rhinitis, nasal polyps, or atopic dermatitis, may be supportive of the diagnosis.

Spirometry should be performed, if possible, whenever a diagnosis of asthma is considered. A chest radiograph is not a required study but can help exclude other diagnoses such as congestive heart failure or in toddlers, foreign-body aspiration. Nonspecific findings of hyperinflation, flattened diaphragms, or increased bronchial wall markings may be the only abnormalities seen with asthma. Other tests such as sweat chloride testing may be needed to exclude other obstructive diseases of the small airways, such as cystic fibrosis. Viral bronchiolitis is the most commonly occurring disease of the small airways and usually does not respond to conventional asthma therapy.

Asthma **management involves classifying the baseline disease severity and identifying and minimizing exposure to triggers.** Classification is made based on spirometry and the patient's symptoms over prior 2 to 4 weeks. The features that are assessed are the frequency of nighttime symptoms, how often the rescue medication is needed, and how much symptoms limit daily activities. Severity is defined as either intermittent or persistent; persistent asthma is further divided into mild, moderate, or severe. Exacerbations of asthma can be any level of severity. Pharmacotherapy for the child's asthma symptoms follows NHLBI guidelines (http://www.nhlbi.nih.gov/guidelines/asthma/asthsumm.pdf).

Pharmacotherapy for asthma includes quick-relief medications for the acute symptoms and exacerbations, as well as long-term controller medications. **Short-acting β-adrenergic agonists or SABAs (ie, albuterol, levalbuterol) rapidly reverse bronchoconstriction via β_2-receptors on bronchial smooth muscle cells; they do not significantly inhibit the LPR.** These agents also can be used immediately prior to exercise or exposure to allergens to minimize the acute asthmatic response. Toxicity includes tachycardia and muscle tremor. Increased levels of drug are delivered to the lungs and toxicity is decreased when these medications are delivered through inhalation routes (nebulizer or inhaler). When inhalers are used, a reservoir device ("spacer") is used to maximize the amount of medication delivered to the lungs. Patients must not over-rely on short-acting inhalers because this practice is associated with death in severe asthma attacks.

Anticholinergics (ie, ipratropium) may be useful in the **acute management** of asthma exacerbation but are of **little value in chronic therapy;** they work by inhibiting the vagal reflex at smooth muscles and give additive benefit to SABAs.

The **most potent available anti-inflammatory drugs are corticosteroids,** which are useful for acute exacerbations (oral or intravenous prednisone, prednisolone) and for chronic therapy (inhaled corticosteroids). They **block the late phase reaction** and reduce hyperresponsive airways. The inhaled route is best for chronic therapy so that adverse effects on bone mineral density, growth, and immune function are minimized while maximal amounts of the drug can be delivered to the lungs.

Other long-term controller medications include **mast cell stabilizers** (cromolyn, nedocromil) and **leukotriene modifiers** (montelukast), which act by reducing the immune response to allergen exposure. They **become effective after 2 to 4 weeks of therapy.**

CASE CORRELATION

- See also Case 10 (Failure to Thrive). Any chronic condition (such as poorly controlled asthma) may result in failure to thrive. Differentiating asthma from pneumonia (Case 14) requires a thorough personal and family history, careful physical examination, and selected testing such as chest radiographs. In some cases viral pneumonia may be a trigger for asthma. Difficult to control or atypical presentations of asthma, especially in a child with failure to thrive, should prompt a consideration of tracheoesophageal atresia (Case 7) or cystic fibrosis (Case 18).

COMPREHENSION QUESTIONS

20.1 A 12-year-old asthmatic girl presents to the ED with tachypnea, intracostal retractions, perioral cyanosis, and minimal wheezing. You administer oxygen, inhaled albuterol, and intravenous prednisone. Upon reassessment, wheezing increases in all fields, and the child's color has improved. Which of the following is the appropriate explanation for these findings?

A. The girl is not having an asthma attack.

B. The girl is not responding to the albuterol, and her symptoms are worsening.

C. The girl is responding to the albuterol, and her symptoms are improving.

D. The girl did not receive enough albuterol.

E. The albuterol was inadvertently left out of the inhalation treatment, and the girl received only saline.

20.2 Which of the following is NOT an essential medication for acute asthma exacerbations?

A. Montelukast

B. Albuterol

C. Prednisone

D. Ipratropium

E. Levalbuterol

20.3 A 6-year-old girl comes to clinic with her mother for a refill of her albuterol inhaler. She has been using the albuterol 4 days per week, and about once per week her mother hears her coughing at night and has her use the inhaler. The girl reports she gets tired quicker at recess compared to her friends. What information do you need to tell the mother?

A. A chest radiograph is needed.

B. The dose of albuterol needs to be increased.

C. You will prescribe a long-acting β-adrenergic agonist.

D. You will change her medication to levalbuterol.

E. Her child has mild persistent asthma and needs a daily controller medication.

20.4 A 15-year-old adolescent boy with asthma uses his albuterol inhaler shortly after he mows the lawn because of a mild feeling of chest "tightness." He later returns home early from dinner at a friend's house when he has the sudden onset of wheezing, cough, and chest pain. Which of the following is the most likely explanation for these circumstances?

A. He likely aspirated a piece of grass.

B. His albuterol inhaler must be empty.

C. His albuterol inhaler must be outdated.

D. He is having a late-phase reaction.

E. He has been exposed to a new allergen that is more irritating than grass.

ANSWERS

20.1 **C.** This child presented in severe respiratory distress. Her improved color indicates reversible symptoms, confirming the diagnosis of asthma. Increased wheezing is auscultated after albuterol treatment because lung areas previously obstructed are now opening, allowing additional airflow. Less-experienced examiners may misinterpret lack of air movement as "clear" breath sounds, further delaying appropriate medical management.

20.2 **A.** Montelukast is a leukotriene modifier that is used in the long-term control of asthma. The other medications are used in acute asthma exacerbations.

20.3 **E.** It is essential to define the severity of every patient's asthma to determine the appropriate management. This patient's frequency of daily inhaler use, nighttime use, and level of limitation from symptoms classifies her as mild persistent asthma and a controller medication is indicated. Changing the dose or type of β-adrenergic agonist will not improve her symptoms and are not appropriate management for her severity of asthma. Chest radiographs are not used to define asthma severity.

20.4 **D.** A late-phase reaction typically occurs 2 to 4 hours after an initial wheezing episode. It is caused by accumulation of inflammatory cells in the airway.

CLINICAL PEARLS

▶ Asthma is characterized by episodic airflow obstruction that is at least partially reversible and may manifest as cough, dyspnea on exertion, chest pain, or wheezing.

▶ Acute asthma symptoms are managed with short-acting β-adrenergic agonists that rapidly reverse the bronchoconstriction.

▶ The late-phase reaction begins 2 to 4 hours after allergen exposure and is responsible for the chronic inflammation seen in asthma.

▶ Acute and long-term management of asthma is guided by the level of severity and the characteristics of any accompanying exacerbations.

REFERENCES

Centers for Disease Control and Prevention. Asthma's impact on the nation. http://www.cdc.gov/asthma/nhis/2013/table3-1.htm. Accessed June 25, 2015.

Hershey GKK. Asthma. In: Rudolph CD, Rudolph AM, Lister GE, First LR, Gershon AA, eds. *Rudolph's Pediatrics*. 22nd ed. New York, NY: McGraw-Hill; 2011:1962-1973.

Liu AH, Covar RA, Spahn JD, Leung DYM. Childhood asthma. In: Kliegman RM, Stanton BF, St. Geme III J, Schor N, Behrman R, eds. *Nelson Textbook of Pediatrics*. 19th ed. Philadelphia, PA: WB Saunders; 2011:780-801.

National Heart, Lung and Blood Institute. National Asthma Education and Prevention Program, Expert Panel Report 3: guidelines for the diagnosis and management of asthma, 2007. http://www.nhlbi.nih.gov/guidelines/asthma/asthsumm.pdf. Accessed August 31, 2014.

A 3-month-old boy is discovered not breathing in his crib this morning. Cardio-pulmonary resuscitation was begun by the parents and was continued by para-medics en route to the hospital. You continue to try to revive the child in the emergency center, but pronounce him dead after 20 minutes of resuscitation. You review the history with the family and examine the child, but you are unable to detect a cause of death.

▶ How should you manage this situation in the emergency department?
▶ What is the most likely diagnosis?
▶ What is the next step in the evaluation?

ANSWERS TO CASE 21:

Sudden Infant Death Syndrome

Summary: A 3-month-old boy discovered not breathing by his parents.

- **First step:** Tell the boy's parents that despite everyone's best efforts, their son has died. Ask the parents if they would like you to call a friend, family member, religious leader, or other support person. Provide them with a quiet room where they can be left alone.

- **Most likely diagnosis:** Sudden infant death syndrome (SIDS) is the most likely diagnosis, assuming that the parents' story is true. Infanticide must be considered, as well as the possibility of an underlying congenital or metabolic disorder.

- **Next step:** Discuss with the parents that routine protocol is followed after an unexplained infant death. A coroner will perform an autopsy and police investigators will examine the parents' home for clues related to the death. Emphasize that these measures can help to bring closure for the family and may yield important information for preventing future child deaths should the couple have more children.

ANALYSIS

Objectives

1. Know the definition of SIDS.

2. Know the factors that are associated with SIDS.

3. Know how to counsel parents about SIDS risk–reducing measures.

Considerations

Sudden infant death syndrome is one of the most tragic and frustrating medical diagnoses. When the family is in the emergency center, other possible causes of death (eg, child abuse or inherited disorders) cannot be excluded. Your role is to remain objective about these other possibilities yet sympathetic to the parents' grieving. Meticulous documentation of the history and physical examination findings is imperative.

| APPROACH TO: |
| Sudden Infant Death Syndrome |

DEFINITIONS

SUDDEN INFANT DEATH SYNDROME (SIDS): The sudden death of an infant that cannot be explained by results of a postmortem examination, death scene investigation, and historical information.

APPARENT LIFE-THREATENING EVENT (ALTE): An abrupt change in an infant's condition that is observed by a caregiver and perceived as life threatening. The change will involve either the infant's breathing, tone, color, or mental status. Myriad conditions may be responsible for this symptom, including cardiac, respiratory, central nervous system (CNS), metabolic, infectious, and gastrointestinal causes. In approximately 50% of cases a cause is never known.

APNEA: Cessation of breathing for at least 20 seconds that may be accompanied by bradycardia or cyanosis.

CLINICAL APPROACH

Sudden infant death syndrome is the most common cause of death in infants between the ages of 1 week and 1 year. The majority of SIDS deaths occur between 1 and 5 months of age, with a **peak incidence between 2 and 4 months** of age; it is more common in winter. SIDS is more common among **African American and Native American infants;** whether these latter associations result from ethnicity or reflect other environmental factors is unclear.

No cause of SIDS has been identified. Epidemiologic studies suggest that the following are independent SIDS risk factors: **prone or side sleep position,** sleeping on a **soft surface, bed sharing,** pre- and postnatal exposure to tobacco smoke, maternal prenatal use of opiates, **overheating,** late or no prenatal care, young maternal age, **prematurity** and/or low birth weight, and male gender. The incidence of SIDS has decreased dramatically in areas with public education campaigns targeted at limiting prone sleep positioning. **Breast-feeding, immunizations, and pacifier use seem to reduce the risk** of SIDS; to promote successful breast-feeding, the introduction of a pacifier is not recommended until the baby is 3 to 4 weeks of age. Home monitors and products marketed to reduce SIDS have no role in protection.

The investigation of the unexpected infant death includes a clinical history, a postmortem examination, and a death scene investigation. In some infants, autopsy reveals mild pulmonary edema and scattered intrathoracic petechiae; these findings are supportive but not diagnostic of SIDS.

Sudden unexpected infant deaths (SUIDs) may have an explainable cause such as a **congenital condition** (cardiac arrhythmia, structural heart disease, metabolic disorder) or an **acquired condition** (infection, intentional trauma, or accidental such as asphyxiation). It can also have an **unexplainable cause,** of which **SIDS** is the most common.

Infants who have experienced an ALTE may be at risk for sudden death. The evaluation of an ALTE is guided by the history and physical examination.

Laboratory studies often include a complete blood count because leukocytosis could suggest an **infectious** etiology, as well as testing for RSV, pertussis, or other respiratory tract pathogens. A comprehensive metabolic panel may uncover a **metabolic** etiology. **A report of feeding difficulties or emesis leads to consideration of upper gastrointestinal studies such as imaging, swallowing evaluation, pH probe, whereas unusual posturing or movements would prompt an electroencephalogram (EEG).** If a murmur is detected, an electrocardiogram, chest x-ray (CXR), or echocardiogram may be considered to look for arrhythmias such as prolonged QT syndrome or a structural cardiac defect.

COMPREHENSION QUESTIONS

21.1 Which of the following features makes sudden infant death syndrome (SIDS) likely as the cause of a sudden death?

   A. An infant found with a bulging fontanelle and facial bruise.

   B. An 18-month-old girl who had a prior sibling that at 1 year of age also died suddenly and unexpectedly.

   C. A 5-month-old infant with dysmorphic features and an enlarged heart found on postmortem examination.

   D. A 3-month-old boy whose parents smoke in the home but were using a high-efficiency particulate arrestance (HEPA) air purifier in his room, a baby monitor, placing him on his side to sleep so he wouldn't aspirate any refluxed formula, and using a special foam wedge pillow to keep him in that position.

   E. All the above features make SIDS likely as the cause of a sudden death.

21.2 A mother presents to the emergency room with her 6-month-old daughter late at night after she noticed her to be breathing fast for 1 minute, then seemed to stop breathing for 1 minute, and became limp, pale, and unresponsive. The mother attempted to give mouth-to-mouth breaths for a few seconds and her daughter then began to cry and her breathing and appearance normalized. Your next best step is to:

   A. Perform a thorough history and physical examination, obtain basic laboratory tests, and admit to the hospital for workup of an ALTE.

   B. Reassure the mother that her infant looks healthy and because the symptoms have resolved, discharge home.

   C. Perform a complete blood count (CBC), chest x-ray (CXR), and discharge home if all are normal.

   D. Instruct the mother to follow-up with the pediatrician to get an apnea monitor and pulse oximeter so that she will know if similar symptoms occur again and if they are actually life threatening.

   E. Tell the mother this was a near SIDS event and instruct her on measures to prevent SIDS.

21.3 You are going to counsel parents of a newborn about prevention of SIDS. Which of the following statements about ways to reduce SIDS is accurate?

A. Infants should sleep in the same bed as the parent or on their chest so they can be closely monitored for apnea.

B. Infants should sleep on their back on a firm mattress with no accompanying soft bedding or objects, including no devices advertised to maintain the sleep position.

C. Pacifiers should be avoided because they can obstruct the baby's airflow during respiration.

D. Keep the infant dressed in several layers and covered with a heavy blanket.

E. Infants should be given acetaminophen before their scheduled vaccines in order to prevent an undetected febrile seizure and resulting SIDS.

21.4 The investigation of an unexpected infant death includes a history, a postmortem examination, and which of the following?

A. DNA studies

B. Maternal drug screen

C. Analysis of parental electrocardiograms

D. A death scene investigation

E. Stool studies

ANSWERS

21.1 **D.** Unfortunately, no specific product has been proven to reduce the risk of SIDS. The child's age, gender, and exposure to tobacco smoke are the main features that make SIDS a possible cause of death. Physical signs of any trauma make intentional injury and infanticide the most likely causes of death, whereas anatomic defects make cardiac or metabolic causes likely. The occurrence of a genetic susceptibility to SIDS within a family is exceedingly rare and SIDS cannot be the diagnosis if the patient is not an infant, that is, older than 12 months.

21.2 **A.** This clinical scenario is typical for an ALTE and is defined by the caregiver's history. It is not required to have other equipment or laboratory test results indicate an abnormality to meet the definition for the symptom. It requires evaluation to find the etiology.

21.3 **B.** The decline in SIDS has been attributed to the change in sleep position emphasizing infants be placed on their back. Other protective factors include pacifier use and vaccination. Risk factors associated with SIDS are bed sharing, prone sleep position, and overheating.

21.4 **D.** A death scene investigation is crucial to rule out trauma, both intentional and accidental.

CLINICAL PEARLS

▶ Sudden infant death syndrome (SIDS) is a diagnosis of exclusion assigned only after the postmortem investigation, postnatal history, and crime scene investigation fail to yield another explanation.

▶ Prone sleep position, bed sharing, overheating, and exposure to cigarette smoke are significant risk factors for SIDS that can be preventable.

▶ An apparent life-threatening event (ALTE) is an abrupt, observed change in an infant's condition that can be caused by myriad etiologies and requires evaluation for the precipitating cause.

REFERENCES

Corwin MJ. Apparent life-threatening events and SIDS. In: Rudolph CD, Rudolph AM, Lister GE, First LR, Gershon AA, eds. *Rudolph's Pediatrics*. 22nd ed. New York, NY: McGraw-Hill; 2011:451-454.

Hunt CE, Hauck FR. Sudden infant death syndrome. In: Kliegman RM, Stanton BF, St. Geme III J, Schor N, Behrman R, eds. *Nelson Textbook of Pediatrics*. 19th ed. Philadelphia, PA: WB Saunders; 2011:1421-1429.

Moon RY. Task Force on Sudden Infant Death Syndrome. SIDS and other sleep-related infant deaths: expansion of recommendations for a safe infant sleeping environment. *Pediatrics*. 2011;128: 1030-1036.

A 2-month-old girl is seen in the pediatric office for her well-child checkup. Her mother reports she previously breast-fed 20 minutes every 2 to 3 hours but now is requiring 40 minutes to breast-feed with a frequency of every 4 hours. She sweats with all the feeds but does not turn blue. She continues to produce her normal quantity of wet diapers and stools. On physical examination, the girl is awake, alert, has subdiaphragmatic retractions, abdominal breathing; her respiratory rate is 58 breaths/min and the pulse is 175 beats/min. Oxygen saturation measured on her right hand is 98%. You hear a 2/6 holosystolic murmur along the left sternal border. The murmur is harsh, low-pitched, and does not radiate. The lung fields have scattered crackles bilaterally.

▶ What is the most likely diagnosis?
▶ What is the treatment for this condition?

ANSWERS TO CASE 22:
Ventricular Septal Defect

Summary: A 2-month-old infant presents with respiratory distress and a 2/6 holo-systolic murmur.

- **Most likely diagnosis:** Ventricular septal defect (VSD)
- **Treatment:** Medical management and possibly surgical closure in the future

ANALYSIS

Objectives

1. Recognize the presenting signs and symptoms of VSD.
2. Know the major acyanotic congenital heart lesions (Table 22–1).
3. Know the tests used to investigate acyanotic heart lesions.

Considerations

An acyanotic heart lesion is suspected in this child who has a new heart murmur without cyanosis. Because pulmonary vascular resistance falls in the weeks following birth, blood flows from the high-pressured left ventricle across the VSD to the right ventricle. Flow across this opening produces turbulence that may be heard as a murmur, usually by 2 to 6 months of age because pulmonary vascular pressures reach normal levels by that time. This child's VSD is of sufficient size to result in congestive heart failure.

APPROACH TO:
Acyanotic Heart Lesions

DEFINITIONS

EISENMENGER SYNDROME: Pulmonary hypertension (HTN) resulting in right-to-left shunting of blood. This occurs due to increased pulmonary blood flow from left-to-right shunts such as large VSDs, atrioventricular canal lesions, and patent ductus arteriosus (PDA). Transplant is the only cure.

LEFT-TO-RIGHT SHUNT: Flow of blood from the systemic circulation into the pulmonary circulation across an anomalous connection, such as a PDA. Such lesions result in pulmonary congestion, but they typically do not cause cyanosis. Systemic hypoperfusion may result if the cause is an obstructive lesion (such as pulmonic or aortic valve stenosis, coarctation of the aorta).

WIDENED PULSE PRESSURE: An increase in the difference between systolic and diastolic pressures, resulting in a bounding arterial pulse. Many conditions may

Table 22–1 • ACYANOTIC CONGENITAL HEART LESIONS			
Lesion	Physical Examination	CXR	ECG
VSD	• Holosystolic murmur at left lower sternal border	• Normal if a small shunt • Cardiomegaly • Enlarged left atrium and left ventricle • Increased pulmonary vascular markings	• Normal if a small shunt • Biventricular hypertrophy • Left axis deviation
ASD	• Fixed, widely split S2	• Enlarged right ventricle • Prominent pulmonary arteries • Increased pulmonary vascular markings	• Right ventricular hypertrophy • Right axis deviation
PDA	• Widened pulse pressure • Continuous machinery-like murmur at second intercostal space	• Increased pulmonary vascular markings	• Biventricular hypertrophy • Right axis deviation
Coarctation of aorta	• Systolic murmur in the left axilla	• Cardiomegaly • Normal to increased pulmonary vascularity	• Right ventricular hypertrophy • Right bundle branch block • Right axis deviation

Abbreviations: ASD, atrial septal defect; CXR, chest x-ray; ECG, electrocardiogram; PDA, patent ductus arteriosus; VSD, ventricular septal defect.

cause this finding, including fever, hyperthyroidism, anemia, arteriovenous fistulas, and PDA.

CLINICAL APPROACH

Congenital cardiac defects are first categorized according to the presence of cyanosis; this can be deciphered by pulse oximetry and a complete physical examination. Further classification is by determining radiographical evidence of increased, normal, or decreased pulmonary vascular markings. Lastly, an electrocardiogram (ECG) provides voltage data to determine if there is right, left, or biventricular hypertrophy. The majority of acyanotic lesions result in a change in *volume* load, usually from the systemic circulation to the pulmonary circulation (the so-called left-to-right shunt). If untreated, defects that affect volume load can eventually result in increased pulmonary vascular pressure, causing reversal of blood flow across the defect and clinical cyanosis. Such lesions include VSD, atrial septal defects (ASDs), and PDA. Other forms of acyanotic defects cause changes in *pressure* and are obstructive lesions; this group includes pulmonic and aortic valve stenosis and coarctation of the aorta.

Ventricular septal defects are the most common heart lesion in children, accounting for 25% of all congenital heart defects and affecting 3 to 6 of every 1000 live term births (Figure 22–1). Most VSDs are small with left-to-right shunting and

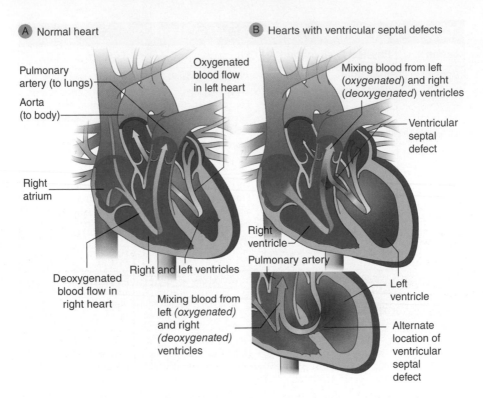

Figure 22–1. Image A shows the structure and blood flow inside a normal heart. Image B shows two common locations for a ventricular septal defect. The defect allows oxygen-rich blood from the left ventricle to mix with oxygen-poor blood in the right ventricle. (*From the National Institutes of Health. http://www.nhlbi.nih.gov/health/health-topics/topics/chd/types.html. Accessed July 4, 2015.*)

are located in the membranous portion of the ventricular septum. Children with **small VSDs** (<5 mm) usually are asymptomatic, and a **harsh, holosystolic murmur is heard at the left lower sternal border.** The **murmur of a large VSD may be less harsh** because of the absence of a significant pressure gradient across the defect. Large lesions are accompanied by **dyspnea, feeding difficulties, growth failure, and profuse perspiration,** and they may lead to recurrent infections and **cardiac failure.** Infants with large VSDs generally are not cyanotic, but they may become dusky during feeding or protracted crying. A VSD may not be detected in the first few weeks of life because of high right-sided pressures but become audible as pulmonary vascular resistance drops and left-to-right shunting of blood increases across the defect. In children with significant VSDs, chest radiography shows cardiomegaly with an enlarged left atrium (LA) and ventricle (LV) and increased pulmonary vascular markings. The ECG shows biventricular hypertrophy. With a small VSD, the ECG and chest x-ray (CXR) are usually normal.

Most small VSDs close spontaneously by 6 to 12 months of life, especially if they occur in the muscular septum. Medical management is reserved for infants who are symptomatic from larger VSDs. Medications include diuretics (eg, furosemide and afterload reduction agents [eg, an angiotensin-converting enzyme inhibitor]). Affected infants also need adequate caloric intake and may require feeding by naso-gastric or gastrostomy tubes. Most children with large VSDs develop pulmonary vascular resistance after 1 year of age and usually undergo surgical closure to pre-vent irreversible pulmonary vascular disease (**Eisenmenger syndrome**) which can occur by 2 years of age.

Children with ASDs usually have no symptoms but large defects may cause mild growth failure, frequent upper respiratory tract infections, and exercise intolerance. Physical findings include a widely split second heart sound that does not vary with respiration ("fixed splitting"), and a systolic murmur at the left upper and midster-nal borders caused by high-volume blood flow from the right ventricle into the normal pulmonary artery; the murmur is not blood flowing across the ASD itself. A lower left sternal border diastolic murmur produced by increased flow across the tricuspid valve may be present. The chest radiograph reveals an enlarged right atrium, right ventricle, and pulmonary artery and increased pulmonary vascular-ity; ECG shows right ventricular hypertrophy and sometimes right-axis deviation. Atrial septal defects are well tolerated during childhood but can lead to pulmonary HTN in adulthood or atrial arrhythmias from atrial enlargement.

Patent ductus arteriosus is most commonly seen in preterm infants. In utero, the ductus arteriosus shunts blood from the quiescent lungs through the pulmonary artery to the descending aorta. Shortly after birth, pulmonary resistance begins to fall, and vasoconstriction of the ductus occurs. Ductus closure in term infants usu-ally occurs within 10 to 15 hours of birth and almost always by 2 days of age. Clo-sure is delayed in premature infants, perhaps because of impaired vasoconstrictor response to increased oxygen tension. Failure of the ductus to close allows shunting of blood from the systemic circulation to the pulmonary circulation, with resul-tant myocardial stress, pulmonary vascular congestion, and respiratory difficulty. A small PDA usually results in no symptoms but is still closed medically (usually with indomethacin) or surgically (if medical therapy fails or is contraindicated) due to risk of infective endarteritis and paradoxical emboli. An infant with a large PDA typi-cally has a systolic or continuous "machinery-like" heart murmur, an active precor-dium, and a widened pulse pressure. Closure of a large PDA is done to prevent heart failure and Eisenmenger syndrome.

Coarctation of the aorta consists of a narrowing of the aorta, and although it can occur anywhere along its path from the transverse arch to the iliac bifurca-tion, it most commonly occurs just below the origin of the left subclavian artery. If the narrowing is severe enough, symptoms may appear in the neonatal period. Classic findings are weak or absent pulses in the lower extremities along with lower systolic blood pressure and pulse oximetry in the legs compared to the arms. Coarcta-tion can be *ductus dependent*, meaning a PDA is required to maintain blood flow to the systemic circulation. Symptoms of the coarctation may then not appear until the ductus begins to close, at which point loss of lower extremity perfusion, severe acidosis, and cardiovascular collapse occur. An infusion of prostaglandin E would be required to maintain the patent ductus until definitive repair could be done. Echocardiogram with color Doppler can usually identify the site of the coarctation. Otherwise, computed tomography (CT), magnetic resonance imaging (MRI), or cardiac catheterization is needed.

CASE CORRELATION

• See also Case 10 (Failure to Thrive). Any chronic condition (such as heart defects) may result in failure to thrive. One of the complications of an infant of a diabetic mother (Case 2) is an increased risk of heart defects, most commonly hypertrophic cardiomyopathy. The child with tracheoesophageal atresia (Case 7) may have also have VACTERL or VATER (vertebral abnormality, anal imperforation, tracheoesophageal fistula, radial and renal anomaly) association, CHARGE (coloboma, heart defect, atresia choanae, retarded growth and development, genital abnormality, and ear abnormality) association, DiGeorge syndrome, and trisomy 18, 21, and 13, all of which have association with cardiac malformations.

COMPREHENSION QUESTIONS

22.1 Which of the following is NOT an important part of the initial evaluation of a heart murmur?

A. Chest radiograph (CXR)

B. Arterial blood gas (ABG)

C. Echocardiogram

D. Pulse oximetry

E. Electrocardiogram (ECG)

22.2 A 3-month-old boy arrives in the emergency room in December with tachypnea and retractions. His mother reports he has nasal congestion, cough, and is not able to feed well. On auscultation, you note fine crackles and an end-expiratory wheeze with every intermittent wheeze. He is tachycardic to 190, and a 2/6 harsh holosystolic murmur is identified along the left sternal border. CXR shows cardiomegaly and increased pulmonary vascular markings. During venipuncture and IV insertion, he is crying vigorously and has an episode in which he appears slightly dusky. Which medication is indicated?

A. Albuterol

B. Racemic epinephrine

C. Indomethacin

D. Prostaglandin

E. Furosemide

22.3 Which of the following statements is true about a ventricular septal defect (VSD)?

A. A murmur may not be present at birth.

B. Surgical repair is always required.

C. A continuous machinery-like murmur is characteristic.

D. A larger defect will have a louder murmur than a small defect.

E. A normal ECG excludes the presence of a VSD.

22.4 A previously healthy term infant suddenly develops respiratory distress on day 3 of life. An echocardiogram reveals coarctation of the aorta. Which of the following is the most appropriate treatment for immediate stabilization of this infant?

A. Digoxin

B. Furosemide

C. Albuterol

D. Racemic epinephrine

E. Prostaglandin therapy

ANSWERS

22.1 **B.** An arterial blood gas gives information about the patient's oxygenation status but does not help identify if a heart murmur is pathologic.

22.2 **E.** This child is exhibiting congestive heart failure. Based on the accompanying murmur and CXR, the most likely etiology is a large VSD. Furosemide decreases the pulmonary congestion.

22.3 **A.** The murmur of a VSD is due to turbulent blood flow across the defect. When pulmonary vascular resistance is high enough, blood cannot flow from left to right across the defect. Once the pulmonary pressure drops to normal levels, which is typically by 2 to 6 months of age, the murmur becomes audible. The murmur is holosystolic and usually smaller defects create more turbulence which in turn, produces a louder murmur. Only large defects require surgical repair. The ECG is usually normal for small VSDs.

22.4 **E.** This infant's symptoms started when his ductus arteriosus began to close. A continuous intravenous infusion of prostaglandin will keep the ductus open and allow blood flow to reach past the area of coarctation and perfuse the lower portion of the body. Surgery provides definitive repair.

CLINICAL PEARLS

▶ Acyanotic heart lesions are characterized by shunting of blood from the systemic circulation to the pulmonary circulation ("left-to-right shunt").

▶ The most common congenital acyanotic heart lesion is the ventricular septal defect. Atrial septal defect, patent ductus arteriosus, coarctation of the aorta, and pulmonary valve stenosis are other acyanotic lesions.

▶ Left-to-right shunts eventually can reverse direction (right-to-left) and cause cyanosis if pulmonary hypertension develops (Eisenmenger syndrome).

REFERENCES

Bernstein D. Acyanotic congenital heart disease: the left-to-right shunt lesions. In: Kliegman RM, Stanton BF, St. Geme III J, Schor N, Behrman R, eds. *Nelson Textbook of Pediatrics*. 19th ed. Philadelphia, PA: WB Saunders; 2011:1551-1561.

Bernstein D. Acyanotic congenital heart disease: the obstructive lesions. In: Kliegman RM, Stanton BF, St. Geme III J, Schor N, Behrman R, eds. *Nelson Textbook of Pediatrics*. 19th ed. Philadelphia, PA: WB Saunders; 2011:1561-1570.

Clyman RI. Patent ductus arteriosus and ductus venosus. In: Rudolph CD, Rudolph AM, Lister GE, First LR, Gershon AA, eds. *Rudolph's Pediatrics*. 22nd ed. New York, NY: McGraw-Hill; 2011: 238-242.

A 4-week-old boy presents to the emergency room with a 5-day history of progressively increased work of breathing and poor feeding. He is diaphoretic, has a respiratory rate of 68 breaths/min with subcostal retractions, pulse of 190 beats/min, oxygen saturation of 85%, and a widened pulse pressure. His gingiva and buccal mucosa appear blue. Rales are heard over both lung fields. An early systolic click followed by a systolic ejection murmur at the left sternal border and a single S2 are heard. The precordium is hyperdynamic, and the femoral pulses are bounding. The liver span is enlarged. Chest radiograph shows cardiomegaly and increased pulmonary vascularity. Emergent echocardiography shows a single arterial cardiac outflow tract that is receiving blood from both ventricles.

▶ What is the most likely diagnosis?
▶ What is the best management for this condition?

ANSWERS TO CASE 23:

Truncus Arteriosus

Summary: A 4-week-old infant develops signs of congestive heart failure (tachypnea, dyspnea, diaphoresis, cardiomegaly, pulmonary vascular congestion, and hepatomegaly). He has central cyanosis and hypoxia along with features suggesting a cardiac malformation (a murmur, a systolic click, and a single S2).

- **Most likely diagnosis:** Truncus arteriosus, a type of cyanotic congenital heart disease (CHD).

- **Best management:** Medications to reduce the congestive heart failure: digoxin, diuretics to reduce preload (furosemide, chlorothiazide), afterload reducers (angiotensin-converting enzyme inhibitors), and inotropes (dopamine, dobutamine). Ultimately surgical correction is needed.

ANALYSIS

Objectives

1. Know the major types of cyanotic CHD and their most common clinical presentations.

2. Understand the management of cyanotic CHD.

Considerations

This infant has truncus arteriosus, an uncommon cardiac defect, in which a single arterial trunk arises from the normally formed ventricles. The single trunk typically straddles a defect in the outlet portion of the intraventricular septum and a single valve at the outflow tract is found (Figure 23–1). The main pulmonary artery and ascending aorta arise from the common arterial trunk. Cyanosis results from the mixing of the systemic and pulmonary blood flow that occurs across the ventricular septal defect and within the single arterial trunk. The condition can be complicated by the presence of an interrupted aortic arch and aberrant coronary arteries. Clinically apparent cyanosis and heart failure may not be present until after the first weeks of life because pulmonary vascular resistance is high after birth but drops to normal levels by 2 to 6 months of age. When the pulmonary resistance drops below the systemic pressure, increased blood flow to the pulmonary system occurs, leading to pulmonary congestion, increased myocardial work, and subsequent heart failure.

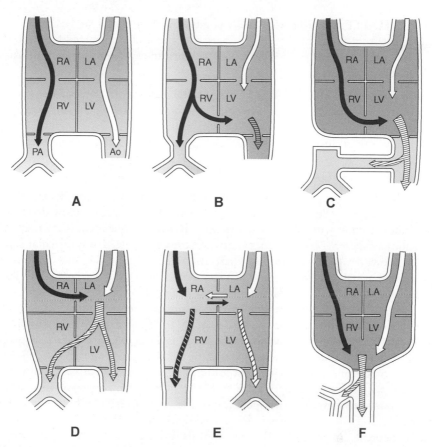

Figure 23–1. Schematic drawing of circulation of various cardiac defects: (A) normal circulation, (B) tetralogy of Fallot, (C) pulmonary atresia, (D) tricuspid atresia, (E) transposition of the great arteries, (F) truncus arteriosus. Black arrows indicate deoxygenated blood, cross-hatched arrows indicate mixed blood, and white arrows indicate oxygenated blood. *Abbreviations: LA, left atrium; LV, left ventricle; RA, right atrium; RV, right ventricle.*

APPROACH TO:
Cyanotic Congenital Heart Disease

DEFINITIONS

CYANOSIS: Bluish discoloration of the skin and mucous membranes caused by insufficient saturation of the blood with oxygen. Peripheral cyanosis (acrocyanosis) is common in neonates and involves the extremities only; it may be normal. Central cyanosis is always abnormal and is seen on the tongue, gingiva, and buccal mucosa.

DUCTUS-DEPENDENT LESIONS: Cardiac defects that are incompatible with life in the absence of a patent ductus arteriosus (PDA).

RIGHT-TO-LEFT CARDIAC SHUNT: Abnormal flow of blood across a cardiac defect from the right side of the heart containing deoxygenated blood to the left side of the heart where it is then pumped into the systemic circulation. These lesions result in cyanosis.

CONOTRUNCAL HEART DEFECTS: Malformations of the cardiac outflow tracts (aorta and main pulmonary artery). Common types include truncus arteriosus, tetralogy of Fallot (TOF), pulmonary atresia, and interrupted aortic arch. These are commonly seen in chromosome 22q11.2 deletions such as DiGeorge syndrome.

CLINICAL APPROACH

Cyanotic CHD mainly comprises cardiac anomalies that either allow deoxygenated blood to bypass the lungs and enter the systemic circulation, or allow deoxygenated blood to mix with blood that has already been oxygenated as it enters the systemic circulation. Mixing occurs via an accompanying atrial or ventricular septal defect. However, in the anomalies where the right ventricle does not connect to the pulmonary circulation, a PDA is needed to conduct the deoxygenated blood to the lungs. These cardiac lesions are termed ductus dependent and often manifest earlier than the anomalies that are ductus independent because ductal closure normally occurs on the first or second day of life in term infants. The distinction is important because intravenous **prostaglandin E$_1$ is given to keep the ductus open** in ductal-dependent lesions and allows for infant stabilization prior to more definitive surgical correction. Ductal-dependent lesions include tricuspid atresia, pulmonary valve atresia, severe pulmonary valve stenosis, TOF if the accompanying pulmonary stenosis is severe, and transposition of the great arteries without ventricular inversion (D-TGA). Hypoplastic left heart syndrome (HLHS) is also a type of ductus-dependent cyanotic CHD, but cyanosis is due to decreased systemic perfusion rather than mixing of deoxygenated and oxygenated blood.

Cyanosis may not be visible unless oxygen saturation is 85% or less, so pulse oximetry is used to identify its presence. Clubbing will not be encountered until the hypoxia has been present for several months. Any infant with tachypnea, tachycardia, poor feeding, or an abnormal cardiac examination should have pulse oximetry performed. Measurement should be done on the tissues that are perfused by the portion of the aorta that is **proximal to the ductus (the right hand** or an ear lobe) as well as on the tissues that are perfused by the portion of the aorta that is **distal to the ductus (the lower extremity).** If a **difference of more than 3% to 5% is found, then a right-to-left shunt across the ductus may be present.** Further evaluation is then required. Several states have mandated that standard newborn care includes pre- and postductal pulse oximetry in neonates 24 hours after birth to screen for congenital cyanotic heart disease prior to hospital discharge.

Many of the cyanotic heart lesions have a nonspecific murmur caused by the accompanying septal defect or patent ductus arteriosus. The exception is severe **pulmonary valve stenosis with its systolic ejection murmur located at the upper left sternal border.** Abnormal heart sounds may be found in some of the cyanotic CHD lesions: a **single S2 occurs with pulmonary valve atresia or truncus arteriosus; an early systolic ejection click is heard with pulmonary stenosis or truncus arteriosus.**

On chest radiograph, cyanotic CHD is usually characterized by increased pulmonary vascularity and cardiomegaly. Only an atretic tricuspid valve, atretic pulmonary valve, or TOF with its pulmonic valve stenosis will have decreased pulmonary vascularity. Some distinctive radiographic appearances of specific anomalies are described (Table 23–1). The right ventricle hypertrophy (RVH) in **TOF** causes the apical shadow of the heart to point upward, creating a **"boot" or "wooden shoe"** shape to the heart. **D-TGA is described as "an egg of a string"** because the reversed pulmonary artery and aorta give a narrow mediastinal vascular shadow. **Total anomalous pulmonary venous return (TAPVR) can appear as a "snowman,"** which is created by the round supracardiac shadow of a dilated innominate vein and vena cava that are receiving venous blood flow from the body as well as from the pulmonary veins. This finding is usually not seen until after the neonatal period because the prominent thymus of the neonate obscures it. **Electrocardiogram** (ECG) **can be normal,** and many abnormal findings are nonspecific. Right ventricular hypertrophy can be normal for a neonate and biventricular hypertrophy may accompany a ventricular septal defect. However, tricuspid valve atresia may be distinguished by ECG because of its left axis deviation, biatrial enlargement, and absent right ventricle markings (ie, no R waves in leads V1-V3). **Echocardiography** is needed **for definitive diagnosis** of the specific cardiac lesion in any of these conditions.

Treatment of the infant with cyanotic heart disease depends on the specific lesions that are present. Stabilization is the essential first step and usually involves medications. If the lesion is ductal dependent, **prostaglandin E₁** infusion should be started. Other measures include creating an atrial septum via cardiac catheterization, known as atrial septostomy, which is used for TGA before definitive surgery occurs. Surgical management is often performed once the infant is stabilized. Initially, palliative procedures, such as the creation of an aortic pulmonary shunt for tricuspid atresia or TOF, may be required. Complete surgical repair occurs later when the infant has grown. Long-term prognosis varies. After complete surgical repair, 90% of patients with TOF survive to adulthood; however, HLHS remains the most common fatal congenital heart defect.

Table 23–1 • TYPICAL RADIOGRAPHIC FINDINGS OF COMMON HEART LESIONS	
Heart Anomaly	**Radiographic Appearance**
Tetralogy of Fallot	"Boot-shaped" heart and decreased pulmonary vascularity
Pulmonary atresia (with intact ventricular septum)	Decreased pulmonary vascularity
Tricuspid atresia (with normally related great vessels)	Decreased pulmonary vascularity
Epstein anomaly	Heart size may be normal to massive, with normal or decreased pulmonary vascularity
Transposition of the great arteries	"Egg-on-a-string" (narrow mediastinum) with normal to increased pulmonary vascularity
Truncus arteriosus	Cardiomegaly and increased pulmonary vascularity
Total anomalous pulmonary venous return	"Snowman" (supracardiac shadow caused by anomalous pulmonary veins entering the innominate vein and persistent left superior vena cava), and increased pulmonary vascularity
Hypoplastic left heart syndrome	Cardiomegaly and increased pulmonary vascularity

CASE CORRELATION

- See also Case 10 (Failure to Thrive). Any chronic condition (such as heart defects) may result in failure to thrive. One of the complications of an infant of a diabetic mother (Case 2) is an increased risk of heart defects, most commonly hypertrophic cardiomyopathy. The child with tracheoesophageal atresia (Case 7) may also have VACTERL or VATER (vertebral abnormality, anal imperforation, tracheoesophageal fistula, radial and renal anomaly) association, CHARGE (coloboma, heart defect, atresia choanae, retarded growth and development, genital abnormality, and ear abnormality) association, DiGeorge syndrome, and trisomy 18, 21, and 13, all of which have association with cardiac malformations [see also Case 22 (Ventricular Septal Defect) as an example of a typically acyanotic heart defect].

COMPREHENSION QUESTIONS

23.1 A 15-hour-old neonate appears dusky. He is tachycardic and tachypneic but the lung fields are clear to auscultation and he has no murmur. His oxygen saturation is 82% and does not improve with administration of 90% oxygen via oxyhood. A chest radiograph shows slightly increased pulmonary vascularity and a narrow mediastinum. Initial management of this infant's condition should include which of the following?

A. Perform electrocardiogram and increase the administered oxygen concentration to 100%.

B. Perform echocardiogram and begin prostaglandin E_1 infusion.

C. Administer furosemide and repeat the chest radiograph.

D. Perform a karyotype and begin dopamine infusion.

E. Perform electrocardiogram and administer packed red blood cells.

23.2 A 30-hour-old term infant has been feeding normally, has a normal physical examination, and her mother is being discharged. The nurse notifies you that the infant's routine pre- and postductal pulse oximetry readings are 99% on the right hand and 91% on the right foot. Over the past 4 hours, he has repeated the measurements twice and keeps getting the same result. When can you tell the mother that her infant does not have a congenital heart defect?

A. If the pulse oximetry readings on the left foot are 93%

B. If the pulse oximetry readings on all extremities at 48 hours of life are 100%

C. If an echocardiogram is normal

D. If the pulse oximetry readings do not improve after an infusion of prostaglandin E_1 is started

E. If a chest radiograph and electrocardiogram are normal

23.3 Which of the following statements about cyanotic congenital heart disease is true?

A. Newborns will always manifest symptoms before discharge from the hospital.

B. Clubbing is usually the first finding of cyanotic congenital heart disease.

C. Cyanotic congenital heart disease cannot be present unless an infant appears cyanotic.

D. Infants with cyanotic congenital heart disease may require treatment with diuretics and angiotensin-converting enzyme (ACE) inhibitors.

E. Emergent surgical repair is the first step in management for all cyanotic heart defects in the neonatal period.

23.4 Which of the following statements about truncus arteriosus is true?

A. A patent ductus arteriosus is required for survival.

B. A "snowman" appearance on chest radiograph is commonly seen.

C. Characteristic ECG findings allow diagnosis.

D. Symptoms may not be present until after 2 weeks of life.

E. Balloon septostomy is the indicated treatment.

ANSWERS

23.1 **B.** This neonate has transposition of the great arteries (TGA), and as the ductus arteriosus begins to close, he will decompensate further. Urgent echocardiogram can confirm the diagnosis. Prostaglandin E_1 should be started immediately to maintain the patency of the ductus arteriosus and to stabilize his condition. Increasing the oxygen concentration or administering packed red blood cells will not improve his oxygenation if the ductus closes and no conduit for the oxygenated blood to reach the systemic circulation exists. An electrocardiogram is often normal or has nonspecific findings that do not identify the heart defect that is present.

23.2 **C.** This infant has evidence of a ductal shunt that should be investigated further because it can signal the presence of a cardiac defect. A postductal pulse oximetry measurement obtained from either lower extremity that is less than 3% to 5% lower than the preductal measurement is indicative of a ductal shunt. A normal echocardiogram would indicate that the infant does not have a congenital heart defect. A normal chest radiograph, a normal electrocardiogram, and the absence of a ductal shunt do not exclude the presence of a serious congenital cardiac defect; truncus arteriosus is an example. Prostaglandin infusion would only improve systemic oxygenation if the infant had a ductus-dependent lesion and was undergoing closure of the ductus arteriosus.

23.3 **D.** Pharmacological management usually is the first step in stabilizing the infant presenting with heart failure. The presence of a heart defect may not be apparent until either the ductus closes or the pulmonary vascular resistance falls, leading to heart failure. Clubbing requires months to develop. ECG findings in cyanotic congenital heart disease (CHD) are usually non-specific. Surgical intervention is best performed once the infant is stabilized and some defects require palliative procedures before the infant has grown sufficiently to undergo complete repair.

23.4 **D.** Infants with truncus arteriosus may not show symptoms until after 2 weeks of life when the pulmonary vascular resistance drops and creates increased pulmonary blood flow with accompanying symptoms of heart failure. This condition is diagnosed by echocardiography because the ECG findings are nonspecific and similar findings would be seen with many other cardiac defects. A snowman appearance on chest radiography is found with total anomalous pulmonary venous return (TAPVR). Treatment for truncus arteriosus is surgical repair.

CLINICAL PEARLS

▶ Pulse oximetry is a valuable tool for the detection of cyanotic congenital heart defects.

▶ Lesions of congenital heart disease that are incompatible with life except in the presence of a PDA are termed "ductus dependent."

▶ Infusion of Prostaglandin E$_1$ can stabilize infants with ductus-dependent lesions until more definitive surgical correction can be attempted.

▶ Truncus arteriosus presents with heart failure and requires stabilization with diuretics and ACE inhibitors prior to undergoing surgical repair.

REFERENCES

Bernstein D. Cyanotic congenital heart lesions: lesions associated with decreased pulmonary blood flow. In: Kliegman RM, Stanton BF, St. Geme III J, Schor N, Behrman R, eds. *Nelson Textbook of Pediatrics*. 19th ed. Philadelphia, PA: WB Saunders; 2011:1573-1577.

Bernstein D. Cyanotic congenital heart lesions: lesions associated with increased pulmonary blood flow. In: Kliegman RM, Stanton BF, St. Geme III J, Schor N, Behrman R, eds. *Nelson Textbook of Pediatrics*. 19th ed. Philadelphia, PA: WB Saunders; 2011:1585-1593.

Hoffman JIE. Congenital heart disease. In: Rudolph CD, Rudolph AM, Lister GE, First LR, Gershon AA, eds. *Rudolph's Pediatrics*. 22nd ed. New York, NY: McGraw-Hill; 2011:1822-1829.

Teitel DF. Neonate and infant with cardiovascular disease. In: Rudolph CD, Rudolph AM, Lister GE, First LR, Gershon AA, eds. *Rudolph's Pediatrics*. 22nd ed. New York, NY: McGraw-Hill; 2011: 1793-1803.

A 2-year-old girl, born at 32 weeks of gestation, comes to your clinic for an initial visit. Her 1-month stay in the neonatal intensive care unit was complicated by necrotizing enterocolitis (NEC), requiring surgical removal of a small section of her intestine that included the ileocecal valve. She had an uncomplicated postoperative course, and her mother declares she has been developing normally and gaining weight. She has a healthy appetite, a varied diet, and no history of abnormal stooling. Her mother is concerned, though, that she has been getting progressively paler since her last clinic visit with another provider 6 months ago. Physical examination reveals an overall healthy-appearing toddler with normal vital signs. She has pallorous skin and conjunctivae and a well-healed abdominal surgical scar. The remainder of her physical examination is normal. You order a complete blood count (CBC) and a reticulocyte count and find that the hemoglobin is 7 g/dL, the mean corpuscular volume is 110 fL, and the reticulocyte count is 2%.

► What is the most likely cause of this child's anemia?
► How should she be treated?

ANSWERS TO CASE 24:

Macrocytic Anemia (B$_{12}$ Deficiency due to Short Gut Syndrome)

Summary: A 2-year-old former premature infant with history of NEC and intestinal resection presenting with pallor and anemia.

- **Most likely cause:** Vitamin B$_{12}$ deficiency secondary to terminal ileal resection and compromised intestinal absorption

- **Treatment:** Monthly intramuscular vitamin B$_{12}$ supplementation

ANALYSIS

Objectives

1. Describe the typical findings in macrocytic anemia.

2. List the potential causes of macrocytic anemia.

3. Understand the treatment options for macrocytic anemia.

Considerations

Evaluation of a child with suspected anemia involves performing thorough personal and family histories and a comprehensive physical examination. Anemia can result from a variety of disorders, including defective red blood cell production, hemolysis, or blood loss. The clinician's goal, therefore, is to gather historical clues (atypical patient or family dietary histories, family history of blood dyscrasias) and examination findings (splenomegaly, flow murmur, hematochezia) that are important in guiding appropriate diagnostic and therapeutic plans.

APPROACH TO:

Macrocytic Anemia

DEFINITIONS

MEAN CORPUSCULAR VOLUME (MCV): Average size of a red blood cell; large cells are macrocytic; small cells are microcytic.

RETICULOCYTE COUNT: Percentage of red blood cells that are immature (new).

INTRINSIC FACTOR: Glycoprotein secreted in the stomach that binds to vitamin B$_{12}$; the intrinsic factor–vitamin B$_{12}$ complex then attaches to receptors in the distal ileum and is absorbed.

CLINICAL APPROACH

Anemia typically is distinguished by the size of the red blood cells. Children with iron deficiency develop a microcytic anemia and typically have a low MCV; their red blood cells are smaller than normal because of the decreased amount of hemoglobin in each cell. Children who quickly lose a large amount of blood usually have a normocytic anemia; the cells are normal, but there are fewer of them.

Various conditions may result in **macrocytic anemia, usually associated with an elevated MCV. Hypothyroidism, trisomy 21, vitamin B$_{12}$ deficiency, and folate deficiency** often are associated with macrocytic anemia and a low reticulocyte count, because of inadequate bone marrow production. A macrocytic anemia also may be seen with active hemolysis, but usually this anemia is accompanied by an elevated reticulocyte count.

Vitamin B$_{12}$–mediated macrocytic anemia can occur because of dietary deficiency, malabsorption, or inborn errors of metabolism. Vitamin B$_{12}$, an important factor in DNA synthesis, is available in many foods (meats, fish, eggs). A pure dietary deficiency is rare in children, but diets devoid of all animal products may result in a deficiency. **Breast-fed infants of mothers who adhere to a strict vegan diet are at risk for vitamin B$_{12}$ deficiency.** Malabsorption can occur when the terminal ileum is absent, as in this case scenario, or when infectious or inflammatory conditions compromise intestinal function.

Children with the rare condition "juvenile pernicious anemia" are unable to secrete intrinsic factor and become vitamin B$_{12}$ deficient between the ages of 1 and 2 years, when the supply of vitamin B$_{12}$ passed transplacentally from mother to child is exhausted. These children will exhibit worsening irritability, loss of appetite, and decreased activity. Children affected with this condition are at risk for permanent neurologic damage resulting from spinal cord demyelinization. Therapy is intramuscular vitamin B$_{12}$ replacement. High-dose oral replacement may be corrective (limited, inconclusive studies at present) in patients with intrinsic factor deficiency or severe dietary deficiency that cannot be corrected with dietary modification.

A variety of other more unusual causes of vitamin B$_{12}$ deficiency can be listed. The fish tapeworm *Diphyllobothrium latum* uses vitamin B$_{12}$, and intestinal infestation can result in macrocytic anemia. Similarly, any intestinal infectious or inflammatory process, such as parasitic infection or inflammatory bowel disease, could promote vitamin B$_{12}$ deficiency. Infants exclusively fed on goat's milk, nutritionally deficient in both vitamin B$_{12}$ and folate, are at risk not only for vitamin B$_{12}$ deficiency but also brucellosis if the milk is unpasteurized. For infants fed on goat's milk, vitamin and mineral supplementation is required.

Treatment for B$_{12}$ deficiency is guided by the underlying disorder. Eradicating or suppressing a gastrointestinal infection or inflammatory disorder should promote sufficient mucosal repair to permit adequate vitamin B$_{12}$ absorption, and further vitamin B$_{12}$ therapy may not be required. For patients with an inability to produce intrinsic factor and for those with absence or permanent dysfunction of the gastric antrum or terminal ileum (the site of intrinsic factor production and absorption, respectively), monthly parenteral vitamin B$_{12}$ therapy is indicated.

For patients with macrocytosis but normal B_{12} and folate levels, consideration for atypical bone marrow pathology (such as leukemia or myelodysplasia) must be entertained. Referral to a pediatric hematologist would be warranted.

CASE CORRELATION

- See also Case 11 (Megaloblastic Anemia) for the presentation of a nutritionally acquired B_{12} deficiency. Any chronic condition (such as malabsorption) may result in failure to thrive (Case 10) and anemia.

COMPREHENSION QUESTIONS

24.1 You are called to the bedside of a mother who just delivered a healthy term infant and has a question regarding her infant's nutrition. The mother was fed goat's milk as a child and wants to do the same for her infant. Under which of the following conditions is goat's milk acceptable as infant nutrition?

A. Goat's milk proteins are hydrolyzed before feeds.

B. Infants are provided supplemental vitamins and minerals.

C. Goat's milk is freshly obtained from goats.

D. Infants of mothers with milk intolerance should preferentially receive goat's milk.

E. Goat's milk is diluted with water.

24.2 You receive the results of a complete blood count (CBC) you performed in your clinic on a pallorous 9-month-old boy. Other than pallor, no historical or physical examination concerns were noted during the patient's visit. The laboratory technician reports a hemoglobin of 8.6 g/dL, a mean corpuscular volume (MCV) of 105 fL, and platelet count of 98,000/mm^3. You are also told that the white blood cell count is 8500/mm^3 and the differential reveals 47% neutrophils and 42% lymphocytes, and that no atypical lymphocytes are seen. Which of the following is the most appropriate next step in this child's care?

A. Measure serum iron and total iron-binding capacity levels.

B. Begin oral iron supplementation.

C. Measure vitamin B_{12} and folate levels.

D. Begin oral vitamin B_{12} and folate supplementation.

E. Obtain a stat referral to a pediatric hematologist.

24.3 The parents of a previously healthy 3-year-old girl bring the child to your clinic because she is complaining that her tongue hurts. The parents also report that she has appeared weak and listless over the last several months, and has not been eating well. Recently she has exhibited trouble walking. The family usually eats a regular diet, including meats and vegetables. On physical examination, she is pale and tachycardic. Her complete blood count reveals a macrocytic anemia. You suspect a vitamin or mineral deficiency. What additional finding is most likely in this toddler?

A. Red tongue

B. Petechiae and ecchymoses

C. Muscle fasciculation

D. Hair loss

E. Blue sclerae

24.4 A 16-year-old boy presents to your clinic with complaint of short stature. Review of systems reveals a normal, varied diet and a history of multiple episodes of diarrhea per day for the past 2 years. Clinical examination shows a Tanner stage 2 male at fifth percentile for height with multiple perianal skin tags. A CBC reveals a hemoglobin level of 8.8 g/dL and MCV of 115 fL; his retic count is normal. What is the most likely etiology for his anemia?

A. Inborn error of metabolism

B. Insufficient caloric intake

C. Infection-mediated hemolysis

D. Lactose intolerance

E. Malabsorption due to inflammatory bowel disease

ANSWERS

24.1 **B.** Infants drinking goat's milk must have nutritional supplementation with vitamin B_{12}, folate, and iron. Several goat's milk–based formulas including these nutrients are available. Fresh, unpasteurized goat's milk can contain *Brucella ovis* and cause brucellosis. Diluting milk will only serve to dilute the caloric content.

24.2 **C.** This infant has hematologic parameters consistent with macrocytic anemia. The mild thrombocytopenia reported is periodically seen in patients with vitamin B_{12} deficiency and is thought to be related to impaired DNA synthesis and ineffective thrombopoiesis. The results reported are not typical for iron deficiency, and neither an iron panel nor iron supplementation is warranted. At this point, your workup should include checking folate and B_{12} levels; supplementation of these compounds is not yet justified. Myelodysplasia or leukemia is in the differential, but is probably less likely with a normal white blood cell count and differential (no atypical cells); referral to pediatric hematology may ultimately be required, but some preliminary data can be gathered first.

24.3 **A.** A smooth, red, and tender tongue may be observed in juvenile pernicious anemia, a rare autosomal recessive condition in which the child is not able to secrete intrinsic factor and cannot absorb vitamin B_{12}. Supplies of vitamin B_{12} passed to the fetus from the mother typically are sufficient for at least the first 1 to 2 years of life. A deficiency in transcobalamin results in megaloblastic anemia in infancy because transcobalamin is required for B_{12} transport and utilization; therefore, vitamin B_{12} provided by the mother cannot be used effectively. Petechiae may occur with vitamin C or K deficiency, muscle fasciculation with vitamin D and calcium disturbance, and hair loss with zinc deficiency.

24.4 **E.** This patient's scenario of presumed growth arrest, chronic diarrhea, and anemia is most consistent with malabsorption related to possible underlying inflammatory bowel disease (IBD). Crohn disease is a form of IBD that may affect any region of the gastrointestinal tract and lead to significant nutritional deficiency. Although iron deficiency is the most common cause of microcytic anemia in patients with Crohn disease, macrocytic anemia is also possible with this disorder. Chronic inflammation involving the terminal ileum can result in fibrosis, limiting absorption of vitamin B_{12}. In addition, stricture formation, necessitating surgical resection of the terminal ileum, is also a risk factor for the development of anemia.

CLINICAL PEARLS

▶ Vitamin B_{12} dietary deficiency is rare; infants breast-fed by vegan mothers are at risk to become vitamin B_{12} deficient and should receive supplementation.

▶ Infants drinking goat's milk must be supplemented with vitamin B_{12}, folate, and iron.

▶ Vitamin B_{12} deficiency related to gastric antrum or ileal resection requires parenteral vitamin B_{12} supplementation.

▶ Vitamin B_{12} deficiency can lead to permanent neurologic damage.

▶ Inflammatory bowel disease may predispose to anemia due to nutritional deficiencies of either iron (microcytic) or vitamin B_{12} (macrocytic).

REFERENCES

Blanton R. Adult tapeworm infections. In: Kliegman RM, Stanton BF, St. Geme JW, Schor NF, Behrman RE, eds. *Nelson Textbook of Pediatrics.* 19th ed. Philadelphia, PA: WB Saunders; 2011:1232-1234.

Journeycake JM, Yang J, Chan AKC. Normal and abnormal hemostasis. In: Rudolph CD, Rudolph AM, Lister GE, First LR, Gerson AA, eds. *Rudolph's Pediatrics.* 22nd ed. New York, NY: McGraw-Hill; 2011: 1569.

Lerner NB. Megaloblastic anemias. In: Kliegman RM, Stanton BF, St. Geme JW, Schor NF, Behrman RE, eds. *Nelson Textbook of Pediatrics.* 19th ed. Philadelphia, PA: WB Saunders; 2011:1655.

Martin PL. Nutritional anemias. In: McMillan JA, Feigin RD, DeAngelis CD, Warshaw JB, eds. *Oski's Pediatrics: Principles and Practice.* 4th ed. Philadelphia, PA: Lippincott Williams & Wilkins; 2006:1692-1696.

A 3-year-old boy arrives to the emergency department after having suffered a seizure. The family reports that they had moved to Baltimore from the Midwest 3 months ago. The child was the product of a normal pregnancy and delivery, and he had experienced no medical problems until the move. The parents report that he has developed emotional lability, abdominal pain, "achy bones," and intermittent vomiting and constipation. They initially attributed his behavior to the move and to the chaos in their house, which is being extensively renovated.

▶ What is the most likely diagnosis?
▶ What is the best test to diagnose this condition?
▶ What is the best therapy?

ANSWERS TO CASE 25:

Lead Ingestion (Microcytic Anemia)

Summary: A 3-year-old, previously healthy child now living in a home undergoing extensive renovation has developed seizures, neurologic changes, and abdominal complaints.

- **Most likely diagnosis:** Lead toxicity.

- **Best test:** Blood lead level (BLL).

- **Best therapy:** Remove child from lead source and initiate chelation therapy.

ANALYSIS

Objectives

1. Understand the signs, symptoms, and treatment of lead poisoning.

2. Be familiar with the environmental sources of lead.

3. Understand the sources of other environmental exposures.

Considerations

This child is demonstrating signs and symptoms of lead poisoning. In addition, the patient is in the age range (**<5 years**) when BLLs peak and the patient has an overall greater risk of lead toxicity. He may have been exposed to lead-containing dust in the renovation environment, or he may have displayed pica (the eating of nonfood substances such as paint chips, dirt, or clay). Therapy can be initiated immediately while awaiting the blood lead level. During the evaluation and treatment, other children in the home must be screened for elevated lead levels given their shared exposure risk.

Lead exposure sources vary across the United States. In the **northeastern** United States, **older homes** undergoing **renovation** are a common source of exposure. Leaded paint is far less common in other parts of the country. A complete investigation includes a travel history and an accounting of lead exposures through hobbies (such as stained glass), home renovation, welding, radiator repair, furniture refinishing, pottery glazing, and similar activities.

> # APPROACH TO:
> ## Lead Poisoning

DEFINITIONS

CHELATING AGENT: A soluble compound that binds a metal ion (in this case lead) so that the new complex is excreted in the urine.

PLUMBISM: Alternate name for lead poisoning.

CLINICAL APPROACH

The incidence of lead poisoning in the United States has decreased dramatically over the last 20 years because of regulatory interventions by the federal, state, and local government. Previous sources (gasoline, foods, beverage cans) have been eliminated; **lead-containing paint in older homes is now the major source.** Less common sources include foodstuffs from countries where regulations are not strict, traditional ethnic remedies, **glazed pottery, ingestion of leaded items (jewelry, fishing equipment), exposure through burning of lead-containing batteries, or through hobbies involving lead smelting.** Several lines of toys were recalled by the US Consumer Product Safety Commission in 2010 when they were found to be coated with lead-based paint. Though the prevalence of elevated BLLs has declined by 84% in the last 20 years, the local prevalence can differ by 10-fold between communities. Children younger than 5 years are at a greater risk for lead toxicity and its sequela because of increased GI absorption, more frequent hand-to-mouth activity, and a susceptible developing central nervous system (CNS).

The signs and symptoms of lead exposure vary from none (especially at lower lead levels) to those listed in this case. However, symptoms may be seen at low BLLs, and a child with very high BLLs occasionally may be asymptomatic. **Anorexia, hyperirritability, altered sleep pattern, and decreased play are commonly seen. Developmental regression, especially with speech, may also be present.** Abdominal complaints (occasional vomiting, intermittent pain, and constipation) are sometimes noted. **Persistent vomiting, ataxia, altered consciousness, coma, and seizures are signs of encephalopathy.** Permanent, long-term consequences include learning and cognitive deficits and aggressive behavior; with less lead in the environment and decreasing average lead levels, these more subtle findings are now more common than acute lead encephalopathy.

The BLL is the diagnostic test of choice and demonstrates recent ingestion; however, a significant amount of lead is stored in other tissue, most notably bone. BLL, then, does not accurately reflect total body lead load. Other findings (free erythrocyte protoporphyrin, basophilic stippling, glycosuria, hypophosphatemia, long bone "lead lines," and gastrointestinal tract radiopaque flecks) in symptomatic patients are less specific.

Treatment varies depending on the BLL and the patient's symptoms. Admission to the hospital, stabilization, and chelation are appropriate for symptomatic patients. Therapy for asymptomatic patients could involve simple investigation of the child's environment, outpatient chelation, or immediate hospitalization (Table 25–1).

Table 25-1 • SUMMARY OF RECOMMENDATIONS FOR CHILDREN WITH CONFIRMED (VENOUS) ELEVATED BLOOD LEAD LEVELS

Blood Lead Level (µg/dL)				
10-14	**15-19**	**20-44**	**45-69**	**≥70**
Lead education • Dietary • Environmental Follow-up blood lead monitoring	Lead education • Dietary • Environmental Follow-up blood lead monitoring Proceed according to actions for 20-44 µg/dL if: • A follow-up BLL is in this range at least 3 mo after initial venous test Or • BLLs increase	Lead education • Dietary • Environmental Follow-up blood lead monitoring Complete history and physical examination Laboratory work: • Hemoglobin or hematocrit • Iron status Environmental investigation Lead hazard reduction Neurodevelopmental monitoring Abdominal x-ray (if particulate lead ingestion is suspected) with bowel decontamination if indicated	Lead education • Dietary • Environmental Follow-up blood lead monitoring Complete history and physical examination Complete neurological examination Laboratory work: • Hemoglobin or hematocrit • Iron status • Free erythrocyte protoporphyrin (FPP) or zinc protoporphyrin (ZPP) Environmental investigation Lead hazard reduction Neurodevelopmental monitoring Abdominal x-ray with bowel decontamination if indicated Chelation therapy	Hospitalize and commence chelation therapy Proceed according to actions for 45-69 µg/dL

The following actions are NOT recommended at any blood lead level:

- Searching for gingival lead lines
- Testing of neurophysiologic function
- Evaluation of renal function (except during chelation with EDTA)
- Testing of hair, teeth, or fingernails for lead
- Radiographic imaging of long bones
- X-ray fluorescence of long bones

Reproduced from the Centers for Disease Control and Prevention, www.cdc.gov.

Close contact with local health agencies is important; they usually are charged with ensuring that the child's environment is lead free.

Chelation in an asymptomatic child may consist of intramuscular calcium disodium ethylenediaminetetraacetic acid (CaEDTA) or more commonly oral meso-2,3-dimercaptosuccinic acid (DMSA, succimer). Hospitalized symptomatic patients are often treated with 2,3-dimercaptopropanol (British anti-Lewisite [BAL]) and CaEDTA. Fluid balance is tricky; urine output is maintained because CaEDTA is renally excreted, but encephalopathy may be exacerbated with overhydration.

Newer research has cast doubt on the utility of chelation therapy in asymptomatic children with lead levels less than 45 µg/dL. According to the US Preventative Services Task Force, no studies have demonstrated clinical benefits from chelation therapy in asymptomatic children. Lead levels do decrease acutely with chelation therapy, but affected children do not show improvement in long-term cognitive testing. The most recent literature suggests that no "safe" lead level exists; even lead levels less than 10 µg/dL have been shown to have a deleterious impact on neurocognitive development. This evidence places further importance upon the primary prevention of lead exposure in children. Currently, the Centers for Disease Control and Prevention (CDC) identifies children with lead levels above 5 µg/dL as having an elevated lead level and requiring further investigation.

No direct evidence shows that targeted BLL screening actually improves clinical outcomes in patients that are asymptomatic. Universal BLL screening is not recommended and BLL screening should be reserved for children identified to be at higher risk for lead toxicity based on location, history, and questionnaires. Questionnaires to assess the risk of lead exposure query the age of the home or day care center, the possibility of exposure to high-lead environments (battery recycling plant, lead smelter, etc), or environments in which others (siblings, playmates, etc) with elevated BLLs have been identified.

CASE CORRELATION

- See also Case 10 (Failure to Thrive) which may be a manifestation of exposure to toxins such as lead.

COMPREHENSION QUESTIONS

25.1 A developmentally normal 2-year-old child is in your inner city clinic for a well-child checkup. As part of the visit, you obtain a blood lead level and a hemoglobin level in accordance with your state's Medicaid screening guidelines. The following week, the state laboratory calls your clinic to report that the child's blood lead level is 14 μg/dL. Appropriate management of this level should include which of the following actions?

A. Initiate chelation therapy.

B. Perform long bone radiographs.

C. Reassure the parents that no action is required.

D. Repeat the blood lead level in 3 months.

E. Report to the local health department for environmental investigation.

25.2 While evaluating the family in the previous question, you discovered a 3-year-old sibling with a lead level of 50 μg/dL. You reported the case to the local authorities and initiated chelation therapy. All lead sources in the home have since been removed (verified by dust wipe samples), and the parents do not work in occupations prone to lead exposure. After a course of outpatient chelation therapy, the 3-year-old's lead level dropped to 5 μg/dL. Today, however, the child's 3-month follow-up blood lead level is 15 μg/dL. At this point, appropriate management includes which of the following actions?

A. Initiate a course of inpatient parenteral chelation therapy.

B. Perform long bone radiographs.

C. Reassure the parents and repeat a blood lead level in 3 months.

D. Recommend the family move to another home.

E. Repeat a course of outpatient chelation therapy.

25.3 A term newborn infant is admitted to the neonatal ICU after having a seizure in the Well Baby Nursery. Your examination reveals a microcephalic infant with low birth weight who does not respond to sound. In your discussions with the family, you discover this is the parents' first child. They recount odd symptoms that have developed in both of them in the last few months, including fine tremors in their upper extremities and blurry vision. They also note that they both can no longer smell their food and that it "tastes funny." The mother notes that she has had trouble walking straight in the last few weeks, but she attributes that to her pregnancy. Which of the following environmental toxins is most likely to have caused these findings?

A. Inorganic arsenic salts

B. Lead

C. Methyl mercury

D. Orellanine

E. Polychlorinated biphenyls

25.4 A mother brings her 2-year-old son to your clinic for a well-child checkup. He was lost to follow-up in early infancy but has come to clinic today to reestablish care. She reports that overall he has been well except that he seems to have less energy lately. He is a very picky eater and mostly drinks whole milk all day. The mother wants your advice about keeping her son from his new favorite hobby, eating dirt. What is the most appropriate next step?

    A. HEADSS examination

    B. Hemoglobin level and lead exposure questionnaire

    C. Hemoglobin level and blood lead level

    D. Cholesterol screening

    E. Reassurance

ANSWERS

25.1 **D.** The patient's lead screen is mildly elevated. Appropriate management includes educating the parents about potential lead exposures in the environment as well as in the diet. A repeat level should be performed in 3 months. Chelation therapy is currently advised for patients with a blood lead level of 45 µg/dL and above. Environmental investigation is recommended in patients with a blood lead level of 20 µg/dL and above, or if levels remain elevated despite educational efforts. Long bone radiographs are not recommended at any blood lead level.

25.2 **C.** In this case, reassurance is appropriate. Lead deposits in bone, and chelation does not remove all lead from the body. After chelation is complete, lead levels tend to rise again; the source is thought to be the redistribution of lead stored in bone. Repeat chelation is only recommended if the blood lead level rebounds to 45 µg/dL or higher. Moving to another home is not necessary, assuming the health department successfully remediated their current home. Long bone radiographs are not recommended at any blood lead level.

25.3 **C.** Infants exposed in utero to methyl mercury may display low birth weight, microcephaly, and seizures. They also display significant developmental delay and can have vision and hearing impairments. Symptoms in children and adults include ataxia, tremor, dysarthria, memory loss, altered sensorium (including vision, hearing, smell, and taste), dementia, and ultimately death. Acute ingestion of arsenic causes severe gastrointestinal symptoms; chronic exposure causes skin lesions and can cause peripheral neuropathy and encephalopathy. Orellanine is a toxin found in the *Cortinarius* species of mushroom that causes nausea, vomiting, and diarrhea; renal toxicity may occur several days later. Polychlorinated biphenyls (PCBs) cross the placenta and accumulate in breast milk; exposure in utero is thought to cause behavioral problems in later life.

25.4 **B.** This patient is at high risk for iron-deficiency anemia given his insufficient dietary intake and symptoms of pica and lethargy. Screening with a blood hemoglobin level is indicated. BLL screening should be performed in patients with identifiable risk factors such as living in pre-1950 homes, parents with occupational lead exposure, or recent immigration. This history should be elucidated from the family either by interview or questionnaire, with subsequent BLL screening if indicated.

CLINICAL PEARLS

▶ Lead-containing paint in older homes is the major source of lead exposure in the United States.

▶ Behavioral signs of lead toxicity include hyperirritability, altered sleep patterns, decreased play activity, loss of developmental milestones (especially speech), and altered state of consciousness. Physical symptoms include vomiting, intermittent abdominal pain, constipation, ataxia, coma, and seizures.

▶ Chelation therapy in an asymptomatic child with elevated lead levels consists of intramuscular calcium disodium ethylenediaminetetraacetic acid (CaEDTA) or oral meso-2,3-dimercaptosuccinic acid (succimer). Hospitalized patients with symptomatic disease are often treated with 2,3-dimercaptopropanol (BAL) and CaEDTA.

REFERENCES

Advisory Committee on Childhood Lead Poisoning Prevention (ACCLPP). Recommendations for blood lead screening of young children enrolled in medicaid: targeting a group at high risk. *MMWR Recomm Rep.* 2000;49(RR-14):1-13.

Advisory Committee on Childhood Lead Poisoning Prevention, Centers for Disease Control and Prevention. Low level lead exposure harms children: a renewed call for primary prevention. January 4, 2012. http://www.cdc.gov/nceh/lead/acclpp/final_document_010412.pdf. Accessed January 15, 2015.

American Academy of Pediatrics. Lead exposure in children: prevention, detection, and management. *Pediatrics.* 2005;116:1036-1046.

American Academy of Pediatrics. Screening for elevated lead levels in childhood and pregnancy: an updated summary of evidence for the US Preventative Services Task Force. *Pediatrics.* 2006;118:e1867-1895.

American Academy of Pediatrics. Trends in blood lead levels and blood lead testing among US children aged 1 to 5 years, 1988-2004. *Pediatrics.* 2009;123;e376-e385.

Centers for Disease Control and Prevention (CDC) Advisory Committee on Childhood Lead Poisoning Prevention. Interpreting and managing blood lead levels <10 microg/dL in children and reducing childhood exposures to lead: recommendations of CDC's Advisory Committee on Childhood Lead Poisoning Prevention. *MMWR Recomm Rep.* 2007;56(RR08):1-16.

Etzel RA. Environmental pediatrics. In: Rudolph CD, Rudolph AM, Lister GE, First LR, Gershon AA, eds. *Rudolph's Pediatrics.* 22nd ed. New York, NY: McGraw-Hill; 2011:67.

Fenick AM. Screening. In: Rudolph CD, Rudolph AM, Lister GE, First LR, Gershon AA, eds. *Rudolph's Pediatrics.* 22nd ed. New York, NY: McGraw-Hill; 2011:45.

Landriagan PJ, Forman JA. Chemical pollutants. In: Kliegman RM, Stanton BF, St. Geme JW, Schor NF, Behrman RE, eds. *Nelson Textbook of Pediatrics.* 19th ed. Philadelphia, PA: WB Saunders; 2011:2448.

Mahajan PV. Heavy metal intoxication. In: Kliegman RM, Stanton BF, St. Geme JW, Schor NF, Behrman RE, eds. *Nelson Textbook of Pediatrics.* 19th ed. Philadelphia, PA: WB Saunders; 2011:2448.

Markowitz M. Lead poisoning. In: Kliegman RM, Stanton BF, St. Geme JW, Schor NF, Behrman RE, eds. *Nelson Textbook of Pediatrics.* 19th ed. Philadelphia, PA: WB Saunders; 2011:2448-2453.

Sperling MA. Hypoglycemia. In: Kliegman RM, Stanton BF, St. Geme JW, Schor NF, Behrman RE, eds. *Nelson Textbook of Pediatrics.* 19th ed. Philadelphia, PA: WB Saunders; 2011:529.

A 7-year-old previously healthy boy presents to the emergency room with a rash and mouth pain. His mother took him to see his primary care physician (PCP) 1 week prior with a 2-week history of cough, subjective fever, and malaise; he was prescribed amoxicillin for presumed pneumonia. Five days into the antibiotic course, he developed an itchy rash and mouth sores. His mother reports markedly diminished intake over the previous 24 hours, but no emesis or diarrhea. He has no known medication or food allergies. In the emergency room (ER), his temperature is 102°F (38.9°C), heart rate 122 beats/min, blood pressure 119/73 mm Hg, respiratory rate 18 breaths/min, and oxygen saturation 97% on room air. On physical examination, he has bilateral conjunctival injection, ulcers on his tongue and lower lip (Figure 26–1), and purpuric macules and bullous lesions on his torso and extremities. Chest x-ray reveals an infiltrate in the right lower lobe.

► What is the most likely diagnosis?
► What is the next step in evaluation?

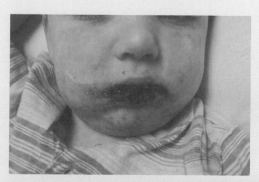
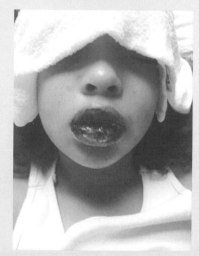

Figure 26–1. Rec going with single pic, boy on left in striped shirt. Closest to scenario, except for age. (*Reproduced, with permission, from Adelaide A. Hebert, MD.*)

ANSWERS TO CASE 26:

Stevens-Johnson Syndrome

Summary: A child with fever, fatigue, and respiratory symptoms, followed by mucosal and skin lesions, while on amoxicillin for presumed bacterial pneumonia.

- **Most likely diagnosis:** Stevens-Johnson syndrome (SJS).

- **Next step in evaluation:** Stop amoxicillin and admit to the hospital for close observation, with additional evaluation and therapeutic considerations to include selected laboratory tests (complete metabolic panel, complete blood count [CBC], blood culture), IV hydration, broad-spectrum antibiotics for typical (pneumococcus, *Staphylococcus aureus*) and atypical (*Mycoplasma pneumoniae*) community-acquired pneumonia (CAP). Ophthalmology should be consulted, and ICU monitoring may be necessary.

ANALYSIS

Objectives

1. Understand SJS risk factors, etiologies, and complications.

2. Identify and manage SJS.

3. Differentiate between SJS and toxic epidermal necrolysis (TEN).

Considerations

Mucosal and cutaneous lesions (conjunctivitis, oral ulcers, cutaneous purpura, and bullae) are strongly suggestive of SJS. Although medications are the most common cause of SJS overall, infections related to viruses and atypical bacteria, such as *M pneumoniae*, typically account for a higher percentage of cases in children than in adults. In this patient, the diagnostic dilemma lies in attempting to define whether SJS is related to the antibiotic or active infection. Irrespective, the first step is to stop any potential offending agent, consider alternative antibacterial treatment for CAP (ceftriaxone, azithromycin), and comprehensively and judiciously evaluate and support him while the syndrome abates.

APPROACH TO:

The Patient with Stevens-Johnson Syndrome

DEFINITIONS

APOPTOSIS: Activation or suppression of a stimulus or trigger, promoting cellular DNA destruction and ultimately cell demise; normal bodily mechanism for eliminating damaged or nonviable cells; also known as "programmed cell death."

NIKOLSKY SIGN: Sign elicited by slight rubbing of the finger against the skin causing separation of the epidermal layer and blister formation; finding in various desquamating syndromes (SJS, TEN, staphylococcal scalded skin syndrome).

SYNECHIAE: Adhesions of the iris to either the cornea or lens; complication of ocular trauma or inflammation of the iris; identified by ophthalmoscope or on slit-lamp examination.

SCORE OF TOXIC EPIDERMAL NECROLYSIS (SCORTEN): Scores the severity of bullous conditions; initially developed for TEN, but also utilized in patients with thermal burns or SJS; involves seven independent risk factors for mortality risk (Table 26–1); as SCORTEN score increases, prognosis worsens and mortality risk increases; ICU placement should be considered for any patient with a SCORTEN score 2 or greater.

CLINICAL APPROACH

The differential for cutaneous syndromes is wide and varied. Characteristics of skin lesions, including shape and location, and associated symptoms may help guide diagnosis. If a rash occurs after medication administration, drug eruption should be included in the differential. SJS and TEN are drug eruptions that present with erythematous or purpuric macules progressing to epidermal sloughing and necrosis. The extent of epidermal detachment differentiates the two syndromes (SJS <10%, SJS/TEN overlap syndrome 10%-30%, TEN >30%).

SJS was first described in the 1920s when two pediatricians jointly published the description of a disorder involving blistering skin and mucosal lesions that occurred after drug administration. The disorder occurs in both children and adults, with medication the usual etiology; but, infections (*Mycoplasma pneumoniae*, Herpes viridae)

Table 26–1 • SCORTEN RISK FACTORS, SCORING AND MORTALITY RATES		
Risk Factor	**Score 0**	**Score 1**
Age	<40 y	>40 y
Associated malignancy	No	Yes
Heart rate (beats/min)	<120	>120
Serum BUN (mg/dL)	<27	>27
Detached or compromised body surface	<10%	>10%
Serum bicarbonate (mEq/L)	>20	<20
Serum glucose (mg/dL)	<250	>250

Number of Risk Factors	**Mortality Rate**
0-1	3.2%
2	12.1%
3	35.3%
4	58.3%
≥5	>90%

account for a higher percentage of SJS in children (~75%-90%). Common inciting agents are antibiotics, nonsteroidal anti-inflammatory agents (NSAIDs), allopurinol, and antiepileptics (carbamazepine, phenytoin, lamotrigine, phenobarbital). Among antibiotics, sulfonamides are the leading agent, followed by penicillins and cephalosporins. Cutaneous lesions typically first occur about 2 weeks after a new medication exposure. If a patient is reexposed to the same medication, SJS findings may occur in as little as 48 hours.

Risk factors for SJS include HIV infection or other underlying immunodeficiency and genetic abnormalities. Some studies suggest a 40- to 100-fold increased risk for SJS after trimethoprim-sulfamethoxazole (Bactrim, Septra) administration in HIV patients when compared to the general population. Patients with select human leucocyte antigen types (HLA-B 1502) are at increased risk for SJS with aromatic antiepileptics, such as carbamazepine, phenytoin, and phenobarbital. Some patients have lower N-acetyltransferase activity in the liver; these "slow acetylators" have longer exposure time to toxic drug metabolites, rendering them at increased risk for SJS. Polymorphism in the interleukin (IL)-4 receptor gene is a genetic variation that may place a patient at risk for SJS by promoting an increased cytokine-driven inflammatory response.

A prodrome of fever and flu-like illness typically occurs a few days to weeks prior to the appearance of mucosal and/or cutaneous lesions in SJS. A prodromal burning sensation or other skin paresthesias, and physical examination findings of erythroderma, tongue swelling, facial edema, and palpable purpura, may herald SJS and should alert the clinician to the possible diagnosis. Skin lesions often begin as ill-defined or target-shaped erythematous macules with purpuric centers. The rash is symmetrical and typically begins on the face and thorax, before extending to other areas (palms and soles typically spared). Epidermal detachment occurs as keratinocytes undergo apoptosis, then vesicles and bullae form. Within days, skin begins to slough and the patient may have a positive Nikolsky sign. Lesions undergo rapid progression of sloughing for 2 to 3 days and then stabilize, while purpuric centers may necrose. Cutaneous findings are typically associated with mucous membrane involvement in two or more areas (eyes, mouth, upper airway, esophagus, gastrointestinal tract, anogenital mucosa). Ocular lesions are the most common mucocutaneous finding, with risk of corneal ulceration, synechiae, and eventual blindness. Every patient with SJS deserves formal ophthalmologic evaluation. Other complications include stomatitis, urethritis, and pulmonary involvement (cough, dyspnea). The syndrome usually is self-limited, and, in the absence of significant complication(s), prodrome onset to resolution usually occurs in 2 to 4 weeks.

SJS is a clinical diagnosis and should be considered in any patient with suggestive history, prodromal symptoms, and characteristic skin findings. Once the diagnosis is considered, the clinician must promptly withdraw the presumed inciting agent. The patient with SJS should be hospitalized, and a **SCORTEN** score assigned for severity and to facilitate level of care. If a patient scores two or above, or lesions are rapidly progressing, prognosis typically is improved if a patient is cared for in an intensive care or burn unit. The management of SJS is similar to the treatment of major burns. Treatment includes supportive care with intravenous fluids and electrolyte replacement as needed, optimal nutrition via early use of nasogastric tube feeds, comprehensive wound care, formal ophthalmologic evaluation and treatment (ocular steroid and/or antibiotic), pain control, and monitoring for possible superimposed infection (*S aureus*, herpes). Systemic antibiotics are indicated for presumed or confirmed bacterial infection, with sepsis the leading etiology for mortality in SJS. Other complications include acute respiratory distress syndrome (ARDS) and multiple organ dysfunction. The use of corticosteroids in the treatment of SJS remains controversial, with little evidence demonstrating their efficacy and possible increased morbidity and poor prognosis observed with their use. Some experts support intravenous immunoglobulin (IVIG) administration in early disease.

COMPREHENSION QUESTIONS

26.1 A 15-year-old girl is prescribed carbamazepine by her pediatric neurologist for generalized tonic-clonic seizures. She had been previously healthy with her only past medical history being an allergy to penicillin. One week later, her younger brother develops an upper respiratory infection. Soon she, too, begins to have similar symptoms of cough and sinus congestion with yellowish rhinorrhea, but no fever, increased work of breathing, or gastrointestinal distress. She restarts an old prescription of intranasal fluticasone for her seasonal allergies. Over the next 2 days her coryza improves, but she then notices an erythematous rash on her calves and forearms. She presents to her pediatrician when the lesions progress to blisters. What is the next best evaluation or treatment step?

A. Prescribe amoxicillin-clavulanate for sinusitis.

B. Obtain chest x-ray to rule out pneumonia.

C. Discontinue carbamazepine.

D. Discontinue fluticasone.

E. Recommend supportive care at home for viral upper respiratory infection.

26.2 A 4-year-old boy presents to your emergency room with dysuria. Symptoms began 2 days ago with crying on urination and penile tip tenderness noted by his mother; his urine output has diminished over the past 24 hours. His mother reports that 2 weeks prior he suffered an ankle sprain, and has experienced occasional leg pain for which she has been giving him ibuprofen one to two times daily. At triage, he has a previously unrecorded temperature of 101.5°F (38.6°C), heart rate of 90 beats/min, blood pressure of 92/68 mm Hg, and respiratory rate of 18 breaths/min. On physical examination, you note conjunctival erythema bilaterally, blisters on the dorsum of his hands and feet, and mucosanguineous urethral discharge and erythema of the distal glans penis. Besides discontinuing his ibuprofen, what other evaluation or intervention would you recommend?

   A. Administer naproxen sodium for his fever.

   B. Consult ophthalmology for urgent ocular examination.

   C. Consult urology for urgent voiding cystourethrogram (VCUG).

   D. Administer intramuscular ceftriaxone for febrile urinary tract infection.

   E. Consult social services for suspected child abuse.

26.3 A 17-year-old boy, with no significant past medical history, presents to the emergency room with a rash, conjunctivitis, and dysuria. His temperature is 102.8°F (39.3°C), heart rate 144 beats/min, blood pressure 132/91 mm Hg, respiratory rate 18 breaths/min, and oxygen saturation 100% on room air. You estimate his rash involves less than 10% of his body surface area. A complete blood count reveals mild leucopenia, and a basic metabolic panel and urinalysis are normal. Your working diagnosis is Stevens-Johnson syndrome. His concerned parents inquire as to his prognosis. What is his mortality risk based on the SCORTEN scale?

   A. <5%

   B. ~10%

   C. ~35%

   D. ~60%

   E. >90%

26.4 You inform the parents of the patient in Question 26.3 that you recommend admission to the hospital. His mother then reports the patient has an uncle who had a similar reaction to allopurinol, and a brother with history of jaundice while on isoniazid (INH) for latent tuberculosis. She inquires whether the patient's family history places her son at increased risk for Stevens-Johnson syndrome (SJS) and whether any other factors might be involved. Which of the following is most likely a risk factor for his SJS?

A. Prior hives on sulfa antibiotic

B. Chronic benzoyl peroxide use for acne

C. Recurring overexposure to sunlight

D. Previous untreated seizure related to febrile illness

E. Abnormal N-acetyltransferase activity

ANSWERS

26.1 **C.** Although viral and atypical bacterial infections account for a higher percentage of SJS in children than in adults, drug administration remains the leading cause of SJS overall; carbamazepine is frequently implicated. In this scenario, the clinician should first perform a thorough medication review and withdraw any possible offending agent (intranasal fluticasone less likely). The patient should then be monitored in a hospital setting, given a high likelihood of progression and development of mucocutaneous lesions. A diagnosis of bacterial pneumonia or sinusitis is not supported in this patient scenario, and supportive care at home alone for viremia would not be standard of care.

26.2 **B.** This patient with likely SJS presents with penile mucosal erosion causing dysuria. Though oculomucocutaneous involvement is most common, possible additional sites include the respiratory tract, oropharynx, esophagus, gastrointestinal tract, and anal and urogenital regions. Conjunctivitis on examination warrants an immediate ophthalmology consult, because serious complications including blindness can occur. Ibuprofen is the likely culprit and should be discontinued immediately. Urology input, evaluation or treatment for urinary tract anomaly or infection, and social work involvement is premature, because the etiology for his penile abnormality is likely mucosal erosion, not infection or trauma.

26.3 **A.** The **SCORTEN** scale is used to assess the severity of symptoms in multiple diseases presenting with bullous lesions, and can be used to guide patient placement in the hospital; higher scores warrant admission to an ICU or burn unit to improve prognosis. According to **SCORTEN** criteria, this patient's only risk factor is tachycardia. With only one risk factor, this patient's mortality rate is 3.2%. He should, however, be closely monitored in an intermediate care unit at the onset.

26.4 **E.** In addition to immunodeficiency and viral infection, some studies have identified various genetic factors that increase risk for SJS. Patients with the haplotype HLA-B 1502 have a propensity to develop SJS due to aromatic antiepileptics such as carbamazepine, phenytoin, and phenobarbital. Some patients have low N-acetyltransferase activity in the liver rendering them "slow acetylators." Because of reduced acetylating capacity, these patients are at increased risk for build-up of toxic drug metabolites. With a positive family history, it is possible he has a genetic factor that makes him a "slow acetylator" and increases his risk for SJS.

CLINICAL PEARLS

▶ Medication administration is the leading cause of Stevens-Johnson syndrome across all age ranges.

▶ SJS lesions are characterized by erythematous macules, with eventual epidermal detachment and mucosal involvement in two or more areas.

▶ Initial step in SJS management is to remove the offending agent, with further management goals being supportive and aimed at preventing complications.

▶ All SJS patients with ocular involvement require ophthalmology consultation.

REFERENCES

Atkinson TP, Boppana S, Theos A, Clements LS, Xiao L, Waites K. Stevens-Johnson syndrome in a boy with macrolide-resistant *Mycoplasma pneumoniae* pneumonia. *Pediatrics.* June 2011;127(6): e1605-e1609. http://pediatrics.aappublications.org/content/127/6/e1605.full.html. Accessed March 6, 2014.

Finkelstein Y, Soon GS, Acuna P, et al. Recurrence and outcomes of Stevens-Johnson syndrome and toxic epidermal necrolysis in children. *Pediatrics.* October 2011;128(4):723-728.

Morelli JG. Stevens-Johnson syndrome. In: Kliegman RM, Stanton BF, St. Geme JW, Schor NF, Behrman RE, eds. *Nelson Textbook of Pediatrics.* 19th ed. Philadelphia, PA: Elsevier Saunders; 2011:2242-2244.

Prendiville J. Drug eruptions. In: Rudolph CD, Rudolph AM, Lister GE, First LR, Gerson AA, eds. *Rudolph's Pediatrics.* 22nd ed. New York, NY: McGraw-Hill; 2011:1277-1279.

A 16-year-old adolescent male resident at the local police department's boot camp was in his normal state of health until this morning when he developed a headache and a fever of 105.8°F (41°C). Over the next 2 hours, he developed a stiff neck and began vomiting. He was brought to the emergency department (ED) when he developed altered mental status. No one else in the facility is ill. In the ED, his heart rate is 135 beats/min, blood pressure 120/70 mm Hg, respiratory rate 25 breaths/min, and temperature 104°F (40°C). He is combative, unaware of his surroundings, and does not follow instructions. Kernig and Brudzinski signs are present.

► What is the most likely diagnosis?
► How would you confirm the diagnosis?
► What treatment is indicated?
► What are possible complications?

ANSWERS TO CASE 27:
Bacterial Meningitis

Summary: A 16-year-old adolescent boy has fever, headache, stiff neck, and altered mental status. He is tachycardic but normotensive.

- **Most likely diagnosis:** Bacterial meningitis
- **Confirm diagnosis:** Lumbar puncture (LP)
- **Treatment:** Intravenous antibiotics
- **Complications:** Deafness, cranial nerve palsies, and, rarely, hemiparesis or global brain injury

ANALYSIS

Objectives

1. Describe the typical presentation of bacterial meningitis.
2. Describe how a patient's age affects the presentation and outcome of bacterial meningitis.
3. List typical pathogens and appropriate treatment strategies by age group.

Considerations

This teen has the typical triad of meningitis symptoms: fever, headache, and a stiff neck; his altered mental status is another often-seen finding. Other causes of mental status changes include viral meningoencephalitis, trauma, intentional or accidental ingestion, and hypoglycemia. Of these alternatives, only viral meningoencephalitis would likely explain the fever and stiff neck.

APPROACH TO:
Bacterial Meningitis

DEFINITIONS

BRUDZINSKI SIGN: A physical finding consistent with meningitis; while the patient is supine, the neck is passively flexed resulting in involuntary knee and hip flexion.

ENCEPHALITIS: Brain parenchyma inflammation causing brain dysfunction.

KERNIG SIGN: A physical finding consistent with meningitis; while the patient is supine, the legs are flexed at the hip and knee at 90° angle resulting in pain with leg extension.

MENINGITIS: Leptomeningeal inflammations, typically infectious, but may also be caused by foreign substances.

CLINICAL APPROACH

The microbiology and clinical presentation of meningitis vary based on the patient's age. The incidence of **neonatal meningitis** is between 0.2 and 0.5 cases per 1000 live births, most commonly due to **group B Streptococcus** (*Streptococcus agalactiae*) which is implicated in roughly 50% of cases. GBS is followed by *Escherichia coli*, accounting for another 20% of cases, and then *Listeria monocytogenes*, responsible for 5% to 10% of cases. Other organisms, including *Citrobacter* sp, *Staphylococcus* sp, group D streptococci, and *Candida* sp, are rare. Infants at increased risk for meningitis include low-birth-weight and preterm infants, and those born to mothers with chorioamnionitis after a prolonged rupture of the amniotic membranes, or by traumatic delivery. Most neonatal bacterial meningitis occurs by hematogenous spread. Clinical symptoms in infants are nonspecific and not the typical triad of headache, fever, and stiff neck. Instead, infants may have thermal instability (often hypothermia), poor feeding, emesis, seizures, irritability, and apnea. Infants may have a bulging fontanelle, and they demonstrate generalized hyper- or hypotonicity.

Bacterial meningitis in older children is usually caused by **Streptococcus pneumoniae or Neisseria meningitidis;** vaccination has essentially eliminated *Haemophilus influenzae* type B. Other rarer causes in this age group include *Pseudomonas aeruginosa*, *Staphylococcus aureus*, *Staphylococcus epidermidis*, *Salmonella* sp, and *Listeria monocytogenes*.

The incidence of pneumococcal meningitis is 1 to 6 cases per 100,000 children per year, more commonly occurring in the winter. It is an **encapsulated pathogen;** children with a **poorly functioning or absent spleen are at higher risk.** Children with **sickle cell disease** have an infection incidence 300 times greater than in unaffected children. Other risk factors include sinusitis, otitis media, pneumonia, and head trauma with subsequent cerebrospinal fluid (CSF) leak.

Neisseria meningitidis colonizes the upper respiratory tract in approximately 15% of normal individuals; carriage rates up to 30% are seen during invasive disease outbreaks. Disease appears to be caused by "new" infection rather than long-term carriage. In the United States, most disease is caused by serotypes B and C. Family members and day care workers in close contact with children having meningitis are at 100- to 1000-fold increased risk for contracting disease. A plethora of other bacterial, viral, fungal, and mycobacterial agents can cause meningitis.

The **classic symptoms of meningitis seen in older children and adults** may be accompanied by **mental status changes, nausea, vomiting, lethargy, restlessness, ataxia, back pain, Kernig and Brudzinski signs, and cranial nerve palsies.** Approximately one-quarter to one-third of patients have a **seizure** during the illness course. Patients with *N meningitidis* can have a petechial or purpuric rash (purpura fulminans), which is associated with septicemia. Patients with septicemia due to *N meningitidis* often are gravely ill and may or may not have associated meningitis.

The **test of choice for suspected meningitis is an LP,** which usually can be performed safely in children with few complications. **Contraindications** include a **skin infection over the planned puncture site,** evidence of or clinical concern for **increased** intracranial pressure, and a critically ill patient who may not tolerate the procedure. Cerebrospinal fluid analysis includes Gram stain and culture, white and red blood cell counts, and protein and glucose analysis. Bacterial antigen screens can be performed in patients already receiving antibiotics before the LP; these antigens may persist for several days, even when the culture is negative. Typical bacterial meningitis findings include an elevated opening pressure, several hundred to thousands of white blood cells with polymorphonuclear cell predominance, and elevated protein and decreased glucose levels.

Treatment strategies vary by patient age, likely pathogens, and local resistance patterns. A CSF Gram stain can guide the decision-making process. In the neonatal period, ampicillin often is combined with a third-generation cephalosporin or an aminoglycoside to cover infections caused by group B *Streptococcus*, *E coli*, and *L monocytogenes*. Neonates in an intensive care unit may be exposed to nosocomial infections; prevalent pathogens in that nursery must be considered.

In some locales, more than half of the pneumococcal isolates are intermediately or highly penicillin resistant; 5% to 10% of the organisms are cephalosporin resistant. Thus, in suspected pneumococcal meningitis, a third-generation cephalosporin combined with vancomycin is often recommended. Most *N meningitidis* strains are susceptible to penicillin or cephalosporins.

Acute meningitis complications may include seizures, cranial nerve palsies, cerebral infarction, cerebral or cerebellar herniation, venous sinus thrombosis, subdural effusions, syndrome of inappropriate antidiuretic hormone (SIADH) secretion with hyponatremia, and central diabetes insipidus. The most common long-term sequela is hearing loss (up to 30% of patients with pneumococcus); patients with bacterial meningitis usually have a hearing evaluation at the conclusion of antibiotic treatment. Mental retardation, neuropsychiatric and learning problems, epilepsy, behavioral problems, vision loss, and hydrocephalus are less commonly seen.

CASE CORRELATION

- See also Case 4 (Group B streptococcal infection) and Case 6 (Neonatal Herpes Simplex Virus Infection) which are common causes of CNS infection in the newborn period. A complication of otitis media (Case 16) is mastoiditis and meningitis. The child with sickle cell disease (Case 13) has an immune deficiency due to splenic auto-infarction and a higher incidence of infection due to encapsulated (pneumococcus) organisms. These children also are prone to stroke which may present with acute onset of neurologic symptoms similar to those of meningitis. Meningitis due to chronic condition such as tuberculosis may present with failure to thrive (Case 10).

COMPREHENSION QUESTIONS

27.1 A 13-year-old boy has a 1-day history of fever and lethargy. Physical examination reveals a lethargic male in no respiratory distress. He has a temperature of 105.8°F (41°C), a heart rate of 135 beats/min, and a blood pressure (BP) of 60/40 mm Hg. He has a stiff neck and a purpuric rash over his trunk. Which of the following is the most appropriate next step in the management of this patient?

A. Computed tomography of the head

B. Intravenous antibiotics

C. Intubation

D. Lumbar puncture (LP)

E. Intravenous fluid resuscitation

27.2 An 8-year-old girl has fever and headache of 2 days duration. Today, her headache was significant enough to keep her home from school. Her highest temperature was 102°F (38.9°C). On examination, you find an alert girl in no respiratory distress. She has a temperature of 101°F (38.3°C), heart rate 121 beats/min, and blood pressure (BP) 100/60 mm Hg. She has nuchal rigidity and mild photophobia. Lumbar puncture reveals a cerebrospinal fluid (CSF) white blood cell count of 60 with lymphocytic predominance, normal protein and glucose counts. The Gram stain is negative for bacteria. Which of the following is the most likely diagnosis?

A. Central nervous system neoplasm

B. Viral (aseptic) meningitis

C. Acute bacterial meningitis

D. Fungal meningitis

E. Tuberculosis meningitis

27.3 A 2-week-old infant develops a temperature to 102°F (38.9°C). Pregnancy and delivery were uncomplicated. The irritable, fussy infant has a heart rate of 170 beats/min and respiratory rate of 40 breaths/min. The anterior fontanelle is full, but he has no nuchal rigidity; the rest of the examination is unremarkable. Which of the following is the most appropriate management of this infant?

A. Encourage oral fluids and office follow-up in 24 hours.

B. Order computed tomography of the head followed by an LP.

C. Perform an LP, blood culture, and urine culture, and admit to the hospital.

D. Prescribe intramuscular ceftriaxone and clinic follow-up in 1 week.

E. Prescribe oral amoxicillin and clinic follow-up in 1 week.

27.4 A 14-year-old boy with history of sickle cell disease complains of fever and stiff neck for 1 day. On examination, he is alert and oriented, but he has nuchal rigidity and a positive Brudzinski sign. The patient's mother refuses lumbar puncture. Which of the following is the most likely organism responsible for this patient's clinical presentation?

    A. *Escherichia coli*

    B. *Streptococcus pneumoniae*

    C. *Listeria monocytogenes*

    D. *Streptococcus agalactiae*

    E. *Staphylococcus aureus*

ANSWERS

27.1 **E.** This patient in the question has meningococcemia. He is in septic shock as evidenced by hypotension and tachycardia. The **ABC** of **A**irway, **B**reathing, and **C**irculation should always take precedence over diagnostic studies. *Neisseria meningitidis* can present as meningococcemia with purpura and shock; in some cases patients will also have meningitis. The LP should be deferred, however, until he is clinically stable. Intubation is not necessary because he is not in respiratory distress. Intravenous fluids through a large-bore catheter to support his cardiovascular status should be administered, followed by IV antibiotics.

27.2 **B.** This girl's history and presentation suggest meningitis. Her diagnostic studies are suggestive of viral or aseptic meningitis because her CSF white blood cell count is less than 100 with lymphocytic predominance and her CSF glucose and protein levels are normal.

27.3 **C.** This infant potentially has a serious bacterial infection, and an evaluation including an LP is performed. Infants do not reliably demonstrate a Kernig or Brudzinski sign; a lack of nuchal rigidity should not preclude an LP. Computed tomography scan before an LP in an infant with an open anterior fontanelle is rarely necessary, because brain herniation is exceedingly rare. A course of oral antibiotics, or a single dose of ceftriaxone, is not sufficient to treat meningitis or septicemia.

27.4 **B.** The child described in this case has a history of sickle cell disease likely causing functional asplenia. Because of his asplenia, he is at increased risk of infection with encapsulated bacteria. Of the organisms listed, only *S pneumoniae* and *S agalactiae* are encapsulated. *Streptococcus pneumoniae* is more common in older children; whereas, *S agalactiae* is more common in neonates.

CLINICAL PEARLS

▶ The typical meningitis presentation in older children consists of fever, headache, and nuchal rigidity.

▶ Nuchal rigidity is not a reliable finding of meningitis until 12 to 18 months of age.

▶ Pneumococcal disease (including meningitis) is more common in patients with functional or anatomic asplenia.

▶ Approximately one-third of meningitis patients have a seizure at some point in the disease.

▶ Typical cerebrospinal fluid findings of bacterial meningitis include elevated protein level, reduced glucose concentration, and several hundred to thousands of white blood cells per cubic millimeter.

REFERENCES

Bernard TJ, Knupp K, Yang ML, et al. Infections and inflammatory disorders of the central nervous system. In: Hay WW, Levin MJ, Sondheimer JM, Deterding RR, eds. *Current Diagnosis & Treatment Pediatrics.* 20th ed. New York, NY: McGraw-Hill; 2011:754-757.

Lebel MH. Meningitis. In: McMillan JA, Feigin RD, DeAngelis CD, Jones MD, eds. *Oski's Pediatrics: Principles and Practice.* 4th ed. Philadelphia, PA: Lippincott Williams & Wilkins; 2006:493-496.

Lepage P, Dan B. Infantile and childhood bacterial meningitis. In: Dulac O, Lassonde M, Sarnat HB, eds. *Handbook of Clinical Neurology.* Vol 112. 3rd series. Brussels, Belgium: Elsevier; 2013:1115-1125.

Maski KP, Ullrich NJ. Meningitis/meningoencephalitis. In: Rudolph CD, Rudolph AM, Lister GE, First LR, Gershon AA, eds. *Rudolph's Pediatrics.* 22nd ed. New York, NY: McGraw-Hill; 2011:2182-2184.

Prober CG, Dyner L. Acute bacterial meningitis beyond the neonatal period. In: Kliegman RM, Stanton BF, St. Geme JW, Schor NF, Behrman RE, eds. *Nelson Textbook of Pediatrics.* 19th ed. Philadelphia, PA: Elsevier; 2011:2087-2095.

Prober CG, Dyner L. Brain abscess. In: Kliegman RM, Stanton BF, St. Geme JW, Schor NF, Behrman RE, eds. *Nelson Textbook of Pediatrics.* 19th ed. Philadelphia, PA: Elsevier; 2011:2098-2099.

You receive a call from the mother of a previously healthy 2-year-old boy. Yesterday, he developed a temperature of 104°F (40°C), cramping abdominal pain, emesis, and frequent watery stools. The mother assumed he had the same gastroenteritis as his aunt and many other children in his day care center. However, today he developed bloody stools with mucus and seemed more irritable. While you are asking about his current hydration status, the mother reports that he is having a seizure. You tell her to call the ambulance and then notify the local hospital's emergency center of his imminent arrival.

- ▶ What is the most likely diagnosis?
- ▶ How can you confirm this diagnosis?
- ▶ What is the best management for this illness?
- ▶ What is the expected course of this illness?

ANSWERS TO CASE 28:
Bacterial Enteritis

Summary: This child was exposed in his day care center and at home to gastro-intestinal (GI) illnesses. He has fever, abdominal pain, and watery diarrhea that progressed to bloody diarrhea with mucus. He had a new-onset seizure.

- **Most likely diagnosis:** Bacterial enteritis with neurologic manifestations.

- **Diagnostic tools:** Fecal leukocytes, fecal blood, and stool culture.

- **Management:** Varies with age and suspected organism; hydration and electro-lyte correction is a priority. *Salmonella* infections are self-limited and generally are not treated with antibiotics except in patients younger than 3 months or in immunocompromised individuals; *Shigella* infections, although self-limited, are generally treated with antibiotics to shorten the illness and decrease organism excretion. Antimotility agents are not used.

- **Course:** Left untreated, most GI infections in healthy children will sponta-neously resolve. Extraintestinal infections are more likely in immunocompro-mised individuals.

ANALYSIS

Objectives

1. Describe the typical clinical presentation of bacterial enteritis.

2. List potential pathogens for gastroenteritis, considering the patient's age.

3. Discuss treatment options and explain when treatment is necessary.

4. Discuss potential complications of bacterial enteritis.

Considerations

Bloody stools can be caused by many diseases, not all of which are infectious. In this child, GI bleeding also could be caused by Meckel diverticulum, intussuscep-tion, Henoch-Schönlein purpura, hemolytic-uremic syndrome, *Clostridium difficile* colitis, and polyps. The description is most consistent, however, with infectious enteritis typical of *Shigella* or *Salmonella*.

APPROACH TO:
Bacterial Enteritis

DEFINITIONS

COLITIS: Inflammation of the colon.

DIARRHEA: Frequent passage of unusually soft or watery stools. Of particular concern would be ill appearance, the passage of blood or dehydration.

DYSENTERY: An intestinal infection resulting in severe bloody diarrhea with mucus.

ENTERITIS: Inflammation of the small intestine, usually resulting in diarrhea; may be because of infection, immune response, or other causes.

CLINICAL APPROACH

Salmonella, Shigella, and *Campylobacter* species are the top three leading causes of bacterial diarrhea worldwide. **Salmonellae organisms** are motile, nonlactose fermenters, facultative anaerobic gram-negative bacilli. They usually enter the body via the GI tract to infect or colonize a wide range of domestic and wild animals, including insects, reptiles, birds, and mammals. Salmonellae cause a number of characteristic clinical infections in humans, more **common in warmer months.** While there are many types of *Salmonella,* they can be divided into two broad categories: nontyphoidal disease (gastroenteritis, meningitis, osteomyelitis, and bacteremia) and typhoid (or enteric) fever, caused primarily by *Salmonella typhi.* Outbreaks usually occur sporadically but can be food related and occur in clusters. Exposure to **poultry and raw eggs** probably is the most common source of human infection. Infection requires the ingestion of many organisms; person-to-person spread is uncommon.

Gastroenteritis is the most common nontyphoidal disease presentation of *Salmonella.* The cardinal features of nausea, vomiting, fever, watery or bloody diarrhea, and cramping usually occur within 8 to 72 hours of ingesting contaminated food or water. Most patients develop a low-grade fever; some have neurologic symptoms (confusion, headache, drowsiness, and seizures). Between 1% and 5% of patients with documented *Salmonella* gastroenteritis develop bacteremia, with subsequent development of a variety of extraintestinal manifestations such as endocarditis, mycotic aneurysm, and osteomyelitis. These findings are more common in immunocompromised patients and in infants.

Shigellae organisms are small gram-negative bacilli. They are motile, nonlactose fermenting facultative anaerobes. Shigellae organisms can survive transit through the stomach because they are less susceptible to acid than other bacteria; for this reason, as few as 10 to 100 organisms can cause disease. Thus, transmission can easily occur via contaminated food and water and via direct person-to-person spread. Infections most commonly occur in warmer months and in patients in their first 10 years of life (peaking in the second and third years). Four *Shigella* species cause human disease: *Shigella dysenteriae, Shigella boydii, Shigella flexneri,* and *Shigella sonnei.* Typically, *Shigella* is an infection of the lower GI tract presenting with high fever, abdominal cramps, and bloody, mucoid diarrhea (often progressing to small bloody stools), and anorexia. Uncommon intestinal complications include proctitis or rectal prolapse, toxic megacolon, intestinal obstruction, and colonic perforation. Systemic complications include bacteremia, reactive arthritis, and hemolytic uremic syndrome (HUS). **Neurologic findings** may include headache, confusion, seizure, or hallucinations. *Shigella* meningitis is infrequent. Rarely, *Shigella* causes a rapidly progressive sepsis-like presentation (lethal toxic encephalopathy or Ekiri syndrome) that quickly results in death.

Definitive determination of the infecting organism (*Salmonella* or *Shigella*) requires stool culture. However, results frequently are negative even in infected test subjects. **Fecal leukocytes usually are positive,** but this nonspecific finding only suggests colonic inflammation. An occult blood assay often is positive. In *Shigella* **infection,** the peripheral white count usually is normal, but a **remarkable left shift** often is seen with more bands than polymorphonuclear cells. *Salmonella* infection usually results in a mild leukocytosis.

Treatment focuses on fluid and electrolyte balance correction. Antibiotic treatment of *Salmonella* **usually is not necessary;** it does not shorten the GI disease course and **may increase the risk of HUS.** Infants younger than 3 months and immunocompromised individuals often are treated with antibiotics for GI infection, because they are at increased risk for disseminated disease. *Shigella* is self-limited as well; if left untreated, diarrhea typically lasts 1 to 2 weeks. However, antibiotics shorten the illness course and decrease the duration organisms are shed. Antimotility agents are not indicated for either *Salmonella* or *Shigella*.

In addition to the previously listed organisms, enteroinvasive *Escherichia coli*, *Campylobacter* sp, and *Yersinia enterocolitica* can cause dysentery, with fever, abdominal cramps, and bloody diarrhea. *Yersinia* can cause an "acute abdomen" picture. Enterohemorrhagic (or Shiga toxin–producing) *E coli* can cause bloody diarrhea but usually no fever. Infection with *Vibrio cholera* produces vomiting and profuse, watery, nonbloody diarrhea with little or no fever.

Hemolytic-uremic syndrome, the most common cause of acute childhood renal failure, develops in 5% to 8% of children with diarrhea caused by enterohemorrhagic *E coli* (O157:H7); it is seen less commonly after *Shigella*, *Salmonella*, and *Yersinia* infections. It usually is seen in children younger than 4 years. The underlying process may be microthrombi, microvascular endothelial cell injury causing microangiopathic hemolytic anemia and consumptive thrombocytopenia. Renal glomerular deposition of an unidentified material leads to capillary wall thickening and subsequent lumen narrowing. The typical presentation occurs 1 to 2 weeks after a diarrheal illness, with acute onset of pallor, irritability, decreased or absent urine output, and even stroke; children may also develop petechiae and edema. Treatment is supportive; some children require dialysis. Most children recover and regain normal renal function; all are followed after infection for hypertension and chronic renal failure.

> ## CASE CORRELATION
>
> - See also Case 15 (Rectal Bleeding) and Case 18 (Cystic Fibrosis) for additional information about patients with conditions that may present similarly to bacterial enteritis.

COMPREHENSION QUESTIONS

28.1 A 2-year-old boy developed emesis and intermittent abdominal pain yesterday, with several small partially formed stools. His parents were not overly concerned because he seemed fine between the pain episodes. Today, however, he has persistent bilious emesis and has had several bloody stools. Examination reveals a lethargic child in mild distress; he is tachycardic and febrile. He has a diffusely tender abdomen with a vague tubular mass in the right upper quadrant. Which of the following is the most appropriate next step in managing this condition?

    A. Computed tomography (CT) of the abdomen

    B. Air contrast enema

    C. Intravenous antibiotics for *Shigella*

    D. Parental reassurance

    E. Stool cultures

28.2 A previously healthy 2-year-old girl had 3 days of bloody diarrhea the previous week that spontaneously resolved. Her mother now thinks she looks pale. On examination, you see that she is afebrile, her heart rate is 150 beats/min, and her blood pressure is 150/80 mm Hg. She is pale and irritable, has lower-extremity pitting edemas, and has scattered petechiae. After appropriate laboratory studies, initial management should include which of the following?

    A. Careful management of fluid and electrolyte balance

    B. Contrast upper gastrointestinal (GI) series with small bowel delay films

    C. Intravenous antibiotics and platelet transfusion

    D. Intravenous steroids and aggressive fluid resuscitation

    E. Intubation and mechanical ventilation

28.3 A family reunion picnic went awry when the majority of attendees developed emesis and watery diarrhea with streaks of blood. Unaffected attendees did not eat the potato salad. A few ill family members are mildly febrile. They come as a group to your clinic, seeking medications. Which of the following is the most appropriate management for their condition?

    A. Antimotility medication

    B. Hydration and careful follow-up

    C. Intramuscular ceftriaxone

    D. Oral amoxicillin

    E. Oral metronidazole

28.4 You are asked to see a 1-month-old infant to provide a second opinion. During a brief, self-limited, and untreated diarrheal episode the previous week, his primary physician ordered a stool assay for *Clostridium difficile* toxin; the result is positive. The infant now is completely asymptomatic, active, smiling, and well hydrated. His physician said treatment was not necessary, but the mother wants treatment. Which of the following is the most appropriate response?

A. *Clostridium difficile* commonly colonizes the intestine of infants; treatment without symptoms is not warranted.

B. The infant should take a 7-day course of oral metronidazole.

C. The infant should take a 10-day course of oral vancomycin.

D. The infant should be admitted to the hospital for intravenous metronidazole.

E. A repeat study to look for the *C difficile* organism is warranted.

ANSWERS

28.1 **B.** This child has an intussusception. He has bloody stools, but he also has bilious emesis, colicky abdominal pain, and a right upper quadrant mass. In experienced hands, an air contrast enema procedure may be diagnostic and therapeutic. Ensure that a surgeon and a prepared operating room are available should the reduction through contrast enema fail or result in intestinal perforation. While a CT scan may diagnose intussusception, an enema is preferred because it can be therapeutic as well as diagnostic.

28.2 **A.** Hemolytic-uremic syndrome may be seen after bloody diarrhea, presenting with anemia, thrombocytopenia, and nephropathy. The child in question is hypertensive and has edema, so large amounts of fluids may be counterproductive. Steroids typically are not helpful. The thrombocytopenia is consumptive; unless the patient is actively bleeding, platelet transfusion is not helpful. Most of the care for such patients is supportive, concentrating on fluids and electrolytes. Early dialysis may be needed. Hypertensive patients should have appropriate control of their blood pressure.

28.3 **B.** This family probably has *Salmonella* food poisoning. Antibiotics are not indicated for this healthy family, and antimotility agents may prolong the illness. Frequent handwashing should be emphasized.

28.4 **A.** *Clostridium difficile* colonizes approximately half of normal healthy infants in the first 12 months. In this infant without a history of antibiotic treatment or current symptoms, treatment is unnecessary. *Clostridium difficile* colitis rarely occurs without a history of recent antibiotic use.

CLINICAL PEARLS

▶ In normal children older than 3 months, isolated intestinal *Salmonella* infections do not require antibiotic treatment; antibiotics do not shorten the course of illness.

▶ Suspected *Shigella* intestinal infections usually are treated to shorten the illness course and to decrease organism shedding.

▶ Hemolytic-uremic syndrome, a potential sequela of bacterial enteritis, is the most common cause of acute renal failure in children.

REFERENCES

Ashkenazi S. Shigella infections in children: new insights. *Semin Pediatr Infect Dis.* 2004;15(4):246.

Bhutta ZA. Acute gastroenteritis in children. In: Kliegman RM, Stanton BF, St. Geme JW, Schor NF, Behrman RE, eds. *Nelson Textbook of Pediatrics.* 19th ed. Philadelphia, PA: Elsevier; 2011:1323-1338.

Brandt M. Intussusception. In: McMillan JA, Feigin RD, DeAngelis CD, Jones MD, eds. *Oski's Pediatrics: Principles and Practice.* 4th ed. Philadelphia, PA: Lippincott Williams & Wilkins; 2006:1938-1940.

Densmore JC, Lal DR. Intussusception. In: Rudolph CD, Rudolph AM, Lister GE, First LR, Gershon AA, eds. *Rudolph's Pediatrics.* 22nd ed. New York, NY: McGraw-Hill; 2011:1428-1429.

Eddy AA. Hemolytic uremic syndrome. In: Rudolph CD, Rudolph AM, Lister GE, First LR, Gershon AA, eds. *Rudolph's Pediatrics.* 22nd ed. New York, NY: McGraw-Hill; 2011:1727-1729.

Guarino A. European Society for Paediatric Gastroenterology, Hepatology, and Nutrition/European Society for Paediatric Infectious Diseases evidence-based guidelines for the management of acute gastroenteritis in children in Europe. *J Pediatr Gastroenterol Nutr.* 2008;46(suppl 2):S81.

Lum GM. Hemolytic uremic syndrome. In: Hay WW, Levin MJ, Sondheimer JM, Deterding RR, eds. *Current Diagnosis & Treatment Pediatrics.* 20th ed. New York, NY: McGraw-Hill; 2011:684.

Ogle JW, Anderson MS. Salmonella gastroenteritis. In: Hay WW, Levin MJ, Sondheimer JM, Deterding RR, eds. *Current Diagnosis & Treatment Pediatrics.* 20th ed. New York, NY: McGraw-Hill; 2011: 1189-1191.

Ogle JW, Anderson MS. Shigellosis (bacillary dysentery). In: Hay WW, Levin MJ, Sondheimer JM, Deterding RR, eds. *Current Diagnosis & Treatment Pediatrics.* 20th ed. New York, NY: McGraw-Hill; 2011:1193-1194.

Patrick ME. Salmonella enteritidis infections, United States, 1985-1999. *Emerg Infect Dis.* 2004;10(1):1.

Pavia AT. *Salmonella, Shigella,* and *Escherichia coli* infections. In: Rudolph CD, Rudolph AM, Lister GE, First LR, Gershon AA, eds. *Rudolph's Pediatrics.* 22nd ed. New York, NY: McGraw-Hill; 2011: 1082-1089.

Pickering LK. *Salmonella* infections. In: McMillan JA, Feigin RD, DeAngelis CD, Jones MD, eds. *Oski's Pediatrics: Principles and Practice.* 4th ed. Philadelphia, PA: Lippincott Williams & Wilkins; 2006:1112-1116.

Sheth RD. Hemolytic-uremic syndrome. In: McMillan JA, Feigin RD, DeAngelis CD, Jones MD, eds. *Oski's Pediatrics: Principles and Practice.* 4th ed. Philadelphia, PA: Lippincott Williams & Wilkins; 2006:2600-2602.

A 5-month-old infant arrives at the emergency center strapped to a backboard with a cervical collar in place. The father was holding him in his lap in the front passenger seat of their vehicle when the driver lost control and crashed into a tree. The child was ejected from the car through the windshield. The paramedics report that his modified Glasgow coma scale (GCS) score was 6 (opens eyes to painful stimuli, moans to painful stimuli, and demonstrates abnormal extension); they intubated him at the scene. He had a self-limited, 2-minute generalized tonic-clonic seizure en route to the hospital.

Your assessment reveals a child with altered mental status. His endotracheal tube is in the correct position, and his arterial blood gas reflects effective oxygenation and ventilation. He is euthermic and tachycardic. He has no evidence of fractures, and his abdominal examination is benign. He has several facial and scalp lacerations. His anterior fontanelle is bulging, his sutures are slightly separated, and his funduscopic examination reveals bilateral retinal hemorrhages.

▶ What is the most likely etiology for this child's altered mental status?
▶ What is the most appropriate study to confirm this etiology?

ANSWERS TO CASE 29:

Subdural Hematoma

Summary: An unrestrained infant is ejected through the windshield. He has altered mental status, experienced brief self-limited seizure activity, and his examination is consistent with increased intracranial pressure (ICP).

- **Most likely diagnosis:** Subdural hematoma

- **Best study:** Emergent computed tomography (CT) of the head

ANALYSIS

Objectives

1. Describe the typical clinical findings in head trauma.

2. Compare the typical findings of subdural hematoma with those of epidural hematoma.

3. Discuss the possible treatment options for intracranial hemorrhage.

Considerations

This child is younger than 1 year, and subdural hematomas are more common in this age group; epidural hematomas are more common in older children. Seizures are more common with subdural hematomas, occurring in 75% of affected patients; seizures occur in less than 25% of epidural hematoma patients. His altered mental status could be due to a simple cerebral concussion, in which case, the CT scan would be normal or show nonspecific changes. The infant's ejection at the crash provides an appropriate mechanism of injury, making other considerations (such as abusive head trauma, formerly known as shaken baby syndrome) less likely. This child's lack of a car seat must also be addressed.

APPROACH TO:

Subdural Hematoma

DEFINITIONS

CONCUSSION: Altered mental state immediately after blunt head trauma; no consistent brain abnormality is seen; can cause retrograde and anterograde memory loss.

EPIDURAL HEMORRHAGE: Bleeding between the dura and the skull; commonly occurs with skull fracture and middle meningeal artery laceration but can result from disruption of dural sinuses or middle meningeal veins (Figure 29–1).

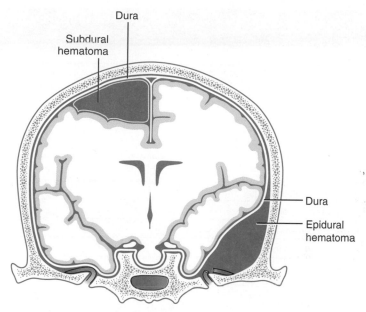

Figure 29–1. Comparison of the anatomic locations of an epidural and subdural hematoma relative to the dura.

GLASGOW COMA SCALE (GCS): A clinical tool developed to assist in head injury severity prediction. For infants and toddlers, several "modified" scales exist that attempt to adapt the verbal portion to reflect language development and modify the motor component to reflect the lack of purposeful movement in early infancy (Table 29–1).

SUBDURAL HEMORRHAGE: Bleeding between the dura and the arachnoid space; occurs with disruption of bridging veins connecting cerebral cortex and dural sinuses (see Figure 29–1).

CLINICAL APPROACH

The child in the case is seriously ill, with evidence of increased ICP and retinal hemorrhages making some form of cerebral hemorrhage likely. Initial management follows the **ABCs** of resuscitation: evaluate the patient's circulatory status by checking pulse and starting cardiopulmonary resuscitation (CPR) if necessary, opening the airway, and giving breaths if needed. Once stable, care can then be directed at his injuries.

Subdural hemorrhage is more common in children younger than 1 year and is far more common than a supratentorial epidural hemorrhage. Approximately one-third of CT-identified subdural hemorrhages have an associated skull fracture; almost all are venous in origin, and approximately three-fourths are bilateral. The CT images typically show a crescentic hematoma. Seizures occur in 60% to 90% of afflicted patients, and retinal hemorrhages are frequently associated. Increased ICP is typical. Subdural hemorrhage is generally associated with less mortality than that seen

Table 29–1 • MODIFIED GLASGOW COMA SCORE FOR CHILDREN YOUNGER THAN 3 YEARS	
Eye opening	
1	None
2	To pain
3	To speech
4	Spontaneous
Verbal communication	
1	No response
2	Incomprehensible sounds
3	Inappropriate words
4	Confused conversation, cries
5	Oriented, cries to indicate needs
Motor response	
1	None
2	Abnormal extension
3	Abnormal flexion
4	Withdraws from pain
5	Localizes pain
6	Spontaneous movement in infants <6 mo and goal-directed movements in children 6-36 mo

with epidural hemorrhage, but long-term morbidity is more significant because the brain parenchyma is more often involved.

Subdural hematomas may be acute, subacute, or chronic. In acute hematomas, symptoms occur in the first 48 hours after injury. Patients with subacute subdural hematoma display symptoms between 3 and 21 days after injury, whereas chronic hematomas cause symptoms after 21 days. **Chronic subdural hematomas are more common in older children** than in infants; symptoms may include chronic emesis, seizures, hypertonicity, irritability, personality changes, inattention, poor weight gain, fever, and anemia. Magnetic resonance imaging is more useful than CT for evaluating subacute and chronic hematomas because the hematoma age can be estimated by signal intensity.

Epidural hemorrhages occur more commonly in older children and adults and are seen more typically in the supratentorial space. **Two-thirds of epidural hemorrhages are associated with skull fracture.** Although most adult epidural hemorrhages are arterial in origin, in children approximately half originate from venous injuries. **Most epidural hemorrhages are unilateral,** are located in the temporoparietal region, and present on CT scan as a lens-like, or biconvex, hematoma. **Fewer than 25% of epidural hematoma patients have seizures,** and retinal hemorrhages are uncommon. **Mortality is greater with epidural hemorrhage than with subdural hemorrhage,** but in survivors, long-term morbidity is low.

Increased ICP, which can be caused by both types of hemorrhages, is important to recognize and treat. In infants with open sutures, symptoms may be nonspecific and include lethargy, vomiting, separated sutures, and a bulging fontanelle. Epidural hematomas are frequently rapidly progressive and may require urgent surgical evacuation with identification of the bleeding source. Subdural hemorrhage usually does not require urgent evacuation but may require evacuation at a later date.

CASE CORRELATION

- See also Case 10 (Failure to Thrive) which also may be seen in a patient who has undergone nonaccidental trauma as a cause of their subdural hematoma. Similarly, Case 21 (Sudden Infant Death Syndrome) requires a thorough investigation of the events surrounding the child's death; unfortunately some cases of apparent sudden infant death syndrome are in reality inflicted trauma with a resultant subdural hematoma.

COMPREHENSION QUESTIONS

29.1 You are the team physician for a local high school football team. During the first quarter of a district playoff game, you watch as your star quarterback is sacked with a helmet-to-helmet tackle. He does not get up from the initial impact. You sprint onto the field with the trainer and assess the injured player. He is breathing and has a steady pulse, but he is unconscious. As you continue your evaluation, he wakes up. He remembers his name but cannot remember the day, his position in the team, or how he got to the game. He has no sensory or motor deficit suggestive of a cervical spine injury, and you assist him off the field. After 15 minutes he is fully oriented and wants to go back in. The coach tells him he is sitting out for the rest of the game. The player appeals to you. Which of the following is the most appropriate management?

   A. Affirm the coach's decision. Tell the player that he will need sequential evaluations before he can come back to practice.

   B. Affirm the coach's decision. Tell the player he can come back and attend regular practice tomorrow.

   C. Refute the coach's decision. Tell the player he can resume playing now.

   D. Refute the coach's decision. Tell the player he can resume playing after half-time.

   E. Strap the player to a backboard and take him to the hospital.

29.2 You see this football player back in clinic 1 week later for medical clearance to return to football practice. He has returned to class and complains of difficulty concentrating, especially in his mathematics class. He reports that he has headaches daily and feels dizzy at times. Despite these symptoms, he is eager to start football practice again so that he can play in next Friday's game. Which of the following is the most appropriate management?

A. Allow the player to return to play without any restrictions.

B. Allow the player to return to practice this week and then return to play the following week.

C. Allow the player to return to practice this week. Follow-up in 1 week to monitor for resolution of symptoms prior to returning to play.

D. Do not allow the player to return to practice this week. Follow-up in 1 week to monitor for resolution of symptoms prior to returning to play.

E. Do not allow the player to return to practice this week. Follow-up in 2 months to monitor for resolution of symptoms prior to returning to play.

29.3 A 17-year-old adolescent girl is brought to the hospital after a motor vehicle crash. She and her boyfriend had been drinking beer and were on their way home when she lost control of the car and hit the side wall of the local police station. She reportedly had a brief loss of consciousness but currently is oriented to name, place, and time. She responds appropriately to your questions. While waiting for her cervical spine series, she vomits and lapses into unconsciousness. She becomes bradycardic and develops irregular respirations. Which of the following brain injuries is most likely in this case?

A. Subdural hemorrhage

B. Epidural hemorrhage

C. Intraventricular hemorrhage

D. Posttraumatic epilepsy

E. Concussion

29.4 Several days after emergent management, the adolescent in Question 29.3 is transferred to your general inpatient ward service from the intensive care unit. She is concerned about her prognosis. Which of the following statements is correct?

A. She will need extensive neuropsychiatric evaluation before she can return to school.

B. She will likely have headaches, fatigue, nausea, and sleep disturbances.

C. She will likely develop seizures and needs 2 years of prophylactic seizure medicine.

D. She can no longer be legally permitted to drive because she has had brain surgery.

E. She should have few long-term problems.

29.5 A 7-month-old child presents to the emergency room after reportedly falling from his high chair. The parents report no loss of consciousness, other trauma, or medical problems. Your examination reveals a few old bruises but no evidence of acute trauma or fracture. He is irritable, so you request a CT scan of the brain without contrast. The pediatric radiologist reports bilateral frontal subdural hematomas and notes two healing skull fractures that she estimates to be approximately 2 weeks old. Which of the following is the best next step in this child's management?

A. Observe him for 6 hours in the emergency center.

B. Assess bleeding time and prothrombin time.

C. Order magnetic resonance imaging of the head.

D. Discharge him from the emergency center with head injury precautions.

E. Order an electroencephalography and a neurology consultation.

ANSWERS

29.1 **A.** Although controversial, the correct answer is for a player who sustains a concussion resulting in loss of consciousness to refrain from play for the remainder of the day. The most recent clinical report from the American Academy of Pediatrics concerning conditions affecting sports participation references the 3rd International Conference on Concussion in Sports from 2008. This report suggests that individualized and frequent reassessment over time, and a stepwise return to play, is more useful than a predetermined length of time to refrain from additional sports. This approach was affirmed in the American Academy of Neurology's concussion guideline update in 2013.

29.2 **D.** There are no standardized guidelines for postconcussive players to return to play. Each player's course should be individualized based on the player's symptoms. A graduated return-to-play schedule should be used that progresses from no activity, to light aerobic exercise, sport-specific exercise, noncontact training drills, full-contact practice, and finally return to play. If the patient develops symptoms with an increase in activity level, activity should be stopped and then returned to the previous level once symptom free. This patient should be followed closely and needs documented medical clearance from a health care provider prior to returning to play.

29.3 **B.** This teen displays the typical adult course of epidural hemorrhage (an initial period of altered mental status [initial concussion], a period of lucidity, and then redevelopment of altered mental status and symptoms of increased ICP [hematoma effect]). Younger children typically do not display this pattern. Immediate neurosurgical evaluation is required.

29.4   **E.** The acute epidural hemorrhage mortality rate is higher than that of acute subdural hemorrhage, but long-term morbidity in survivors is less. The complaints in answer B are common after a subdural hemorrhage. A seizure disorder may preclude driving; a cranial surgery history does not.

29.5   **C.** This child has evidence of old skull fractures with subdural hematomas. Head magnetic resonance imaging would help to determine the hematoma age. If the hematoma blood age correlates with the estimated skull fracture age, child abuse should be considered. Neurology may be helpful later, but an immediate consultation would be of limited benefit before additional data were gathered. Discharge with the information presented in the case is dangerous; the child likely requires hospital admission and the involvement of social services. Bleeding studies are unlikely to be helpful initially but may be required at some point if child abuse is suspected and a court case is anticipated. The child has no history consistent with a bleeding disorder, and a bleeding disorder does not explain the old fractures.

CLINICAL PEARLS

▶ Subdural hemorrhage is more common in children younger than 1 year and in the supratentorial space; seizures and retinal hemorrhages are frequently associated findings, and increased ICP is typical. CT will show crescent-shaped hematoma.

▶ Epidural hemorrhages are more commonly seen in older children and adults. Fewer than 25% of patients have seizures; retinal hemorrhages are uncommon. CT will show lens-shaped hematoma.

▶ Mortality with subdural hemorrhage is generally less than that seen with epidural hemorrhage, but long-term morbidity is more significant with subdural injury because the brain parenchyma is more often involved.

REFERENCES

Berg MD, Schexnayder SM, Chameides L, et al. Part 13: Pediatric basic life support: 2014 American Heart Association Guidelines for Cardiopulmonary Resuscitation and Emergency Cardiovascular Care. *Circulation.* 2010;122:S862-S875.

Halstead ME, Walter KD. The Council on Sports Medicine and Fitness. Sports-related concussion in children and adolescents. *Pediatrics.* 2010;126:597-611.

Harmon KG, Drezner JA, Gammons M, et al. American medical society for sports medicin position statement: concussion in sport. *Br J Sports Med.* 2013;47:15-26.

Giza CC, Kutcher JS, Ashwam S, et al. Summary of evidence-based guideline update: Evaluation and management of concussion in sports. *Neurology.* 2013;80:2250-2257.

Kochanek PM, Bell MJ. Neurologic emergencies and stabilization. In: Kliegman RM, Stanton BF, St. Geme JW, Schor NF, Behrman RE, eds. *Nelson Textbook of Pediatrics.* 19th ed. Philadelphia, PA: Elsevier; 2011:296-301.

McCrory P, Meeuwisse W, Johnston K, et al. Consensus statement on concussion in sport—The 3rd International Conference on Concussion in Sport, held in Zurich, November 2008. *J Clin Neurosci.* 2009;16:755-763.

Prasad MR, Ewing-Cobbs L, Swank PR, Kramer L. Predictors of outcome following traumatic brain injury in young children. *Pediatr Neurosurg.* 2002;36:64-74.

Rosman NP. Acute head trauma. In: McMillan JA, Feigin RD, DeAngelis CD, Jones MD, eds. *Oski's Pediatrics: Principles and Practice.* 4th ed. Philadelphia, PA: Lippincott Williams & Wilkins; 2006:730-746.

Sobeih MM. Trauma to the nervous system. In: Rudolph CD, Rudolph AM, Lister GE, First LR, Gershon AA, eds. *Rudolph's Pediatrics.* 22nd ed. New York, NY: McGraw-Hill; 2011:2158-2164.

Teasdale G, Jennett B. Assessment of coma and impaired consciousness: a practical scale. *Lancet.* 1974;2:81-84.

The emergency department (ED) notifies you that one of your patients is being evaluated for new-onset seizures. The 2-year-old boy was in his normal state of good health until this morning, when he complained of a headache and then fell to the floor. While waiting for the ED physician to come to the phone, you review the patient's chart and find that he has had normal development. His family history is significant for a single seizure of unknown etiology in his father at 4 years of age. According to the ED physician, the boy's mother saw jerking of the left arm and leg along with left eye deviation. This lasted 10 minutes before 911 was called. When the ambulance arrived 5 minutes later, the child continued to have left-sided twitching which only subsided 5 minutes after administration of lorazepam. At this point the child had stopped jerking but was not arousable; his heart rate was 108 beats/min, respiratory rate 16 breaths/min, blood pressure 90/60 mm Hg, and temperature 104°F (40°C). His blood sugar level was 135 mg/dL. By the time the child arrived to the ED, he was awake and he recognized his parents. His physical examination in the ED is significant only for a red bulging immobile tympanic membrane. His complete blood count and urinalysis are normal.

▶ What is the most likely diagnosis?
▶ What is the best management for this condition?
▶ What is the expected course of this condition?

ANSWERS TO CASE 30:

Complex Febrile Seizure

Summary: An otherwise normal 2-year-old boy, with a family history of a single seizure in his father at 4 years of age, has a prolonged, focal seizure associated with an elevated temperature. His examination is now nonfocal. He has completely recovered within 1 to 2 hours of the seizure.

- **Most likely diagnosis:** Complex febrile seizure.

- **Best management:** Parental education, injury prevention during seizures, and fever control.

- **Expected course:** More seizures with fever may occur, but he is likely to "grow out" the condition by 5 to 6 years of age. He is likely to have no sequelae and is expected to have normal development.

ANALYSIS

Objectives

1. Describe a typical febrile seizure.

2. Explain the typical course of febrile seizures.

3. List factors that increase the risk of further seizure activity.

Considerations

This patient likely had a complex febrile seizure. The seizure was prolonged, had focal findings, and was finally interrupted with the administration of a benzodiazepine. The child had an elevated temperature and is between the ages of 6 months and 6 years. He had a short postictal state and then quickly returned to normal. He is old enough to have reliable neck examination findings and has no evidence of meningeal irritation. The father might have had a febrile seizure; data are insufficient to make that conclusion.

APPROACH TO:

Febrile Seizure

DEFINITIONS

EPILEPSY: Recurrent seizure activity; may or may not have identifiable cause.

FEBRILE SEIZURE: A seizure occurring in the absence of central nervous system (CNS) infection with an elevated temperature in a child between the ages of 6 months and 6 years. They can be divided into the following:

SIMPLE FEBRILE SEIZURE: A generalized seizure lasting no more than 15 minutes, with a very short postictal state and no recurrence in 24 hours. The most common type of febrile seizure, making up about 80% of all reported.

COMPLEX FEBRILE SEIZURE: A febrile seizure that is either focal, prolonged, or recurrent. These are less common, making up about 20% of all febrile seizures.

SEIZURE: Abnormal electrical activity of the brain resulting in altered mental status and/or involuntary neuromuscular activity.

CLINICAL APPROACH

A diagnosis of febrile seizure must be made only after considering CNS infection as the cause. **Two classic physical findings** suggest **meningeal** irritation: **Kernig sign** (patient is supine, leg flexed at the hip and knee at 90° angle, pain is induced with leg extension) and **Brudzinski sign** (while supine, passive neck flexion results in involuntary knee and hip flexion). If the **neurologic examination is abnormal** after the seizure, the **seizure occurred several days into the illness,** or if the **child is unable to provide adequate feedback** during a neck examination, a **lumbar puncture (LP) may be necessary.** The meningeal signs described previously usually are **not reliable in children younger than 1 year;** therefore, an **LP is recommended for such patients with fever and seizure** particularly those infants with deficient or unknown immunizations. **Contrast-enhanced brain imaging should occur before LP when a space-occupying lesion, such as a brain abscess, is a possibility.**

Febrile seizures are a uniquely pediatric entity. **Typically occurring between 6 months and 6 years of age,** these convulsions are distressing to the parent but only occasionally pose a threat to the child. Febrile seizures are common, occurring in 2% to 4% of all children; they seem to have a **genetic basis** (many children have a family history of febrile seizure). Febrile seizure risk is increased (10%-20%) when a **first-degree relative** has been diagnosed with the same. Studies suggest that a mutation in the sodium channel SCN1A is a risk factor for febrile seizures.

Febrile seizures frequently are classified as simple or complex; the distinction helps to clarify the recurrence risk and prognosis. **Simple febrile seizures last less than 15 minutes without focal or lateralizing signs or sequelae.** If more than one seizure occurs in a brief period, the total episode lasts less than 30 minutes. A complex febrile seizure lasts for more than 15 minutes and may have lateralizing signs. If several seizures occur in a brief period, the entire episode may last for more than 30 minutes. Children with complex febrile seizures tend to be younger and are more likely to have a history of abnormal development.

The timing of the febrile seizure in relation to the temperature elevation is variable. Whereas many children will have a febrile seizure during the initial temperature upswing (many parents are unaware that the child is ill until the seizure and the subsequent temperature recording), some children will have seizures at other points during the febrile illness.

A febrile seizure usually is self-limited. Seizures lasting longer than 5 minutes may be interrupted with lorazepam or diazepam. Airway management is a priority, because benzodiazepines occasionally cause respiratory depression.

Ongoing seizures unresponsive to lorazepam or diazepam can be interrupted with **fosphenytoin.**

The evaluation of a simple febrile seizure need not be extensive (Figure 30–1). Electroencephalography (EEG) is not recommended unless focal findings were present during or after the seizure, or if the seizure was prolonged. EEG is not predictive of future febrile or afebrile seizures. Laboratory studies (except as needed to determine the cause of fever) and brain imaging usually are not helpful. Imaging may be indicated for a complex febrile seizure or in patients with evidence of increased intracranial pressure. An LP is not routinely indicated, except as outlined earlier.

Prophylactic medications usually are not necessary. In the practice parameter published in 2008, the American Academy of Pediatrics emphasized that prophylactic medications for the usually benign condition of febrile seizures were not routinely useful.

Prognosis is generally good; most children who develop febrile seizures will not develop neurologic or developmental consequences. **Children younger than 12 months at the time of their first seizure have a 50% to 65% chance of having another febrile seizure; older children have a 20% to 30% chance of recurrence.** The chance of developing epilepsy increases from 0.5% in the general population to 1% in the child with a febrile seizure history. Children at highest risk for developing epilepsy following a febrile seizure often have preexisting neurologic problems and have complex febrile seizures; these children have 30 to 50 times the baseline risk of developing epilepsy.

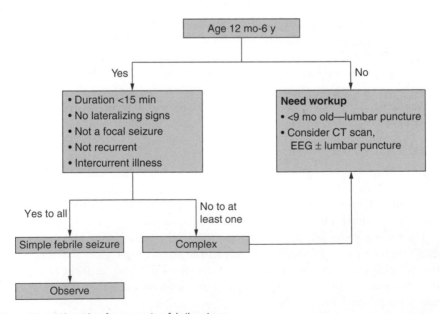

Figure 30–1. Algorithm for managing febrile seizure.

CASE CORRELATION

- Myriad other conditions may result in pediatric seizures. Bacterial Enteritis (Case 28) that is caused by *Shigella sp.* is well known to present as a seizure. Bacterial meningitis (Case 27) can have seizure and fever as a presenting sign and may be a complication of otitis media (Case 16); all children with febrile seizures (especially if the **presentation is atypical as** in the case presented) must have meningitis included on the differential until proven otherwise. Subdural hematoma (Case 29) and other head trauma may result in seizures. The child with sickle cell disease (Case 13) is prone to stroke, which may present with altered mental status and seizure activity. Many patients with cerebral palsy (Case 17) have a lower seizure threshold that may be triggered by fever.

COMPREHENSION QUESTIONS

30.1 Paramedics bring a 7-month-old infant to the ED with seizure activity. The father reports the infant was in a normal state of health until approximately 3 days ago when she developed a febrile illness, diagnosed by her physician as a viral upper respiratory tract infection. Approximately 30 minutes ago she began having left arm jerking, which progressed to whole-body jerking. The episode spontaneously ceased on the way to the hospital. Vital signs include heart rate 90 beats/min, respiratory rate 25 breaths/min, and temperature 100.4°F (38°C). Your examination reveals a sleeping infant in no respiratory distress. The child's anterior fontanelle is full. The oropharynx is clear, and crusted mucus is found in the nares. The tympanic membranes are dark and without normal landmarks. The lungs are clear, and the heart and abdominal examinations are normal. She has a bruise over the occiput and several parallel bruises along the spine. Which of the following is the best next step in management?

A. Computed tomography (CT) of the head

B. Electroencephalogram (EEG)

C. Lumbar puncture

D. Observation

E. Phenobarbital

30.2 A 2-year-old boy who had a simple brief febrile seizure comes to your clinic a day after his ED visit. He is currently afebrile, is happily pulling the sphygmomanometer off the wall, and is taking antibiotics for an ear infection diagnosed the previous day. His mother wants to know what to expect in the future regarding his neurologic status. You correctly tell her which of the following?

A. He has no risk of further seizures because he was age 2 years at the time of his first febrile seizure.

B. He will need to take anticonvulsant medications for 6 to 12 months to prevent further seizure activity.

C. You want to schedule an EEG and a magnetic resonance scan of his head.

D. Although he does have a risk of future febrile convulsions, seizures of his type are generally benign and he is likely to outgrow them.

E. This is an isolated disorder, and his children will not have seizures.

30.3 A 10-month-old boy presents to the ED with a 1-day history of fever to 104°F (40°C), increased irritability, decreased breast-feeding, and refusal of solid foods. The parents brought him in after two 30-second episodes of generalized jerking that occurred over a 20-minute span. Your examination reveals an awake but lethargic infant. The anterior fontanelle is flat, the tympanic membranes and oropharynx are moist and not erythematous, the lungs are clear, and the heart and abdominal examinations are normal. He has no focal neurologic findings. Which of the following is the best next step in management?

A. Intravenous ceftriaxone

B. Admission overnight for observation

C. Computed tomography of the head

D. Discharge from ED to follow up with his primary care provider in 24 hours

E. Lumbar puncture

30.4 The father of a 4-year-old girl calls your clinic to report her second febrile seizure. He states that this seizure was identical to the first one that happened 4 months ago: she developed an elevated temperature and within a short time had a generalized convulsion lasting 90 seconds. She was sleepy for approximately 2 minutes afterward. Upon awaking, she was given ibuprofen. She is now running around the house, chasing the family's chihuahua. The parents wonder if she needs to take anticonvulsants now that she has had another seizure. You should tell the father which of the following?

A. Febrile seizures frequently are recurrent but usually have no significant long-term effect.

B. You will prescribe an anticonvulsant because it will reduce the risk of future epilepsy.

C. You will order an EEG and CT scan of her head to be done on an outpatient basis.

D. He needs to take his daughter to the hospital for inpatient admission.

E. He should stop the ibuprofen and observe the fever curve.

ANSWERS

30.1 **A.** This child's history is worrisome for trauma. The fontanelle is full, bruises are found along the spine and on the occiput, and she has hemotympanum. A CT scan is of paramount importance; this child likely had a seizure from acute intracranial hemorrhage associated with physical abuse. Although this child is febrile and within the proper febrile seizure age range, the history and physical findings are more consistent with a diagnosis other than febrile seizure. Performing a lumbar puncture (LP) in a patient who may have increased intracranial pressure is not advisable, an EEG would probably not reveal the diagnosis, and phenobarbital is not immediately necessary in a patient who is not actively seizing.

30.2 **D.** Part of the anticipatory guidance for parents of children with febrile seizures is to impress upon them that the child may have another febrile seizure; it is similarly important to emphasize the usual benign nature of this condition. In a simple febrile seizure, imaging and EEG generally are not recommended, nor are prophylactic anticonvulsants. Because febrile seizures seem to have a genetic basis, it is possible that your patient's children will also have febrile seizures.

30.3 **E.** Although this child ultimately may be diagnosed as having had a simple febrile seizure, the patient's age (<1 year) precludes a reliable neck examination. An LP is required to evaluate the child for meningitis. Administering antibiotics before the LP (or other cultures are obtained) is inadvisable unless the patient's condition is such that he would not tolerate the procedure.

30.4 **A.** Some children will develop recurrent febrile seizures. Anticonvulsants will decrease the risk of further febrile seizures, but they do not decrease the risk of developing epilepsy. The possible adverse reactions with antiepileptic medications are numerous, including severe allergic reactions and interference with school performance; often the benefit is not worth the risk. Fever reduction with medications is generally encouraged in children with a febrile seizure history. Hospital admission and diagnostic studies are not necessary in simple febrile seizures.

CLINICAL PEARLS

▶ Febrile seizures usually are benign and self-limited. They do not require an extensive diagnostic evaluation unless they are prolonged or focal.

▶ A diagnosis of febrile seizure must be made only after considering the possibility of central nervous system infection as the seizure cause.

▶ Febrile seizures rarely lead to epilepsy; risk factors for nonfebrile seizures include preexisting developmental abnormalities and complex febrile seizures.

REFERENCES

American Academy of Pediatrics; Subcommittee on Febrile Seizures. Neurodiagnostic evaluation of the child with a Simple Febrile Seizure. *Pediatrics.* 2011;127: 389-394.

Bernard TJ, Knupp K, Yang ML, et al. Febrile seizures. In: Hay WW, Levin MJ, Sondheimer JM, Deterding RR, eds. *Current Diagnosis & Treatment Pediatrics.* 20th ed. New York, NY: McGraw-Hill; 2011:720-722.

Mikati MA. Febrile seizures. In: Kliegman RM, Stanton BF, St. Geme JW, Schor NF, Behrman RE, eds. *Nelson Textbook of Pediatrics.* 19th ed. Philadelphia, PA: Elsevier; 2011:2017-2018.

Murray TS, Baltimore RS. Bacterial meningitis. In: Rudolph CD, Rudolph AM, Lister GE, First LR, Gershon AA, eds. *Rudolph's Pediatrics.* 22nd ed. New York, NY: McGraw-Hill; 2011:913-916.

Prober CG, Dyner L. Acute bacterial meningitis beyond the neonatal period. In: Kliegman RM, Stanton BF, St. Geme JW, Schor NF, Behrman RE, eds. *Nelson Textbook of Pediatrics.* 19th ed. Philadelphia, PA: Elsevier; 2011:2087-2095.

Takeoka M. Febrile seizures. In: Rudolph CD, Rudolph AM, Lister GE, First LR, Gershon AA, eds. *Rudolph's Pediatrics.* 22nd ed. New York, NY: McGraw-Hill; 2011:2204-2206.

Parents worry about their 4-year-old son's ability to walk. He began walking at 18 months, but he was clumsy and fell frequently; they were reassured by another pediatrician that he would "outgrow it." He remains clumsier than his peers, falls during simple tasks, and has developed a "waddling" gait. Within the last month he has experienced increasing difficulty arising from a sitting position on the floor, often supporting himself with his hands along the length of his legs. Birth and developmental history was normal until symptoms onset.

▶ What is the most likely diagnosis?
▶ What is the diagnostic test of choice?
▶ What is the mechanism of disease?

ANSWERS TO CASE 31:

Muscular Dystrophy

Summary: A 4-year-old boy has delayed walking, a regression of motor milestones, a waddling gait, clumsiness, and proximal muscle weakness.

- **Most likely diagnosis:** Muscular dystrophy (MD), probably Duchenne type.

- **Diagnostic test:** DNA peripheral blood analysis and/or immunohistochemical detection of abnormal dystrophin on a muscle biopsy tissue section.

- **Mechanism of disease:** Duchenne MD is an **X-linked recessive** trait. An **out of frame mutation** at the Xp21.2 locus encodes for an aberrant form of the protein **dystrophin,** which normally functions to stabilize the muscle membrane proteins.

ANALYSIS

Objectives

1. Know the presentation of children with inherited MD.

2. Understand the inheritance pattern of the common MDs.

3. Understand the progression of MD.

Considerations

This 4-year-old boy exhibits classic signs of Duchenne muscular dystrophy (DMD): **waddling gait** and **progressive proximal muscle weakness.** In addition to the proximal weakness, physical examination may also reveal enlarged calves and toe walking on ambulation. Initial testing includes serum creatine kinase (CK) assessment (elevated from muscle destruction) and DNA analysis of peripheral blood for diagnosis. After the diagnosis of DMD, the family is introduced to support organizations and is offered genetic counseling. Ongoing cardiac evaluation for the development of cardiomyopathy is routine. Medical therapy is supportive.

APPROACH TO:

Muscular Dystrophy

DEFINITIONS

MUSCULAR DYSTROPHY: Inherited disease characterized by progressive weakness and degeneration of the skeletal muscles that control movement.

GOWER SIGN: A description of patients with proximal muscle weakness arising to a standing position. The legs are brought under the torso and weight is shifted to the hands and feet. The hands are walked toward the feet and up the thighs as the patient attempts to rise.

TRENDELENBURG GAIT: A pelvic waddling gait from proximal muscle weakness.

PSEUDOHYPERTROPHY: Enlargement of muscles (ie, calves) secondary to replacement of muscle tissue with fat and connective tissue.

CLINICAL APPROACH

DMD is the most common hereditary neuromuscular degenerative disease, with an incidence **of 1 in 3300 male births;** 30% of cases are new mutations. It is the most severe progressive primary myopathy of childhood.

DMD usually is asymptomatic during infancy, with normal or mildly delayed developmental milestones, but by 3 to 5 years of age patients have increasing lumbar lordosis (gluteal weakness), **frequent falling, difficulty climbing stairs, hip waddle, and proximal muscle weakness (Gower sign). Muscular enlargement, caused by hypertrophy of muscle fibers and infiltration of fat and collagen proliferation,** causes calf, gluteal, and deltoid muscle **pseudohypertrophy** and a "woody" feel of the affected area. Contractures of hip flexors, heel chords, and iliotibial bands develop, limiting joint range of motion. **Cardiomyopathy** with electrocardiography (ECG) findings on the precordial leads of tall R waves on the right and deep Q waves on the left can be seen. Nonprogressive intellectual impairment is common (mean IQ 80); brain atrophy can be seen on brain CT.

Patients generally become wheelchair dependent by 10 and 13 years of age and have rapid progression of scoliosis after the loss of ambulation. Distal muscles remain functional, permitting adequate manual dexterity. Respiratory muscle involvement and the scoliosis result in diminished pulmonary function and recurrent pulmonary infections. Oropharyngeal dysfunction can lead to aspiration, further compromising respiratory capacity.

DNA blood analysis is diagnostic in two-thirds of cases. Muscle biopsy tissue testing for abnormal dystrophin can be performed when blood samples are not diagnostic. Muscle biopsy findings include endomysial connective tissue proliferation, inflammatory cell infiltrates, areas of regeneration interspersed with areas of degeneration, and areas of necrosis. Other laboratory findings include elevated CK levels at least 10 times normal; **in 80% of cases, female carriers have elevated CK levels.** Electromyography (EMG) findings reveal myopathy. Of note, **Becker MD** is an **X-linked recessive** disease caused by a genetic **in-frame mutation** at the Xp21.2 locus, which results in a similar, but less severe disease with later onset than DMD.

Treatment consists of medical therapies to slow disease progression. Orthopedic intervention, including bracing and tendon lengthening, can prolong the duration of ambulation and slow the progression of scoliosis. Caution must be exercised with surgical interventions, because these patients are prone to hyperthermia with anesthesia. Physiotherapy may delay the onset of contractures but is not intended for muscle strengthening because significant exercise can hasten muscle degeneration. The American Academy of Neurology and the Child Neurology Society recommend offering affected boys age 5 and older treatment with prednisone (optimal dosing 0.75 mg/kg/d). It is important that the potential benefits and risks of steroid therapy are discussed with the patient and family. **All DMD patients have some degree of cardiomyopathy;** it does not correlate with the degree of skeletal involvement. Thus, routine cardiac evaluation is required. Early cardiac dysfunction may be responsive to digoxin.

Respiratory failure is often the cause of death. Pulmonary infections are treated early and aggressively; exposure to respiratory illnesses should be limited when possible. Routine immunizations and pneumococcal vaccine are supplemented with yearly influenza vaccine.

The nutritional status of patients is monitored to ensure appropriate caloric intake. Caloric needs are lower for wheelchair-bound patients because of their decreased activity, with careful assessment for adequate intake of calcium and vitamin D; supplementation may be required to minimize osteoporosis. Patients are at risk for depression, often resulting in overeating, weight gain, and added burden to their already limited muscle function.

Another common form of MD is **myotonic muscular dystrophy,** the second most common type of MD in the United States. It is inherited as an **autosomal dominant** trait. Infants born with this condition may have an inverted V-shaped upper lip, thin cheeks, and wasting of the temporalis muscles. The head is abnormally narrow, and the palate is high and arched. In the ensuing years weakness of the distal muscles leads to progressive challenges in walking. A variety of other findings arise including speech difficulties, gastrointestinal tract problems, endocrinopathies, immunologic deficiencies, cataracts, intellectual impairment, and cardiac involvement.

COMPREHENSION QUESTIONS

31.1 The parents of a 3-year-old child are worried about the child's apparent clumsiness with frequent falls and a waddling gait. The child had normal development of motor skills during the first year of life and has normal language development. Which of the following is consistent with Duchenne muscular dystrophy?

A. Female gender

B. Hypertrophy of the quadriceps

C. 22-year-old sister with Becker muscular dystrophy

D. Gower sign

E. Positive antinuclear antibodies in the blood

31.2 Which of the following is the best screening test for the child discussed in Question 31.1?

A. Muscle biopsy

B. Measurement of serum creatinine

C. Electromyogram

D. Blood analysis for antinuclear antibodies

E. Measurement of serum creatine kinase level

31.3 A 12-year-old healthy boy has noticed some muscle weakness. He has experienced increasing difficulty lifting his backpack and walking long distances. He has no trouble with schoolwork, and he continues to play the piano and video games without tiring. His 38-year-old maternal uncle recently became wheelchair bound for unclear reasons. Which of the following is the most likely diagnosis?

A. Cerebral palsy

B. Duchenne muscular dystrophy

C. Myasthenia gravis

D. Becker muscular dystrophy

E. Guillain-Barré syndrome

31.4 A 32-year-old G2 P1 pregnant woman who is at 14 weeks of gestation and is a known carrier of Duchenne muscular dystrophy (DMD) asks a genetic counselor about the possibilities that her unborn child will inherit DMD. The father is healthy. Of the following statements, the genetic counselor would be most accurate in saying:

A. If she had a daughter, she has a 100% chance of having DMD.

B. If she had a daughter, she has a 100% chance of being a carrier of DMD.

C. If she had a son, he has a 50% chance of having DMD.

D. If she had a son, he has a 50% chance of being a carrier of DMD.

E. If she had a son, he has no chance of having DMD.

ANSWERS

31.1 **D.** Duchenne muscular dystrophy is an X-linked recessive disease and is clinically evident only in males. Affected boys may have calf hypertrophy that occurs as a compensation for **proximal muscle weakness.** They will generally develop a Gower sign.

31.2 **E.** A definitive diagnosis can be made by using muscle biopsy tissue, but serum creatine kinase measurement is preferred because it is less invasive and results can be obtained rapidly. Electromyography will reveal nonspecific myopathy.

31.3 **D.** This patient does not have muscle weakness that precludes extended use of distal muscles (hands) or limits his manual dexterity. The child's presentation at age 12 years and a 38-year-old wheelchair-bound maternal uncle suggest a diagnosis of Becker muscular dystrophy.

31.4 **C.** Males have one copy of the X chromosome, while females have two copies of the X chromosome. If mother is a carrier, then she has one copy with a mutation and one functional copy. Therefore, she has a 50% chance of passing the copy with a mutation to her daughters or sons. Daughters who receive the copy with a mutation can only be carriers, whereas sons who receive the copy with a mutation can only have DMD. Therefore, daughters have a 50% chance of being carriers and sons have a 50% chance of having DMD.

CLINICAL PEARLS

▶ Duchenne muscular dystrophy (DMD) is an X-linked recessive disorder.

▶ A Gower sign reflects proximal muscle weakness and is a classic feature of DMD.

▶ Creatine kinase level is elevated in patients with DMD and in many female carriers of the gene.

REFERENCES

Darras BT. Myopathies. In: Rudolph CD, Rudolph AM, Lister GE, First LR, Gershon AA, eds. *Rudolph's Pediatrics*. 22nd ed. New York, NY: McGraw-Hill; 2011:2241-2244.

DeVivo DC, DiMauro S. Hereditary and acquired types of myopathy. In: McMillan JA, Feigin RD, DeAngelis CD, Jones MD, eds. *Oski's Pediatrics: Principles and Practice*. 4th ed. Philadelphia, PA: Lippincott Williams & Wilkins; 2006:2322-2324.

Fenichel GM. Muscular Dystrophies. In: Fenichel GM, ed. *Clinical Pediatric: Neurology A Signs and Symptoms Approach*. 6th ed. Philadelphia, PA: WB Saunders; 2009:183-184.

Sarnat HB. Muscular dystrophies. In: Kliegman RM, Stanton BF, St. Geme JW, Schor NF, Behrman RE, eds. *Nelson Textbook of Pediatrics*. 19th ed. Philadelphia, PA: WB Saunders; 2011:2119-2129.

A mother brings her 11-month-old daughter to the clinic because of a persistent facial rash. The child is restless at night and scratches in her sleep. She is otherwise healthy. Physical examination reveals a well-nourished, healthy-appearing white woman with dry, red, scaly areas on the cheeks, chin, and around the mouth as well as on the extensor surfaces of her extremities. The areas on the cheeks have a plaque-like, weepy appearance. The diaper area is spared. The remainder of the child's examination is normal.

▶ What is the most likely diagnosis?
▶ What is the most appropriate next step in the evaluation?
▶ What is the best management for this condition?

ANSWERS TO CASE 32:

Atopic Dermatitis

Summary: An 11-month-old female infant has dry, red, scaly areas on the extensor surfaces of her skin and on the cheeks, chin, and around the mouth, with sparing of the diaper area.

- **Most likely diagnosis:** Atopic dermatitis.

- **Next step in evaluation:** Further history to determine rash duration and exacerbating factors, and family history for atopic dermatitis, allergic rhinitis, and asthma.

- **Best management:** Use emollients frequently, control pruritus, and consider a topical corticosteroid.

ANALYSIS

Objectives

1. Describe incidence, etiology, and risk factors for atopic dermatitis.

2. Discuss diagnostic criteria and differential diagnoses for atopic dermatitis.

3. Describe treatment and follow-up of atopic dermatitis.

4. Be familiar with other conditions associated with atopic dermatitis.

Considerations

A new rash in an infant can reflect a viral infection, because many viruses have skin manifestations. However, the lack of associated symptomatology such as fever makes infection unlikely. This child's history and examination, however, are consistent with atopic dermatitis. Further history may reveal additional risk factors for allergic disease. Treatment involves avoiding aggravating factors and ensuring intensive skin hydration.

APPROACH TO:

Atopic Dermatitis

DEFINITIONS

ATOPIC DERMATITIS (AD): A patch or plaque of erythematous skin with intense pruritus; the most common eczematous eruption in childhood.

CONTACT DERMATITIS: An adverse reaction of the skin to an outside agent, includes primary irritant dermatitis (irritant diaper rash) and allergic contact dermatitis (poison ivy, nickel allergy).

ECZEMA: General term for a skin condition consisting of acutely inflamed papules and plaques, frequently associated with serous discharge and pruritus; eczematous eruptions include atopic, seborrheic, and contact dermatitides.

EMOLLIENT: Cream or lotion that restores water and lipids to the epidermis; those containing urea or lactic acid are more lubricating and may be more effective; creams lubricate better than lotions.

FLEXURAL AREAS: Areas of repeated flexion and extension, which often perspire on exertion (antecubital fossae, neck, wrists, ankles).

LICHENIFICATION: Epidermal thickening, with normal skin lines resembling a washboard.

SEBORRHEIC DERMATITIS: Self-limited scaly, erythematous, and/or crusty eruption limited to areas of the skin with a high concentration of sebaceous glands (cradle cap).

CLINICAL APPROACH

Atopic dermatitis (eczema) typically is pruritic, recurrent, and flexural in older children and symmetrical in adults. The term *atopy* was coined to describe a group of patients who had a personal or family history of "hay fever," asthma, dry skin, and eczema. More than 15 million American adults and children have atopic dermatitis. The highest incidence is seen among children, and the lifetime prevalence of AD is 20% in children aged 3 to 11 years. Sixty-five percent of patients develop symptoms in the first year of life and 90% before the age of 5 years. The etiology is unknown, but is thought to be related to immune factors. Seventy percent of atopic patients have a family history of asthma, "hay fever," or eczema.

The cause of AD is thought to be multifactorial, involving genetic abnormalities of the epidermal barrier, immune function, environmental exposures, and infection. Recent studies have linked an abnormal epidermal barrier to mutations in the filaggrin (FLG) gene. Abnormal epidermal barrier function results in increased transepidermal fluid losses, leading to the ubiquitous finding of dry skin in AD patients. The abnormal epidermis also allows easier entrance of allergens and bacteria, stimulating an immune reaction.

Atopic dermatitis occurs in three phases: infant (**birth to 2 years**), childhood (**2-12 years**), and adult (**>12 years**). Infants are rarely born with atopic dermatitis, but typically develop the first signs of inflammation during the third month of life. A common scenario is a baby who, during winter months, develops dry, red, scaling cheeks without perioral and paranasal involvement. The chin is often involved; the diaper area is usually spared. The infant is uncomfortable because of intense pruritus and is often restless during sleep. Atopic dermatitis resolves in approximately 50% of infants by the age of 18 months.

The most common finding in the childhood phase is inflammation in flexural areas. Perspiration stimulates burning and itching, initiating an itch-scratch cycle. Initial papules rapidly coalesce into plaques that ultimately become lichenified when scratched. The exudative lesions typical of the infant phase are not common in the childhood phase.

The adult phase begins near the onset of puberty. The reason for the resurgence of inflammation may be related to hormonal changes. Adult phase disease includes flexural inflammation, often accompanied by hand dermatitis, inflammation around the eyes, and lichenification of the anogenital area. White dermographism may be seen, demonstrated by stroking the skin of a patient with AD; after the initial red line develops, a white line replaces it without wheal. Other findings include keratosis pilaris, accentuated palmar creases, small fissures at the base of the earlobe, and Dennie-Morgan creases under the lower eyelid.

Two misconceptions about AD are common. The first is that eczema is an emotional disorder. Patients with skin inflammation lasting for months or years are often irritable, a normal response to a frustrating disorder. The second misconception is that atopic skin disease is precipitated by an allergic reaction. Atopic individuals frequently have respiratory allergies and, when skin tested, are informed that they are "allergic to everything." Individuals with atopy may react with a wheal when challenged with a needle during skin testing, but this is a characteristic of atopic skin and is not necessarily an allergic response. Evidence to date indicates that most cases of AD are precipitated by environmental stress on genetically compromised skin and not by interaction with allergens.

Patient Evaluation

Evaluation of the child with AD involves ruling out other potential causes of the child's rash through a complete personal history (Table 32–1), family history, and physical examination to obtain a proper diagnosis and initiate treatment. Skin is evaluated for locations and nature of affected areas (patches, weepiness, lichenification), extent of skin dryness, and warmth or tenderness (possible secondary infection). Eyes, nose, throat, and chest are examined for evidence of allergic rhinitis or asthma (watery eyes, dark circles under eyes [atopic periorbital hyperpigmentation], runny nose, wheezing).

Laboratory studies are not particularly helpful in diagnosing atopic dermatitis. **A serum immunoglobulin E (IgE) level is often elevated, and there may be eosinophilia on a complete blood count (CBC).** Culture of the skin is performed if bacterial superinfection is suspected.

The differential diagnosis includes seborrheic dermatitis (cradle cap), which usually begins on the scalp in the first few months of life and may involve the ears, nose, eyebrows, and eyelids. The greasy brown scales of seborrheic dermatitis are in contrast to the erythematous, weeping, crusted lesions of infantile atopic dermatitis. Other considerations include scabies, irritant dermatitis (perioral fruit juice dermatitis), allergic

Table 32–1 • QUESTIONS TO ASK WHEN INVESTIGATING RASHES
How long have the symptoms been present? Were there previous episodes of similar outbreaks?
How itchy are the affected areas? Is the child irritable or awakening at night because of itching and scratching?
Do symptoms appear to get worse with exposure to cold weather, wool, perspiration, or stress?
Do other family members have eczema, asthma, or allergic diseases?
Has the child had fever or other signs of infection?

contact dermatitis (poison ivy), and eczematoid dermatitis (infectious lesion near a draining ear). Rare conditions might include ichthyosis, severe combined immune deficiency (SCID), Wiskott-Aldrich syndrome (eczema, thrombocytopenia, and immunodeficiency), zinc deficiency, and drug reactions. Selective testing to elucidate a specific metabolic or genetic abnormality might be indicated (peripheral leukocytes and immunoglobulins in primary immunodeficiency, cytogenetic studies in Wiskott-Aldrich syndrome).

Treatment

Treatment goals include preserving and restoring the skin barrier by using emollients, eliminating inflammation and infection with medications, reducing scratching through antipruritic use, and controlling exacerbating factors. Some recommend limiting bathing to brief baths or showers of moderate temperature with mild and preferably nonsoap cleansers (Cetaphil). Drying soaps (Ivory) are avoided. Lubricants (Eucerin) are applied immediately after bathing and air- or pat-drying. Some products contain urea (Nutraplus) or lactic acid (Lac-Hydrin); they have special hydrating qualities and may be more effective than other moisturizers. Lotions and creams may sting shortly after application due to bases or specific ingredients, such as lactic acid. If itching and stinging continue with each application, another product should be selected.

Topical corticosteroids used to control inflammation vary in potency; percentage is not an indication of potency. Lower-potency preparations (glucocorticoid groups VI and VII) can be used for longer periods to treat chronic symptoms involving the trunk and extremities. Lower-potency steroids are generally used for infants and can be added to moisturizers to cover large areas of affected skin. The lower-dose steroids have no associated adverse endocrinological side effects. Fluticasone propionate 0.5% cream (Cutivate) and desonide 0.05% gel (Desonate) are the only Food and Drug Administration (FDA)-approved topical corticosteroid creams for infants as young as 3 months. **Fluorinated corticosteroids are generally avoided on the face, genitalia, and the intertriginous area because they may depigment and thin the skin.** Higher-potency steroids (glucocorticoid groups I and II) are used only for short periods and on lichenified areas; the face and skin folds are avoided. Ointment preparations are generally preferable because they result in better penetration of the corticosteroid, thus reducing the incidence of irritant and hypersensitivity reactions. Application is usually once to twice daily, dependent upon the preparation used. **The lowest effective potency steroid preparation should be used.** Lubrication often is continued after corticosteroids are discontinued.

Tacrolimus 0.03% (Protopic) and pimecrolimus 1% (Elidel) are nonsteroidal, immunomodulator topicals FDA approved for the treatment of AD in children 2 years and older. These agents are recommended for short-term and long-term intermittent therapy, on a twice-daily basis, in patients not adequately responsive to, or intolerant of, conventional therapy. Both carry FDA "black box" warnings concerning their possible association with malignancies (skin, lymph nodes) when used for extended periods of time. **Their exact role for use in children is under investigation; consultation with a pediatric dermatologist may be indicated.**

Oral antihistamines are used to reduce itching. Because symptoms of AD are often worse at night, sedating oral antihistamines (hydroxyzine, diphenhydramine) may offer an advantage over nonsedating agents. Less-sedating agents include loratadine (Claritin) and cetirizine (Zyrtec). Doxepin (Sinequan) has tricyclic antidepressant and antihistamine effects and may be useful in some cases in older children. Topical antihistamines (Caladryl) are avoided because of the potential for skin irritation or toxicity due to absorption. Fingernails should be cut short to prevent further skin damage through scratching.

Patients with secondary bacterial infections (*Staphylococcus* or *Streptococcus* sp) often require antibiotic therapy. Topical antibiotic therapy with mupirocin (Bactroban) may be used for limited areas of infection or in the nose to reduce chronic *Staphylococcus aureus* carriage. Oral antibiotics are indicated for more extensive areas of infection. First-generation cephalosporins, erythromycin, penicillinase-resistant penicillins, or clindamycin are chosen based on local susceptibility patterns. Patients with evidence of superinfection with herpes simplex virus (HSV) require oral or intravenous acyclovir. An alternative oral HSV nucleoside analogue, valacyclovir (Valtrex), is FDA approved in children 2 years and older. Intravenous acyclovir preferentially should be administered in infants and considered in older children with documented severe or disseminated HSV or those with "toxicity" (marked irritability, hemodynamic instability) and suspected HSV.

The role of food allergies in the management of AD is controversial. Dietary manipulation in a child (usually less than about 3 years of age) with a strong history of exacerbation of symptoms upon exposure to a particular food may be helpful. A 4- to 6-week trial excluding eggs and milk in children, followed by a rechallenge, may be justified, especially in a child who does not respond to first-line treatment.

Consultation with a pediatric dermatologist may be warranted for patients with an unclear diagnosis, who fail to respond to treatment, or who have extensive skin involvement. Consultation also may be appropriate for patients with ocular or serious infectious complications, for patients requiring steroid therapy, and for patients with atypical HSV superinfection.

Other skin eruptions can be confused with atopic dermatitis. Contact dermatitis is the reaction of skin to an outside agent. This category of eczematous eruptions includes both **primary irritant contact dermatitis** and **allergic contact dermatitis**. Primary irritant dermatitis can be caused by harsh detergents and soaps, bubble baths, saliva, urine, and feces. Examples of primary irritant contact dermatitis in the pediatric population include diaper dermatitis, lip-licker's dermatitis, and shin guard dermatitis seen in soccer and hockey players. Allergic contact dermatitis is a delayed T-cell hypersensitivity reaction (type IV) that occurs 7 to 14 days after initial exposure and 1 to 4 days after subsequent exposures. The most common cause is exposure to plants of the genus *Toxicodendron* that includes poison oak, ivy, and sumac. Also common in the pediatric population is nickel allergy, causing irritation below the umbilicus, where nickel-containing buckles or snaps make contact, and on pinnae from nickel ear piercings. Allergic contact dermatitis can also trigger an "id" reaction of widespread pruritic papules in nonexposed areas.

CASE CORRELATION

- See also Case 20 (Asthma) for a discussion about asthma which is often allergy based.

COMPREHENSION QUESTIONS

32.1 A mother brings her 2-week-old son to the clinic for a well-baby visit. Her only concern is a rash on his face and scalp that began a week earlier. Examination reveals a healthy white male child with normal vital signs and a normal examination except for yellowish, waxy-appearing, adherent plaques on the scalp, forehead, cheeks, and nasolabial folds. Which of the following therapies is appropriate for this condition?

A. High-potency steroid

B. Mupirocin

C. Acyclovir

D. Ketoconazole

E. Tacrolimus

32.2 An otherwise healthy 8-year-old girl, with normal growth and development and no recurring rash history, arrives at your clinic complaining about very itchy lesions on her chest, abdomen, and arms. The dermatitis started with a few red, raised areas on her chest 3 days ago, and then quickly spread. They appear to come and go in different areas. Physical examination reveals many ovoid, red, and raised eruptions on her torso and arms. Some are confluent, many are warm to touch or tender, and a few are weepy, crusty, or scaly with excoriations nearby. She is afebrile and the rest of her examination is unremarkable. Which of the following is the most important medical historical clue for achieving an accurate diagnosis?

A. Her infant brother has severe eczema.

B. She just completed an unidentified oral antibiotic course for her first bladder infection.

C. Her mother has recurring "spider bites" that often require drainage and antibiotics.

D. She had many ear infections as a toddler, and a few required repeat antibiotic courses.

E. Her father had allergies and asthma as a child.

32.3 A father brings his 4-month-old daughter to an emergency room for worsening skin rash and fever. He reports that his daughter usually has weepy, red lesions on her face that are relatively well controlled with bathing her with gentle soaps, using topical emollients and steroids, and occasionally giving her an oral antihistamine at the direction of her pediatrician. Over the previous few days, however, the rash has gotten progressively worse and the child has become "sicker." Your physical examination reveals a lethargic child with an oral temperature of 103°F (39.4°C). The child's cheeks are red and contain numerous red, punched-out, and umbilicated vesicles; some lesions are pustular. Which of the following would you prescribe?

A. Intravenous acyclovir

B. Intramuscular ceftriaxone

C. Topical bacitracin

D. Intravenous methylprednisolone

E. Topical acyclovir

32.4 An 8-month-old child has refractory eczema that was first noticed at 2 months of age. His past medical history reveals multiple episodes of otitis media and pneumonia, and he has now developed severe nose bleeds. You suspect a primary immunodeficiency. Which of the following is the next best test in your evaluation?

A. Sweat chloride test

B. Chest computed tomography (CT)

C. Complete blood count (CBC)

D. CD4 cell count

E. Referral to ear, nose, and throat (ENT) for nasal endoscopy

ANSWERS

32.1 **D.** Seborrheic dermatitis presents in infancy and adolescence. The chronic, symmetrical eruption, characterized by overproduction of sebum, affects the scalp, forehead, retroauricular region, auditory meatus, eyebrows, cheeks, and nasolabial folds. More commonly known as "cradle cap" in infants, this self-limited eruption typically develops between 2 and 3 months of age primarily on the scalp. The scale is yellow and waxy, and typically comes off with daily shampooing. The scale may be loosened with a small amount of oil. In infants who do not respond to shampooing with baby shampoo, an antidandruff shampoo containing antifungal medication (Nizoral) or selenium may help, as will low-to-medium-potency topical corticosteroids.

32.2 **B.** This patient's symptoms and rash are most consistent with acute urticaria and possible bacterial superinfection from scratching. The most likely etiology for her hives is her recent antibiotic use. Her family's atopic history is important, but her current rash and her past benign skin history are inconsistent with eczema. Recurring ear infections in the context of a patient with no failure to thrive or serious, difficult-to-eradicate infections make immune system dysfunction and associated dermatitides less likely. Her mother's "spider bites," requiring drainage and antibiotics, infer possible colonization and infection with methicillin-resistant *Staphylococcus aureus*. The patient herself may be an asymptomatic nasal or skin carrier and have seeded excoriations when scratching.

32.3 **A.** Atopic infants may develop rapid onset of diffuse cutaneous herpes simplex. The disease is most common in areas of active or recently healed atopic dermatitis, particularly the face. High fever and adenopathy occur 2 to 3 days after the onset of vesiculation. Viral septicemia can be fatal. Eczema herpeticum of the young infant is a medical emergency. The child should be admitted immediately for intravenous acyclovir.

32.4 **C.** This patient most likely has Wiskott-Aldrich syndrome, an X-linked condition with recurrent infections, thrombocytopenia, and eczema. Infections and bleeding usually are noted in the first 6 months of life. Potential infections include otitis media and pneumonia caused by poor antibody response to capsular polysaccharides, and fungal and viral septicemias caused by T-cell dysfunction. A complete blood count could aid diagnosis; thrombocytopenia usually is in the 15,000 to 30,000/mm^3 range, and platelets are typically small. In addition to eczema, these children have autoimmune disorders and a high incidence of lymphoma and other malignancies.

CLINICAL PEARLS

▶ Atopic dermatitis is a chronic, itchy disease that often begins in childhood. In infancy, the itchy eruption is found on the face and cheeks; by childhood, the rash is noted in flexural areas.

▶ Baseline therapy for atopic dermatitis is avoidance of drying soaps and replenishment of skin hydration with emollients; topical steroids may be required.

REFERENCES

Buckley RH. Immunodeficiency with thrombocytopenia (Wiskott-Aldrich syndrome). In: McMillan JA, Feigin RD, DeAngelis CD, Jones MD, eds. *Oski's Pediatrics: Principles and Practice*. 4th ed. Philadelphia, PA: Lippincott Williams & Wilkins; 2006:2467-2468.

Chatila TA. Wiskott-Aldrich syndrome. In: Rudolph CD, Rudolph AM, Lister GE, First LR, Gerson AA, eds. *Rudolph's Pediatrics*. 22nd ed. New York, NY: McGraw-Hill; 2011:761-762.

Holland KE. Atopic dermatitis. In: Rudolph CD, Rudolph AM, Lister GE, First LR, Gerson AA, eds. *Rudolph's Pediatrics*. 22nd ed. New York, NY: McGraw-Hill; 2011:1257-1259.

Leung DYM. Atopic dermatitis (atopic eczema). In: Kliegman RM, Stanton BF, St. Geme JW, Schor NF, Behrman RE, eds. *Nelson Textbook of Pediatrics*. 19th ed. Philadelphia, PA: Elsevier Saunders; 2011:801-807.

Sampson HA. Atopic dermatitis. In: McMillan JA, Feigin RD, DeAngelis CD, Jones MD, eds. *Oski's Pediatrics: Principles and Practice*. 4th ed. Philadelphia, PA: Lippincott Williams & Wilkins; 2006: 2423-2427.

A father reports his 3-year-old daughter has decreased energy, loss of appetite, and an enlarging abdomen over the past few weeks. Intermittent emesis began yesterday. Physical examination reveals pallor, proptosis, periorbital discoloration, and a large, irregular abdominal mass along her left flank that crosses the midline. Her vital signs and the remainder of her examination are normal.

▶ What is the most likely diagnosis?
▶ What is the next step in evaluation?

ANSWERS TO CASE 33:

Neuroblastoma

Summary: A toddler with fatigue, decreased appetite, periorbital discoloration, and a multiquadrant abdominal mass.

- **Most likely diagnosis:** Neuroblastoma.

- **Next step in evaluation:** Select laboratory testing and imaging to ascertain tumor genetic characteristics, location and extent, and impact on surrounding structures. Resultant staging and risk stratification help guide decision making regarding perisurgical chemotherapy and/or irradiation.

ANALYSIS

Objectives

1. Recognize the signs and symptoms of neuroblastoma.

2. Describe the diagnosis and treatment of neuroblastoma.

Considerations

Neuroblastoma origin and progression vary from patient to patient, and a mass may not always be readily apparent on examination. It often is accompanied by nonspecific findings influenced by tumor location and disease extent. Clinicians must perform thorough histories and comprehensive examinations to evaluate for syndromes associated with neuroblastoma. Timely and accurate diagnosis to diminish the potential for metastatic disease at discovery is an important goal.

APPROACH TO:

Suspected Neuroblastoma

DEFINITIONS

HORNER SYNDROME: Characterized by eyelid ptosis and sluggish pupillary reflex; related to sympathetic nervous system dysfunction (specifically the superior cervical ganglion).

PARANEOPLASTIC SYNDROME: Characterized by hypertension, flushing, sweating, and secretory diarrhea; related to tumor production of catecholamines and vasoactive intestinal peptide.

OPSOCLONUS-MYOCLONUS SYNDROME: Characterized by chaotic eye movements and myoclonic jerks; described as "dancing eyes, dancing feet" related to autoantibodies produced against neuronal elements.

CLINICAL APPROACH

The differential diagnosis for abdominal mass or pain in children is wide and varied, and includes both benign and reactive processes. Some of these conditions may need little more than supportive care, while other conditions mandate timely and thorough assessment and intervention. Included in the list of possible abdominal conditions are palpable stool in the constipated toddler, genitourinary tract abnormalities in the infant with urinary tract outlet obstruction, and reactive hepatosplenomegaly or mesenteric lymphadenopathy in the teenager with infectious mononucleosis.

One etiology for abdominal mass that warrants swift recognition is neuroblastoma, an embryonal cancer of the peripheral sympathetic nervous system composed of primitive neuroendocrine tissue. Its etiology is poorly understood, but believed to be multifactorial. It is the third most common pediatric malignancy, with 90% of cases diagnosed before age 5 years. It is the most prevalent solid, extracranial tumor in children and accounts for more than half of all cancers in infancy. Most arise in the abdomen from the adrenal gland, with other origins including intrathoracic and paraspinal neuronal ganglia.

Signs and symptoms related to neuroblastoma depend on tumor location. Cervical ganglia tumors may cause Horner syndrome, intrathoracic tumors (most commonly seen in infancy) may be associated with wheezing and respiratory distress, and paraspinal tumors may cause compressive neuralgias, back pain, and urinary or stool retention. Abdominal masses are typically firm, nodular, nontender, and cross the midline. Retroperitoneal tumors may be difficult to palpate, and a large mass may go undetected until metastatic symptoms arise. Dependent on a tumor's location and impact on surrounding structures, intrathoracic or paraspinal decompressive surgery may emergently be required.

Metastatic disease typically involves the long bones and skull, lymph nodes, liver, and skin. Findings may include fever, irritability, failure to thrive, and lymphadenopathy. Bluish skin discoloration (most often seen in infancy) represents subcutaneous infiltration. Pulmonary involvement can promote increased work of breathing, dyspnea, and pneumonia. Bone marrow involvement may cause bone pain and pancytopenia; petechiae, bruising, pallor, and fatigue may occur. If the orbital bones are involved, **proptosis and bluish periorbital discoloration, described as "raccoon eyes,"** may be noted. Many consider this finding **pathognomonic for neuroblastoma**. Some patients develop paraneoplastic syndrome related to tumor neuroendocrine mediators, or opsoclonus-myoclonus syndrome (an autoimmune-mediated phenomenon that may be characterized by cerebellar ataxia without cerebellar tumor involvement).

The major differential diagnostic consideration is Wilms tumor. These tumors typically are associated with hematuria, hypertension, and a localized abdominal mass that is smooth, well-defined, and rarely crosses the midline. In general, patients with neuroblastoma are slightly younger and sicker than patients with Wilms tumor.

Computed tomography (CT) or magnetic resonance imaging (MRI) is useful in identifying and assessing the extent of neuroblastoma. Characteristic findings may include calcifications or hemorrhage. Laboratory markers include **elevated urinary vanillylmandelic acid (VMA) and homovanillic acid (HVA) levels** (catecholamine metabolites), and are observed in approximately 95% of neuroblastoma patients. Other markers include elevated enolase, ferritin, and lactate dehydrogenase levels. Pathologic diagnosis usually is achieved via tissue analysis from tumor biopsy or resection. In select cases, neuroblastoma may be diagnosed at presentation, without tissue analysis, if neuroblasts are found in the bone marrow and accompanied by elevated urine VMA or HVA levels. If metastatic disease is suspected, further evaluation might include CT or MRI of the abdomen and chest, as well as bone scan and bone marrow aspiration and biopsy.

Treatment involves surgical excision of the tumor, usually after chemotherapy and/or radiotherapy to decrease tumor size. Combined multiagent chemotherapy and radiotherapy often is used in patients with advanced-stage neuroblastoma, while surgical excision alone may suffice for low-staged tumors. Staging is classically dependent on tumor location and extent, with risk assessment and therapeutic decision making based on variables such as age at diagnosis and staging (eg, stage 2 disease localized to the abdomen of a 1-year-old requiring only limited postexcision chemotherapy versus stage 4 disease with bony metastases in a toddler mandating multiagent chemotherapy and bone marrow transplantation). Other therapies under investigation include monoclonal antibody immunotherapy and radionuclide therapy.

Overall cure rates for neuroblastoma can exceed 90%, with 5-year survival rates for low- to moderate-risk patients ranging from 95% to 100% and high-risk from 45% to 50%. Of note, **infants typically have a better prognosis than older children**. Select features, such as skeletal metastases or N-*myc* oncogene amplification at the cellular level, often denote a poor prognosis.

CASE CORRELATION

- See also Case 10 (Failure to Thrive) which can present with any chronic medical condition. While neuroblastoma is classically described as presenting with an abdominal mass, pancytopenia and bone pain similar to leukemia (Case 19) are other possibilities.

COMPREHENSION QUESTIONS

33.1 A mother recently feels a mass in the abdomen of her 4-year-old son during a bath and brings him to your clinic for evaluation. He has no history of emesis, abnormal stooling, or abdominal pain. Physical examination reveals a resting blood pressure of 130/88 mm Hg, heart rate of 82 beats/min, pallor, and a firm left-sided abdominal mass that doesn't cross the midline. Which of the following is the most likely explanation for these findings?

A. Constipation

B. Intussusception

C. Neuroblastoma

D. Wilms tumor

E. Volvulus

33.2 A 1-week-old infant presents with a right midquadrant abdominal mass and decreased urinary output. There has been no temperature lability, irritability, or abnormal stooling or urine appearance. Which of the following tests would be most helpful in determining the etiology of this infant's abdominal mass?

A. Complete blood count

B. Abdominal ultrasound

C. Urinary catecholamines

D. Abdominal computed tomography (CT)

E. Barium enema

33.3 A father presents his otherwise healthy 15-month-old daughter to the emergency center with cough, post-tussive emesis, and subjective fever over the past 3 days. He also thinks her abdomen has been hurting her. Diarrhea started yesterday, with "regular" stooling prior to this illness. She has been drinking well and recently had a wet diaper. Physical examination reveals normal vital signs, congested nares, shoddy neck lymphadenopathy, and a mildly distended and apparently tender abdomen without obvious guarding. Which of the following is the next best step in your evaluation?

A. Obtain abdominal computed tomography (CT).

B. Biopsy lymph node.

C. Collect 24-hour urine for catecholamines.

D. Admit to the hospital for exploratory laparotomy.

E. Reassure parent and await spontaneous resolution.

33.4 During a routine preventive health visit for a 3-year-old boy, you incidentally note an irregular abdominal mass involving both lower quadrants. His mother denies having noted this previously and declares her son to be generally healthy. There has been neither gastrointestinal distress nor apparent abdominal pain. Beyond the abdominal mass and pallorous conjunctivae, his vital signs and physical examination are normal. Which of the following tests would be most helpful in determining the etiology of his abdominal mass?

A. Abdominal radiograph

B. Chest radiograph

C. Urinary catecholamines

D. Complete blood count

E. Urine myoglobin

ANSWERS

33.1 **D.** The scenario presented is typical for Wilms tumor. Beyond abdominal imaging, checking a urinalysis for hematuria, metabolic panel for renal or hepatic dysfunction, and complete blood count for anemia should be considered in the workup of Wilms tumor.

33.2 **B.** This infant most likely has a urinary tract obstruction. In the newborn, a palpable abdominal mass is commonly a hydronephrotic or multicystic dysplastic kidney, and typically can be easily identified by ultrasound (differentiates solid versus cystic masses, easily attainable in infants, involves no radiation exposure).

33.3 **E.** Upper respiratory tract infection symptoms, neck lymphadenopathy, and diarrhea are consistent with viremia; viral-mediated mesenteric lymph node enlargement can occur and cause nonspecific abdominal pain. Parental reassurance is adequate in this otherwise healthy child with classic viremia signs. An abdominal CT scan may show diffuse, mildly enlarged lymph nodes in mesenteric lymphadenitis, but imaging is rarely warranted unless an etiology for abdominal pain remains elusive.

33.4 **C.** This boy's history and examination are consistent with neuroblastoma. Given the vast majority of neuroblastoma patients have elevated urinary catecholamines, a 24-hour quantitative assessment of these metabolites should be confirmatory.

CLINICAL PEARLS

▶ Neuroblastoma may present with an abdominal mass, pallor, proptosis, and periorbital discoloration, with many considering proptosis and "raccoon eyes" to be pathognomonic for the disease.

▶ Masses are often discovered incidentally by a family member or on routine physical examination.

▶ Patients with neuroblastoma are slightly younger and appear sicker than patients with Wilms tumor.

▶ Approximately 95% of neuroblastoma patients have elevated levels of the catecholamine metabolites, vanillylmandelic acid and homovanillic acid.

REFERENCES

Anderson PM, Dhamne CA, Huff V. Neoplasms of the kidney. In: Kliegman RM, Stanton BF, St. Geme JW, Schor NF, Behrman RE, eds. *Nelson Textbook of Pediatrics*. 19th ed. Philadelphia, PA: WB Saunders; 2011:1757-1760.

Ater JL, Worth LL. Neuroblastoma. In: Chan KW, Raney Jr RB, eds. *MD Anderson Cancer Care Series: Pediatric Oncology*. New York, NY: Springer Science+Business Media; 2005:82-95.

Hogarty MD, Brodeur GM. Neuroblastoma. In: Rudolph CD, Rudolph AM, Lister GE, First LR, Gerson AA, eds. *Rudolph's Pediatrics*. 22nd ed. New York, NY: McGraw-Hill; 2011:1647-1651.

Strother DR, Russell HV. Neuroblastoma. In: McMillan JA, Feigin RD, DeAngelis CD, Warshaw JB, eds. *Oski's Pediatrics: Principles and Practice*. 4th ed. Philadelphia, PA: Lippincott Williams & Wilkins; 2006:1778-1781.

A full-term 1-week-old boy presents with bilious vomiting and lethargy. His mother notes a normal prenatal course and uncomplicated delivery. On physical examination he is noted to have significant abdominal distension and blood in his diaper.

▶ What is the most likely diagnosis?
▶ What is the best management for this condition?

ANSWERS TO CASE 34:

Malrotation

Summary: A full-term 1-week-old boy presents with bilious vomiting and lethargy. He is noted to have significant abdominal distension and blood in his diaper.

- **Most likely diagnosis:** Malrotation with volvulus

- **Best treatment:** Surgical intervention to remove any necrotic bowel and to ensure adequate blood supply to surviving intestine

ANALYSIS

Objectives

1. Know the presentation of malrotation with volvulus.

2. Understand the treatment of malrotation.

3. Be familiar with the differential diagnosis of acute abdominal pain in children.

Considerations

In this neonate with bilious emesis, a variety of etiologies are possible (Table 34–1). The clues to the diagnosis are bilious emesis due to intestinal obstruction, abdominal distension, blood per rectum, and lethargy. The most important next step is surgical intervention to prevent death and loss of viable intestine.

Table 34–1 • COMMON ETIOLOGIES OF ACUTE ABDOMINAL PAIN IN INFANTS AND YOUNG CHILDREN	
Condition	Signs and Symptoms
Abdominal migraines	Recurrent abdominal pain with emesis
Appendicitis	Right lower quadrant pain, abdominal guarding, and rebound tenderness
Bacterial enterocolitis	Diarrhea (may be bloody), fever, vomiting
Cholecystitis	Right upper quadrant pain, which may extend subscapular
Diabetes mellitus	History of polydipsia, polyuria, and weight loss
Henoch-Schönlein purpura	Purpuric lesions, joint pain, blood in urine, and guaiac-positive stools
Hepatitis	Right upper quadrant pain and jaundice
Incarcerated hernia (inguinal)	Inguinal mass, lower abdominal or groin pain, emesis
Intussusception	Colicky abdominal pain and currant jelly stools
Malrotation (with volvulus)	Abdominal distention, bilious vomiting, blood per rectum, usually presents in infancy
Nephrolithiasis	Hematuria, colicky abdominal pain
Pancreatitis	(Severe) epigastric abdominal pain, fever, and persistent vomiting
Pneumonia (esp. left lower)	Fever, cough, rales on auscultation of the chest
Small-bowel obstruction	Emesis, frequent history of prior abdominal surgery
Streptococcal pharyngitis	Fever, sore throat, headache
Testicular torsion	Testicular pain and edema
Urinary tract infection	Fever, vomiting, and diarrhea in infants; back pain in older children

APPROACH TO:

Malrotation

DEFINITIONS

VOLVULUS: Twisting of the mesentery of the small intestine and superior mesenteric artery leading to decreased vascular perfusion, which results in ischemia and ultimately bowel necrosis.

INTUSSUSCEPTION: A condition in which a proximal portion of the gastrointestinal tract telescopes into an adjacent distal portion. The most common location is ileocolic portion of the bowel.

CLINICAL APPROACH

Malrotation occurs when intestinal rotation is incomplete during fetal development. During normal fetal development in the first trimester, the growing intestine exits the abdominal cavity, elongates, and ultimately rotates 270° in a counterclockwise manner before returning into the abdomen. Following normal intestinal rotation, the duodenojejunal junction (ligament of Treitz) is fixed to the posterior body wall to the left of the spine. In cases of malrotation, the ligament of Treitz is located on the right side and the intestine may use the small portion of attached mesentery as an axis to turn (volvulus) leading to ischemia and possible necrosis.

Although individuals with intestinal malrotation may present from birth to adulthood, most cases occur in infants younger than 1 year. The classic presentation is that of an infant with abdominal distension, tenderness, and bilious vomiting due to intestinal obstruction. With prolonged ischemia the bowel becomes necrotic and the patient may have melena or hematemesis, and may develop peritonitis, acidosis, and sepsis. Without surgical intervention, the risk of mortality is significant. Patients with malrotation and either partial or intermittent volvulus may present with recurrent abdominal pain, or lymphatic congestion leading to failure to thrive because of malabsorption, protein losing enteropathy, or chylous ascites. Individuals may also have asymptomatic malrotation as an incidental finding.

Abdominal radiographs may be normal or have nonspecific findings in cases of volvulus; thus, an upper gastrointestinal contrast series is the test of choice. The characteristic finding in cases of volvulus is a "corkscrew" pattern of the duodenum or "bird's beak" of the second or third portions of the duodenum. In cases of malrotation with or without volvulus, abnormal position (right sided) of the ligament of Treitz or malposition of the colon may be noted with contrast radiography.

Prior to **emergent** surgical intervention, the initial management of patients with malrotation and volvulus includes appropriate evaluation of fluid status because patients may have significant fluid loss with electrolyte abnormalities. In the ill-appearing infant, placement of a nasogastric tube to aid gastrointestinal decompression, and initiation of parenteral antibiotic, in order to address potential sepsis are indicated. Exploratory laparotomy is performed and bowel viability assessed. Areas of necrotic bowel are removed and Ladd procedure of disengaging bowel with anomalous fixation and appendectomy are performed. Complications include short gut syndrome if a significant portion of necrotic bowel is removed, and adhesions may develop leading to obstruction. Because of the significant mortality and morbidity associated with volvulus, asymptomatic patients with malrotation require surgical intervention.

CASE CORRELATION

- Rectal bleeding (Case 15) may be a finding somewhat late in the course of a patient who has malrotation. Abdominal pain can be seen with lead poisoning (Case 25) along with other findings of behavior changes, achy joints, and encephalopathy. Bacterial enteritis (Case 28) may present with bloody stools, fever, and abdominal pain; this diagnosis should be on the differential while further evaluation is underway.

COMPREHENSION QUESTIONS

34.1 Malrotation with volvulus is most likely to be present in which of the following patients?

A. A healthy 15-month-old with severe paroxysmal abdominal pain and vomiting

B. A 15-year-old sexually active girl with lower abdominal pain

C. A 3-day-old term infant with bilious emesis, lethargy, and abdominal distension

D. A 4-day-old premature baby (33-week gestation) who has recently started nasogastric feeds; he now has abdominal distention, bloody stools, and thrombocytopenia

E. A 7-year-old non-toxic-appearing girl with abdominal pain, vomiting, fever, and diarrhea

34.2 An ill-appearing 7-day-old boy presents with 72 hours of bilious vomiting, abdominal pain, and abdominal distension. Which of the following is the most helpful to establish a diagnosis?

A. Order an abdominal ultrasonography.

B. Order a computed tomography scan of the abdomen.

C. Order an upper gastrointestinal (GI) contrast series.

D. Order a barium enema.

E. Order a chest radiograph.

34.3 A 6-week-old male infant has projectile emesis after feeding. He has an olive-shaped abdominal mass on abdominal examination. Which of the following statements is accurate?

A. He likely has hypochloremic metabolic alkalosis.

B. He likely has metabolic acidosis.

C. This condition is more common in female infants.

D. He should be restarted on feeds when the vomiting resolves.

E. He likely will develop diarrhea.

34.4 At 3 weeks of life a former 33-week gestation infant develops poor feeding, abdominal distension, vomiting, and bloody stools. He has also had several apneic episodes and temperature instability overnight. Which of the following abnormalities would you expect to see on imaging?

A. "Double bubble" sign

B. Absence of colonic gas

C. Decreased or absent air in the rectum with dilated loops of bowel proximally

D. Air in the wall of the small intestine

E. Target sign

ANSWERS

34.1 **C.** The 3-day-old term infant with bilious emesis and abdominal distension has classic presenting features of malrotation with volvulus. The 15-month-old child with paroxysmal abdominal pain is most likely to have intussusception. The adolescent girl is evaluated for ectopic pregnancy, pelvic inflammatory disease, appendicitis, ovarian torsion, and ruptured ovarian cyst. The premature infant might have necrotizing enterocolitis, whereas the 7-year-old girl most likely has gastroenteritis.

34.2 **C.** Order an upper GI contrast series. Prior to emergent surgical intervention, the initial management of patients with malrotation and volvulus includes appropriate evaluation of fluid status because patients may have significant fluid loss with electrolyte abnormalities. In the ill-appearing infant, placement of a nasogastric tube to aid gastrointestinal decompression, and initiation of parenteral antibiotic, in order to address potential sepsis are indicated.

34.3 **A.** This infant has the features of pyloric stenosis, a condition four times more common in males and more common in first-born children. Affected infants usually present between the third and eighth weeks of life with increasing projectile emesis. Abdominal examination may reveal an olive-shaped mass and visible peristaltic waves. Serum electrolyte levels usually reveal hypochloremic metabolic alkalosis. Ultrasonography is useful in confirming the diagnosis.

34.4 **D.** Necrotizing enterocolitis (NEC) can be mistaken for malrotation in young premature infants. Pneumatosis intestinalis (air in the wall of the small bowel) is a characteristic radiographing finding and aids in distinguishing NEC from malrotation and other abdominal pathology.

CLINICAL PEARLS

▶ Treatment of malrotation with volvulus includes emergent surgical intervention.

▶ Classic features of intussusception are fever, intermittent colicky abdominal pain, currant jelly stools, and a sausage-like abdominal mass.

▶ Classic features of pyloric stenosis include projectile vomiting, an olive-shaped abdominal mass, and **hypochloremic metabolic alkalosis.**

▶ Classic features of NEC include abdominally related findings of distension, vomiting, bloody stools, and systemic signs such as temperature instability, thrombocytopenia, poor feeding, apnea, and respiratory failure.

REFERENCES

Aiken JJ. Malrotation and volvulus. In: Rudolph CD, Rudolph AM, Lister GE, First LR, Gershon AA, eds. *Rudolph's Pediatrics*. 22nd ed. New York, NY: McGraw-Hill; 2011:1417-1419.

Bales C, Liacouras CA. Intestinal atresia, stenosis, and malrotation. In: Kliegman RM, Stanton BF, St. Geme JW, Schor NF, Behrman RE, eds. *Nelson Textbook of Pediatrics*. 19th ed. Philadelphia, PA: WB Saunders; 2011:1277-1281.

Brandt ML. Intussusception. In: McMillan JA, Feigin RD, DeAngelis CD, Jones MD, eds. *Oski's Pediatrics: Principles and Practice*. 4th ed. Philadelphia, PA: Lippincott Williams & Wilkins; 2006:1938-1940.

Chu A, Liacouras CA. Ileus, adhesions, intussusception, and closed-loop obstructions. In: Kliegman RM, Stanton BF, St. Geme JW, Schor NF, Behrman RE, eds. *Nelson Textbook of Pediatrics*. 19th ed. Philadelphia, PA: WB Saunders; 2011:1287-1289.

Hunter AK, Liacouras CA. Hypertrophic pyloric stenosis. In: Kliegman RM, Stanton BF, St. Geme JW, Schor NF, Behrman RE, eds. *Nelson Textbook of Pediatrics*. 19th ed. Philadelphia, PA: WB Saunders; 2011:1274-1275.

McEvoy CF. Developmental disorders of gastrointestinal function. In: McMillan JA, Feigin RD, DeAngelis CD, Jones MD, eds. *Oski's Pediatrics: Principles and Practice*. 4th ed. Philadelphia, PA: Lippincott Williams & Wilkins; 2006:371-375.

Nazarey P, Sato TT. Gastrointestinal obstruction. In: Rudolph CD, Rudolph AM, Lister GE, First LR, Gershon AA eds. *Rudolph's Pediatrics*. 22nd ed. New York, NY: McGraw-Hill; 2011:1394-1396.

A 3700-g male infant is born at 38 weeks of gestation after a pregnancy with limited prenatal care. The infant is noted after birth to have a dribbling urinary stream and a lower abdominal mass. Postnatal ultrasonography (USG) reveals bilateral hydronephrosis with bladder wall hypertrophy and an enlarged urethra.

▶ What is the most likely diagnosis?
▶ What is the most appropriate next test?

ANSWERS TO CASE 35:
Posterior Urethral Valves

Summary: A term newborn male has evidence of severe urinary obstruction.

- **Most likely diagnosis:** Posterior urethral valves (PUVs)
- **Most appropriate next test:** Renal USG

ANALYSIS

Objectives

1. Know the various presentations of patients with PUV.

2. Know the possible long-term sequelae associated with PUV.

3. Be familiar with common abdominal masses in the newborn period.

Considerations

Many conditions cause abdominal masses in the newborn (Table 35–1). In this infant's case, the dribbling urinary stream suggests PUV. An abdominal USG is a useful and noninvasive tool to aid in the diagnosis.

Table 35–1 • ABDOMINAL MASSES CAUSING DISTENTION	
Hepatic enlargement	**Adrenal masses**
• Cardiac failure, arrhythmias	• Adrenal hemorrhage
• Hepatic tumors (mesenchymal hamartoma, hemangioma, hemangioendothelioma, metastatic tumors such as neuroblastoma)	• Neuroblastoma
	Renal mass
	• Multicystic or polycystic kidney
• Metabolic disorders (storage diseases [lysosomal or carbohydrate], tyrosinemia, galactosemia)	• Hydronephrosis (posterior urethral valves, ureterovesical or ureteropelvic junction obstruction)
• Beckwith-Wiedemann syndrome	• Renal vein thrombosis
• Congenital infections (cytomegalic inclusion disease, syphilis, toxoplasmosis, rubella)	**Retroperitoneal masses**
	• Neuroblastoma
Pelvic masses	• Wilms tumor
• Ovarian cyst (follicular, dermoid, teratoma)	• Mesoblastic nephroma
• Hydrocolpos, hydrometrocolpos	• Sacrococcygeal teratoma
• Imperforate hymen	• Lymphangioma
• Vaginal atresia/stenosis	**Gastrointestinal masses**
• Cloaca	• Duplication
	• Mesenteric cyst

Data from Seashore JH. Distended abdomen. In: McMillan JA, DeAngelis CD, Feigin RD, Warshaw JB, eds. Oski's Pediatrics. 3rd ed. Philadelphia, PA: Lippincott Williams & Wilkins; 1999:323.

> # APPROACH TO:
> ## Posterior Urethral Valves

DEFINITIONS

VESICOURETERAL REFLUX (VUR): Retrograde urine flow from the bladder into the ureter(s) and, if severe, into the kidney. In general this condition is more common in females and may lead to recurrent urinary tract infections (UTIs) and diminished renal function. Depending on the degree of reflux, treatment ranges from antibiotic prophylaxis to surgical intervention.

VOIDING CYSTOURETHROGRAM (VCUG): A radiographic study in which a catheter is placed in the bladder and contrast is instilled. Upon voiding, the urethra is visualized and, in cases of VUR, the ureters are outlined.

CLINICAL APPROACH

Fetal USG assists in the prenatal diagnosis of urinary tract obstruction. Sonographic findings include **bilateral hydronephrosis with bladder distention with a "keyhole" appearance,** particularly in a male fetus. In severe cases, oligohydramnios is found and may lead to poor fetal lung development with pulmonary insufficiency and congenital contractures. Prenatal USG leads to the diagnosis in most cases of PUV.

Urethral valves are leaflets of tissue located in the lumen of the distal urethra from the prostate to the external sphincter. **Posterior urethral valves are the most common cause of severe urinary tract obstruction in boys,** occurring in 1 of every 5000 to 8000 newborn male infants; 25% to 30% ultimately have end-stage renal disease or chronic renal insufficiency. Neonates may present with respiratory distress secondary to lung hypoplasia from oligohydramnios, distended bladders, poor or dribbling urinary streams, palpable kidneys, reduced renal function, or UTI. Older infants have failure to thrive, renal dysfunction, or UTI. Older boys may present with voiding difficulty, such as diurnal enuresis or frequency. Posterior urethral valve is confirmed with VCUG or postnatal USG. The evaluation of the boy who has UTI includes VCUG and renal USG. Radionuclide scans are done to assess the renal parenchyma and the degree of obstruction. The diagnosis is confirmed with cystoscopy which allows for direct visualization of the PUV and ablation.

Immediate relief of PUV obstruction includes bladder catheterization through the urethra with a small feeding tube. If UTI is suspected, antimicrobial therapy is initiated. Serum electrolytes, blood urea nitrogen (BUN), and creatinine levels are measured with correction as needed. Hemodynamic status is monitored because sepsis or renal failure can lead to cardiovascular collapse.

After acute obstruction is relieved and the patient has been stabilized, endoscopic transurethral valve ablation may be performed if the serum creatinine level is normal and urethral size permits. If the serum creatinine remains elevated, the urethral lumen is too narrow, or the UTI does not respond to antibiotics, emergent vesicostomy may be necessary. Following ablation, VUR and persistent hydroureteronephrosis may occur.

FOLLOW-UP

After surgery, patients require surveillance of renal function and for possible UTI. Many patients will have polyuria because of diminished ability to concentrate the urine and are at greater risk for dehydration.

Routine care for boys with a history of PUV includes regular monitoring with urinalysis, renal USG, serum electrolyte levels, BUN, creatinine, blood pressure, and linear growth. They may have prolonged diurnal enuresis and may require urodynamic studies to evaluate their voiding. Renal insufficiency is common, and some may require renal transplantation.

COMPREHENSION QUESTIONS

35.1 A 3-month-old boy presents with fever without a source. As part of his evaluation a urinalysis is performed; a urinary tract infection (UTI) is suspected. Which of the following is the best next step?

A. If the urine culture reveals UTI, renal ultrasonography (USG) and voiding cystourethrogram (VCUG) should be performed.

B. VCUG should be performed only after a second UTI is diagnosed.

C. Antibiotics should be initiated after urine culture and sensitivities are obtained.

D. Renal biopsy should be performed.

E. Preferred methods of collection for urine culture for this infant include midstream clean-catch and bag urine.

35.2 An expectant mother accompanies her son for a routine visit. She states that she was told that her unborn child may have posterior urethral valves. Which of the following statements is true about the condition?

A. It occurs with equal frequency in males and females.

B. The unborn child will need a CT scan immediately after birth.

C. No postnatal evaluation or follow-up is required if the neonate has a normal respiratory function at birth.

D. The risk of end-stage renal disease or chronic renal insufficiency is 25% to 30%.

E. Use of prophylactic antibiotic therapy may preclude the need for more invasive treatment.

35.3 In which of the following neonates should the diagnosis of posterior urethral valves be considered?

A. A newborn with abdominal distension and respiratory distress with poor lung volumes on chest radiograph (CXR).

B. A newborn with abdominal distension bloody stools and air in the portal venous system on CXR.

C. A newborn with frequent episodes of apnea and bradycardia who is hypothermic.

D. A newborn with increased work of breathing with feedings, frequent desaturations, and perioral cyanosis.

E. A newborn who is large for gestational age and appears jittery on examination.

35.4 A 5 year old presents to clinic with abdominal pain and vomiting for the past 3 days. He has been afebrile but the mother reports strong smelling urine during that time. A urinalysis is obtained via catheterized sample and is significant for large leukocyte esterase and nitrates. The specimen is sent for culture and grows more than 100,000 CFU gram-negative rods. The mother denies any previous history of UTI. Which of the following is the next appropriate step in management for this patient?

A. Obtain a voiding cystourethrogram.

B. Obtain a cystoscopy.

C. Obtain a radionuclide scan using 99mTc dimercaptosuccinic acid (DMSA) scan to assess the extent of renal parenchymal damage.

D. Prescribe antimicrobial based on sensitivity.

ANSWERS

35.1 **A.** For any male infant with a UTI, evaluation of anatomy and function is necessary. The preferred methods of urine collection include bladder catheterization and suprapubic bladder aspiration. Antimicrobial therapy is started empirically while awaiting urine culture and sensitivity results.

35.2 **D.** The risk of end-stage renal disease or chronic renal insufficiency is 25% to 30%. Postnatal evaluation includes VCUG or postnatal USG.

35.3 **A.** Posterior urethral valves can cause oligohydramnios, which can lead to lung hypoplasia. Some infants may even have urinary retention in the bladder or urinary ascites. Lung hypoplasia will cause respiratory distress and will be evident on chest radiograph. Abdominal distension, bloody stools, and portal venous air should raise suspicion for necrotizing enterocolitis. This typically occurs in premature infants after feedings have been initiated. Infant sepsis can have very subtle signs, such as frequent episodes of apnea and bradycardia as well as feeding intolerance. In infants fever should always prompt a workup for sepsis; however, hypothermia can be a sign of sepsis in a newborn as well. Infants who present with increased work of breathing with feeds and cyanosis should undergo evaluation for cyanotic heart disease. These infants can appear cyanotic when agitated or when stressed because of intracardiac shunting. Infants who appear jittery on examination should be evaluated for hypoglycemia. Infant who are small for gestational age, large for gestational age, or infants of diabetic mother are at increased risk for developing hypoglycemia within the first few hours of life.

35.4 **D.** Older children who do not have a previous history of UTIs can be treated on an outpatient basis with oral antibiotics. However, children aged 2 to 24 months, children with recurrent UTIs, febrile UTIs, or pyelonephritis should undergo evaluation for vesicoureteral reflux in addition to being treated with antimicrobials. These patients should undergo renal ultrasound to assess for renal anomalies. Patients with abnormalities on renal ultrasound should then have a VCUG to assess for vesicoureteral reflux where the presence of posterior urethral valves can be identified. If posterior urethral valves are detected on VCUG, a cystoscopy should be done to confirm the diagnosis and allow for ablation.

CLINICAL PEARLS

▶ Posterior urethral valve occurs exclusively in males.

▶ Boys with posterior urethral valve are at risk for end-stage renal disease, even after appropriate therapy.

REFERENCES

Braga LHP, Bägli DJ. Urologic abnormalities of the genitourinary tract. In: Rudolph CD, Rudolph AM, Lister GE, First LR, Gershon AA, eds. *Rudolph's Pediatrics.* 22nd ed. New York, NY: McGraw-Hill; 2011:1741-1743.

Elder JS. Posterior urethral valves. In: Kliegman RM, Stanton BF, St. Geme JW, Schor NF, Behrman RE, eds. *Nelson Textbook of Pediatrics.* 19th ed. Philadelphia, PA: WB Saunders; 2011:1845-1846.

Gonzales ET, Roth DR. Urinary tract infection. In: McMillan JA, Feigin RD, DeAngelis CD, Jones MD, eds. *Oski's Pediatrics: Principles and Practice.* 4th ed. Philadelphia, PA: Lippincott Williams & Wilkins; 2006:1836-1840.

Krasinski KM. Urinary tract infections. In: Rudolph CD, Rudolph AM, Lister GE, First LR, Gershon AA, eds. *Rudolph's Pediatrics.* 22nd ed. New York, NY: McGraw-Hill; 2011:950-956.

Maria S, Finnel E, Carroll AE, Downs SM. Technical report—Diagnosis and management of an initial UTI in febrile infants and young children. *Pediatrics*. 2011;128 (3):e749-e770.

Roth DR, Gonzales ET. Disorders of renal development and anomalies of the collecting system, bladder, penis, and scrotum. In: McMillan JA, Feigin RD, DeAngelis CD, Jones, MD, eds. *Oski's Pediatrics: Principles and Practice*. 4th ed. Philadelphia, PA: Lippincott Williams & Wilkins; 2006:1823-1826.

Sand-Loud N, Rappaport LA. Enuresis. In: McMillan JA, Feigin RD, DeAngelis CD, Jones, MD, eds. *Oski's Pediatrics: Principles and Practice*. 4th ed. Philadelphia, PA: Lippincott Williams & Wilkins; 2006:670-672.

Seashore JH. Distended abdomen. In: McMillan JA, DeAngelis CD, Feigin RD, Warshaw JB, eds. *Oski's Pediatrics: Principles and Practice*. 3rd ed. Philadelphia, PA: Lippincott Williams & Wilkins; 1999: 321-325.

A 2.5-year-old boy is seen by his pediatrician with a 1-day history of refusing to use his left arm. His father states that the patient and his older sister were cared for by a babysitter the previous day. The babysitter said she had been playing with the children in the front yard, when the patient ran after a ball that was rolling toward the street. She grabbed the patient's left forearm and pulled him away from the street. Thereafter, the patient was irritable and holding his left arm close to his body with the elbow in a flexed position. On physical examination, the child has no bony tenderness, erythema or swelling of the joints, but on passive motion, the child resists and cries in pain.

▶ What is the diagnosis?
▶ What is the diagnostic test of choice?
▶ What is the best treatment?

ANSWERS TO CASE 36:

Nursemaid's Elbow (Subluxation of Radial Head)

Summary: A 2.5-year-old boy was pulled by the arm. He now holds his left arm close to his body with the elbow in a flexed position and resists movement of the arm.

- **Most likely diagnosis:** Nursemaid's elbow, subluxation of the radial head.

- **Best test for diagnosis:** None (radiographs not necessary with this classic presentation).

- **Treatment:** Supinate the forearm with the elbow in flexed position while applying pressure over the radial head. A "click" may be felt when the annular ligament is freed from the joint.

ANALYSIS

Objectives

1. Learn the classic presentation of nursemaid's elbow.

2. Know the maneuver to treat nursemaid's elbow.

3. Determine when childhood injuries should raise suspicion for abuse.

Considerations

This child's presentation is classic for nursemaid's elbow. However, in the setting of any injury to a child, nonaccidental trauma should be included in the differential diagnosis.

APPROACH TO:

Nursemaid's Elbow

DEFINITIONS

NURSEMAID'S ELBOW: Subluxation of the radial head

SUBLUXATION: A partial dislocation

NONACCIDENTAL TRAUMA: Damage, such as a bruise, burn or fracture, deliberately inflicted on a child or an old person

CLINICAL APPROACH

Nursemaid's elbow (subluxation of the radial head) is the most common elbow injury in childhood. It occurs when sudden traction is applied to an extended arm. It occurs most frequently in children aged 1 to 4 years. Caregivers typically give a history of pulling the child from the ground, swinging the child by their arms, or holding the child by the arm as the child is trying to pull away. Initially, the child will cry and **hold the affected arm close to their body with the elbow flexed and forearm pronated.** An older child may complain of joint pain in the elbow, forearm, or wrist. On physical examination, an absence of bony tenderness and swelling are noted. Passive movement of the affected arm results in pain, and the child will resist movement of the arm.

Pathologically, the annular ligament is torn at the attachment site to the radius bone when sudden traction is placed on the child's arm. The radial head slips through the tear, and when the pulling motion has ceased, the radial head recoils with a small portion of the annular ligament trapped between the radius and humerus. Any movement of the elbow thereafter is painful.

With a classic history and physical examination findings of an absence of tenderness and swelling with simultaneous resistance to supination, the diagnosis of nursemaid's elbow can be made without radiographs. Treatment involves the physician **supinating the child's forearm with the elbow in flexed position while applying pressure over the radial head.** If the maneuver is successful, a "click" may be heard when the annular ligament goes back into place as it is released from the joint space. The child may experience initial pain during the maneuver with rapid relief and an expected return of normal function in 10 to 15 minutes.

Nonaccidental trauma must be considered in cases of pediatric injury. One fracture induced by violently yanking a child by their arm and causing hyperextension at the elbow is called a three-point bending fracture (compression/distraction fracture). There will be soft tissue swelling on physical examination, and a radiograph will reveal a linear lucency in the distal humerus.

Signs of abuse are as follows:

- History is not consistent with type or degree of injury
  - A 3-year-old girl tripped and fell, breaking her arm in three places
- History of how the injury occurred is vague
  - The child is "just clumsy"
- History changes when given to different health care personnel or with repetitive questioning
- Inconsistent history when parents or caretakers are interviewed separately
- History is not consistent with development of child
  - A 6-week-old baby crawled over to heater, knocked it off the table, and burned himself
- Repeated doctor or emergency room (ER) visits for "accidents"
- Poor compliance with well-child visits

> **CASE CORRELATION**
>
> - The patient with nursemaid's elbow should have a history that is of a new-onset arm pain and reduced movement. The patient with these symptoms who also has failure to thrive (Case 10) or bruising may represent nonaccidental trauma for which a subdural hematoma (Case 29) should be entertained. See also Case 38 (Child Abuse).

COMPREHENSION QUESTIONS

36.1 In what position does the patient with nursemaid's elbow hold his arm? And how does the physician maneuver the child's arm for treatment of nursemaid's elbow?

   A. Flexed and pronated, supinate

   B. Flexed and supinated, pronate

   C. Extended and pronated, supinate

   D. Extended and supinated, pronate

36.2 The mother of an anxious 4-year-old girl presents to the pediatrician's office with a chief complaint of the patient not moving her right arm. The mother gives a history of the patient's father swinging her by her arms earlier in the day. The patient suddenly yelled out in pain while the father was swinging her. She clutched her arm close to her abdomen and would not allow anyone to touch it. On physical examination, the girl resists movement of her right arm. The affected arm is without tenderness to palpation or swelling. The girl has not been febrile. The doctor attempts to supinate the affected arm with the elbow in flexed position. She attempts three times but fails to hear a click and the child is still in pain and holding her arm close to her body. Which of the following is the most appropriate next step in her management?

   A. Reattempt reduction maneuvers until a click is heard and patient can move her arm.

   B. Aspirate the joint fluid for suspected infection.

   C. Radiograph of the right arm.

   D. MRI of the right arm.

   E. Inform Child Protective Services.

36.3 A 3-month-old boy presents to the emergency room with his father with a complaint of right arm swelling. The father states he fell asleep on the couch and when he awoke the patient was crying and lying next to the playpen in which he had been placed earlier. Which of the following is the most appropriate next step in the management of this child?

    A. Splint the arm and discharge the patient.

    B. Obtain radiographs of the right arm only.

    C. Supinate the affected arm with the elbow in flexed position.

    D. Order a skeletal survey.

    E. Inform Child Protective Services.

36.4 A 5-year-old boy presents to the emergency room with his mother with a complaint of left shoulder pain and fever for a week. Vitals include temperature of 102.3°F (39.1°C), heart rate 95 beats/min, respiratory rate 24 breaths/min, and blood pressure 96/54 mm Hg. On physical examination, the left shoulder is warm and tender to palpation, and has decreased range of motion. Laboratory test results were drawn and were positive for white blood cell (WBC) count of 17,000/μL, erythrocyte sedimentation rate (ESR) of 46 mm/h, and C-reactive protein (CRP) of 18 mg/L. What is the diagnosis?

    A. Transient synovitis

    B. Septic arthritis

    C. Humerus fracture

    D. Shoulder dislocation

ANSWERS

36.1 **A.** A child with nursemaid's elbow holds the arm close to his body with the elbow flexed and forearm pronated. Treatment consists of supinating the child's forearm with the elbow in a flexed position while applying pressure over the radial head.

36.2 **C.** Initial management includes two to four attempts about 15 minutes apart in an attempt to reduce the annular ligament. Should the expected improvement not be seen, radiographs of the affected extremity are indicated.

36.3 **D.** A 3-month-old child would not be able to climb out of a playpen to sustain the injuries his father stated. A high likelihood for child abuse in this scenario exists. The next step is to perform a detailed history and physical examination, followed by a skeletal survey (full-body radiographs) to assess for old or new injuries in the infant. If further questions remain, admission to the hospital and notification to Child Protective Services are indicated.

36.4 **B.** This patient has a fever, high WBC count, elevated ESR and CRP, and physical examination positive for a warm and tender joint. There is an infectious process occurring. To distinguish septic arthritis from transient synovitis, the Kocher criteria are used: fever, refusal to move joint or bear weight, WBC greater than 12,000/μL, and ESR greater than 40 mm/h. This is an orthopedic emergency. The next step is to aspirate the joint and send laboratory tests on the joint aspirate.

CLINICAL PEARLS

▶ Nursemaid's elbow can be diagnosed by history and physical examination alone, with no need for imaging.

▶ The classic description of nursemaid's elbow is initial crying at the time of the injury with the child holding the affected arm with the elbow flexed and forearm pronated. On physical examination, an absence of bony tenderness and swelling are noted. Passive movement of the affected arm results in pain, and the child will resist movement of the arm.

▶ Treatment of nursemaid's elbow is to supinate the affected arm with the elbow in flexed position.

▶ Have a high index of suspicion for childhood injuries caused by abuse, especially if the history does not match the degree of injury.

REFERENCES

Campo, TM. A case of subluxation of the radial head: nursemaid's elbow. *Advanced Emergency Nursing Journal.* Vol 33. No. 1. Philadelphia, PA: Lippincott Williams & Wilkins; 2011:8-14.

Carrigan, RB. Orthopedics. In: Kliegman RM, Stanton BF, St. Geme JW, Schor NF, Behrman RE, eds. *Nelson Textbook of Pediatrics.* 19th ed. Philadelphia, PA: WB Saunders; 2011:2384.

Davis HW, Carrasco MM. Child abuse and neglect. In: Zitelli BS, McIntire SC, Nowalk AJ, eds. *Atlas of Pediatric Physical Diagnosis.* 6th ed. Philadelphia, PA: Elsevier Saunders; 2012:181-207.

Deeney VF, Arnold J, Moreland MS, Ward WT, Davis HW. Orthopedics. In: Zitelli BS, McIntire SC and Nowalk AJ, eds. *Atlas of Pediatric Physical Diagnosis.* 6th ed. Philadelphia, PA: Elsevier Saunders; 2012:837-838.

Ezaki M. Nursemaid's elbow. In: Rudolph CD, Rudolph AM, Lister GE, First LR, Gershon AA, eds. *Rudolph's Pediatrics.* 22nd ed. New York, NY: McGraw-Hill;2011:866.

Reece RM. Child maltreatment. In: McMillan JA, Feigin RD, DeAngelis CD, Jones MD, eds. *Oski's Pediatrics: Principles and Practice.* 4th ed. Philadelphia, PA: Lippincott Williams & Wilkins; 2006:147-160.

Sponseller PD. Bone, joint, and muscle problems. In: McMillan JA, Feigin RD, DeAngelis CD, Jones MD, eds. *Oski's Pediatrics: Principles and Practice.* 4th ed. Philadelphia, PA: Lippincott Williams & Wilkins; 2006:2493.

A previously healthy 3-year-old boy presents with sudden onset of rash. His mother says he had been playing when she noticed small red spots and a large purple area on his skin. He has had no fever, upper respiratory tract infection (URI) symptoms, weight loss, bone pain, or diarrhea, and he is not taking medications. Three weeks previously, he had a mild illness that self-resolved after 48 hours. He is playful on examination, but he has multiple petechiae and purpuric lesions on his upper and lower extremities and on his trunk. He has no adenopathy, splenomegaly, or mucosal bleeding. His white blood cell (WBC) count is 8500/mm^3, hemoglobin level is 14 mg/dL, and his platelet count is 20,000/mm^3.

▶ What is the most likely diagnosis?
▶ What is the next step in management?

ANSWERS TO CASE 37:

Immune Thrombocytopenic Purpura

Summary: A healthy 3-year-old develops thrombocytopenia, petechiae, and purpuric lesions. He is well appearing but recently had a febrile illness. His WBC count and hemoglobin levels are normal.

- **Most likely diagnosis:** Immune thrombocytopenic purpura (ITP)

- **Next step in management:** Evaluation of his peripheral blood smear

ANALYSIS

Objectives

1. Know the most common causes of childhood thrombocytopenia.

2. Understand the natural history of ITP.

Considerations

This 3-year-old has purpuric lesions and petechiae resulting from thrombocytopenia. He lacks the systemic signs of illness expected with disseminated intravascular coagulation or hemolytic-uremic syndrome (HUS). Because his hemoglobin level and WBC count are normal, bone marrow infiltration is less likely the cause of his thrombocytopenia. A peripheral blood smear is examined to identify large normal platelets, but in diminished numbers. Children with ITP have relatively normal peripheral blood smears without evidence of leukemic or microangiopathic processes. This child has a platelet count of 20,000/mm^3 and lacks evidence of active bleeding; the next step is close observation. In the setting of typical ITP, bone marrow aspiration is not necessary. However, if this child had an abnormal WBC count or differential, or other signs or symptoms on history and physical examination suggestive of a bone marrow failure syndrome or malignancy (eg, prolonged fever, lymphadenopathy, organomegaly), a bone marrow aspirate would be indicated.

APPROACH TO:
Thrombocytopenia

DEFINITIONS

THROMBOCYTOPENIA: Platelet count less than $150,000/mm^3$. Normal platelet count is 150,000 to $450,000/mm^3$. Causes of thrombocytopenic include decreased platelet production, platelet sequestration, or increased platelet destruction.

HEMOLYTIC-UREMIC SYNDROME (HUS): A syndrome of nephropathy, thrombocytopenia, and microangiopathic hemolytic anemia. It is associated with *Escherichia coli* 0157:H7, *Shigella*, and *Salmonella*. A prodrome of bloody diarrhea is common.

THROMBOTIC-THROMBOCYTOPENIC PURPURA: Pentad of fever, microangiopathic hemolytic anemia, thrombocytopenia, abnormal renal function, and central nervous system (CNS) changes. This condition is clinically similar to HUS, although usually presenting in adolescents.

HENOCH-SCHÖNLEIN PURPURA (HSP): A syndrome of small-vessel vasculitis in young children. The syndrome may have dermatologic (petechial/purpuric rash), renal (nephritis), gastrointestinal (abdominal pain, gastrointestinal bleeding, intussusception), and joint involvement (arthritis).

IMMUNE THROMBOCYTOPENIC PURPURA (ITP): A condition of increased platelet destruction by circulating antiplatelet antibodies, most frequently antiglycoprotein IIb/IIIa.

CLINICAL APPROACH

Acute ITP is the most common cause of thrombocytopenia in an otherwise well child usually aged 2 to 4 years. The evidence suggests an immunologic etiology triggered by a preceding viral illness with subsequent development of an autoantibody directed against the platelet surface resulting in a destructive thrombocytopenia. Acute ITP occurs with an equal gender distribution. Young children usually present with acute onset of petechiae and purpura, and often a history of a viral illness 1 to 4 weeks previously. Bleeding from the gingivae and other mucous membranes may occur if platelet levels are severely low (typically $<10,000/mm^3$). Examination findings most often include petechiae and purpura, especially in trauma areas. If significant lymphadenopathy or organomegaly is found, other causes for thrombocytopenia are considered.

Laboratory findings of ITP include thrombocytopenia, which can be severe ($<20,000/mm^3$), but the platelet size is normal or increased. The WBC count and hemoglobin level are normal (unless excessive bleeding has occurred). Prothrombin time (PT) and activated partial thromboplastin time (aPTT) are normal. The peripheral blood smear may reveal enlarged platelets that are diminished in number; immature WBCs and abnormal red cell morphology are absent. Generally, bone marrow aspiration is unnecessary. If the peripheral blood smear is concerning, the WBC count is abnormal, or adenopathy or organomegaly is present, **bone marrow evaluation** aids in proper diagnosis, demonstrating an **increased number of megakaryocytes** in ITP.

The most serious ITP complication, **intracranial hemorrhage,** occurs in less than 1% of affected children. Patients with severe thrombocytopenia (<20,000/mm³), extensive mucosal bleeding, severe complications (eg, massive gastrointestinal bleeds), or without a protective environment may require medical intervention.

Most cases of ITP (70%-80%) are self-limited with good outcomes. Treatment is typically not initiated and close observation alone is a well-accepted treatment option for patients with minimal or mild symptoms. In the cases of ITP with significant bleeding, treatment can be initiated to decrease platelet destruction. Options include **intravenous immunoglobulin** for 1 to 2 days, **intravenous anti-D therapy,** or a 2- to 3-week course of **systemic corticosteroids.** Platelet transfusion is reserved for life-threatening bleeding. **Splenectomy** may be considered in children with **serious complications not responding to other therapies. After splenectomy, pneumococcal vaccine and penicillin prophylaxis** are required because of risk for sepsis.

Within a month of presentation, more than half of untreated children have complete resolution of their thrombocytopenia and up to another 30% have resolution by 6 months. Persistence beyond 6 months is considered chronic ITP.

Approximately 20% of ITP patients have chronic thrombocytopenia lasting for more than 6 months, occurring more commonly in older children and in females; it may be part of other autoimmune disease or may occur with infection such as human immunodeficiency virus (HIV) or Epstein-Barr virus (EBV). The ITP treatment options listed previously are available for chronic ITP patients; the goal remains prevention of serious thrombocytopenia complications.

Many pharmacologic agents may cause immune-mediated thrombocytopenia, including penicillins, trimethoprim-sulfamethoxazole, digoxin, quinine, quinidine, cimetidine, benzodiazepine, and heparin. The measles, mumps, and rubella (MMR) vaccine is associated with thrombocytopenia and is used cautiously in ITP patients.

CASE CORRELATION

- See also Case 19 (Leukemia) which also presents with thrombocytopenia. Typically in ITP, however, the blood abnormalities are limited to one cell line (platelets), whereas in leukemia the abnormalities exist across all three hematologic cell lines.

COMPREHENSION QUESTIONS

37.1 A 2-year-old girl has a rash. She was well until 2 weeks prior when she had fever and upper respiratory tract infection (URI) symptoms that resolved without treatment. On examination, she has petechiae on her upper and lower extremities and trunk. Her platelet count is 25,000/mm^3. Her white blood cell (WBC) count is 9000/mm^3 and hemoglobin level is 11 mg/dL. Which of the following is the best next step in management?

A. Obtain a review of the peripheral blood smear.

B. Administer intravenous immunoglobulin.

C. Send a blood culture and begin empiric antimicrobial therapy.

D. Order a platelet transfusion.

E. Arrange for bone marrow biopsy.

37.2 A 14-year-old adolescent girl has a rash on her arms and legs. She was diagnosed with a urinary tract infection 4 days ago, which is being treated with trimethoprim-sulfamethoxazole. She denies fever, vomiting, diarrhea, headache, and dysuria. On examination she has multiple upper- and lower-extremity petechiae. Her WBC count is 7000/mm^3 and hemoglobin level is 13 mg/dL; her platelet count is 35,000/mm^3. Which of the following is the best next step in management?

A. Send blood for antinuclear antibody (ANA).

B. Send a repeat urinalysis.

C. Discontinue the trimethoprim-sulfamethoxazole.

D. Obtain HIV testing.

E. Administer intravenous immunoglobulin.

37.3 A 7-year-old boy has a rash on his lower extremities and pain in his right knee. He has had a low-grade fever and abdominal pain, and he has felt tired. He is nontoxic appearing, but he has palpable petechiae on his lower extremities and buttocks. His right knee is mildly edematous and he can bear weight on his right leg, but complains of pain. His prothrombin time (PT), partial thromboplastin time (PTT), and platelet counts are normal. Which of the following is the best next step in management?

A. Begin a course of systemic corticosteroids.

B. Begin empiric antimicrobial therapy for sepsis.

C. Obtain a urinalysis and provide supportive care.

D. Perform aspiration of the synovial fluid in his right knee.

E. Administer intravenous immunoglobulin.

37.4 A 3-year-old boy has pallor, lethargy, and decreased urine output. He was well until the preceding week, when he had fever, vomiting, and bloody diarrhea (now resolved). On examination, he is lethargic and has hepatosplenomegaly and scattered petechiae. Urinalysis reveals hematuria and proteinuria. Which of the following statements about his condition is accurate?

A. A complete blood (cell) count (CBC) is likely to reveal thrombocytosis.

B. Initial therapy includes systemic corticosteroids.

C. Empiric antimicrobial therapy for sepsis should be initiated.

D. An emergent oncology consultation for probable leukemia should be arranged.

E. Peripheral blood smear is likely to reveal helmet cells and burr cells.

ANSWERS

37.1 **A.** This child has the classic immune thrombocytopenic purpura (ITP) features of isolated thrombocytopenia in a well-appearing child. An examination and peripheral blood smear are necessary. If no lymphadenopathy or organomegaly is found, the peripheral blood smear is normal, and there is no evidence of severe bleeding, initial management includes close observation and a protective environment.

37.2 **C.** The thrombocytopenia may be because of the trimethoprim-sulfamethoxazole; the medicine is discontinued and her platelet count is monitored. If thrombocytopenia continues, she may have ITP and should be followed for the development of chronic ITP. Chronic ITP occurs in older children (female predominance); it may be seen with autoimmune disease such as systemic lupus erythematosus or with chronic infections including HIV.

37.3 **C.** This child has signs and symptoms of Henoch-Schönlein purpura (HSP), a vasculitis of the small vessels with renal, gastrointestinal, joint, and dermatologic involvement. Initial therapy consists of hydration and pain control. With renal involvement, urinalysis reveals red blood cells (RBCs), WBCs, casts, or protein. Gastrointestinal complications include hemorrhage, obstruction, and intussusception; abdominal pain requires careful evaluation.

37.4 **E.** This child has features of hemolytic-uremic syndrome (HUS), which frequently follows a bout of gastroenteritis; it has been associated with *Escherichia coli* 0157:H7, *Shigella*, and *Salmonella*. Patients have pallor, lethargy, and decreased urine output; some have hepatosplenomegaly, petechiae, and edema. Laboratory findings include hemolytic anemia and thrombocytopenia; peripheral blood smear demonstrates helmet cells, burr cells, and fragmented RBCs. Acute renal failure is manifested by hematuria, proteinuria, and an elevated serum creatinine level. Management is supportive with careful monitoring of renal and hematologic parameters; dialysis may be required.

CLINICAL PEARLS

► Idiopathic thrombocytopenic purpura is the most common cause of acute thrombocytopenia in a well young child.

► Approximately 70% to 80% of children with idiopathic thrombocytopenic purpura have spontaneous resolution within 6 months.

► Hemolytic-uremic syndrome consists of nephropathy, thrombocytopenia, and microangiopathic hemolytic anemia; it is associated with *E coli* 0157:H7 and *Shigella*.

REFERENCES

Casalla JF, Pelidis MA, Takemoto CM. Disorders of platelets. In: McMillan JA, Feigin RD, DeAngelis CD, Jones MD, eds. *Oski's Pediatrics: Principles and Practice*. 4th ed. Philadelphia, PA: Lippincott Williams & Wilkins; 2006:1731-1736.

Davis ID, Avner ED. Hemolytic-uremic syndrome. In: Kliegman RM, Behrman RE, Jenson HB, Stanton BF, eds. *Nelson Textbook of Pediatrics*. 18th ed. Philadelphia, PA: WB Saunders; 2007:2181-2182.

Devarajan P. Hemolytic uremic syndrome (HUS). In: Rudolph CD, Rudolph AM, Lister GE, First LR, Gershon AA, eds. *Rudolph's Pediatrics*. 22nd ed. New York, NY: McGraw-Hill; 2011:1727-1729.

Devarajan P. Henoch-Schönlein purpura (HSP) nephritis. In: Rudolph CD, Rudolph AM, Lister GE, First LR, Gershon AA, eds. *Rudolph's Pediatrics*. 22nd ed. New York, NY: McGraw-Hill; 2011: 1720-1721.

Higuchi LM, Sundel RP. Henoch-Schönlein syndrome. In: McMillan JA, Feigin RD, DeAngelis CD, Jones MD, eds. *Oski's Pediatrics: Principles and Practice*. 4th ed. Philadelphia, PA: Lippincott Williams & Wilkins; 2006:2559-2562.

Neunert CE, Yee DL. Disorders of platelets. In: Rudolph CD, Rudolph AM, Lister GE, First LR, Gershon AA, eds. *Rudolph's Pediatrics*. 22nd ed. New York, NY: McGraw-Hill; 2011:1581-1584.

Scott JP, Montgomery RR. Hemolytic-uremic syndrome. In: Kliegman RM, Stanton BF, St. Geme JW, Schor NF, Behrman RE, eds. *Nelson Textbook of Pediatrics*. 19th ed. Philadelphia, PA: WB Saunders; 2011:1718.

Scott JP, Montgomery RR. Idiopathic (autoimmune) thrombocytopenic purpura. In: Kliegman RM, Stanton BF, St. Geme JW, Schor NF, Behrman RE, eds. *Nelson Textbook of Pediatrics*. 19th ed. Philadelphia, PA: WB Saunders; 2011:1714-1718.

Sheth RD. Hemolytic-uremic syndrome. In: McMillan JA, Feigin RD, DeAngelis CD, Jones MD, eds. *Oski's Pediatrics: Principles and Practice*. 4th ed. Philadelphia, PA: Lippincott Williams & Wilkins; 2006:2600-2602.

Van Why SK, Avner ED. Hemolytic-uremic syndrome. In: Kliegman RM, Stanton BF, St. Geme JW, Schor NF, Behrman RE, eds. *Nelson Textbook of Pediatrics*. 19th ed. Philadelphia, PA: WB Saunders; 2011:1791-1794.

CASE 38

A 4-month-old boy presents with irritability for 7 days. He lives with his mother, step father, 21-month-old sister, and 3-year-old brother. On physical examination, the infant has right thigh swelling and tenderness. Radiographs of the right lower extremity reveal a femur fracture.

▶ What is the most likely diagnosis?
▶ What is the next step in the management of this child?

ANSWERS TO CASE 38:

Child Abuse

Summary: A 4-month-old boy presents with a 7-day history of irritability. The infant has no history of trauma. A right transverse femur fracture is present.

- **Most likely diagnosis:** Physical abuse.
- **Next step:** Obtain a skeletal survey.

ANALYSIS

Objectives

1. Understand the importance of reporting suspected child maltreatment.

2. Recognize that child abuse is suspected if significant inconsistencies exist between the physical injury and the trauma history. It is imperative that the child's developmental level be assessed regarding the child's possible role in an accidental injury.

Considerations

The lack of trauma history is very concerning in this infant who is not mobile. The mother's delay in seeking medical care for 7 days from symptom onset is concerning. Cases of suspected abuse are reported to Child Protective Services (CPS) and/or law enforcement. Thus, the next steps are to obtain a complete skeletal survey to detect other bony injuries and to report this child's possible abuse case to CPS. The infant's siblings require medical evaluations and it is imperative that all the children are in a safe environment while the index child is evaluated.

APPROACH TO:

Child Abuse

DEFINITIONS

CHILD PROTECTIVE SERVICES (CPS): Local governmental agency responsible for investigating suspected child maltreatment cases.

CLASSIC METAPHYSEAL LESION: A fracture of the long bones that is considered pathognomonic for inflicted injury. Other names for this type of fracture are the "corner fracture," the "bucket handle fracture," and the "metaphyseal fragmentation fracture." The fracture occurs at the primary spongiosa region of the ends of the long bones and has the appearance of a bone fragment.

MEDICAL CHILD ABUSE (PREVIOUSLY REFFERED TO AS MUNCHAU-SEN SYNDROME BY PROXY OR CONDITION FALSIFICATION): Abuse in which the caretaker falsifies symptoms or inflicts injury upon a child to necessitate medical intervention.

ABUSIVE HEAD TRAUMA (SHAKEN BABY OR SHAKEN IMPACT SYN-DROME): Brain injury resulting from violent shaking of the infant or shaking the infant followed by collision of the head against a hard surface. Infants may present with seizures, respiratory arrest, a bulging fontanelle, or irritability. Intracranial injury is found with computed tomography (CT) or magnetic resonance imaging (MRI), and **retinal hemorrhages** may be visualized on fundoscopy. Skeletal injuries such as rib fractures or classic metaphyseal lesions may also be present.

CLINICAL APPROACH

Child maltreatment is common, with approximately 1 million substantiated cases per year in the United States. Child maltreatment includes neglect and physical, sexual, and emotional abuse; children often suffer from more than one type. **Neglect is the most common form of child maltreatment and consists of failure to provide adequate nutrition, shelter, supervision, or medical care.** Physical abuse accounts for approximately 20% of cases, occurring when caregivers inflict excessive physical injury. Although the definition of "appropriate" corporal punishment is argued (the American Academy of Pediatrics advises against all forms of corporal punishment but state laws vary on the issue), physical abuse is considered when marks (eg, bruising, lacerations, burns, or fractures) result. Sexual abuse occurs in 10% of substantiated maltreatment cases.

Medical child abuse is a less common form of child abuse. Affected children are hospitalized repeatedly with undiagnosed or vague conditions. Children may also have underlying medical conditions with abnormally frequent or persistent symptoms. The hospitalization is remarkable for a caretaker who takes great interest in the medical staff and interventions and often times has some type of medical background. The caretaker forms relationships with health care providers and is often noted to be an exemplary parent. Munchausen syndrome by proxy ranges from fabricating symptoms to actual poisoning or suffocations.

Reporting of cases of child maltreatment has been mandated since the 1960s, resulting in increased public and medical awareness. Health care providers legally are required to report suspected abuse to CPS or law enforcement.

Medical evaluation of suspected child maltreatment cases includes obtaining a medical history and a family assessment, conducting a thorough physical examination, obtaining appropriate diagnostic testing, and interviewing the child and the family. Routine medical history includes information about illnesses, hospitalizations, injuries, and pertinent family history. History should be carefully documented within the medical record because discrepancies to different providers or by different caretakers may provide vital information. A **developmental history** helps determine if the events described by a family are a plausible explanation for injuries (eg, a 10-month-old child is unable to climb into a bathtub, turn on the water, and sustain second-degree burns only to the buttocks). Documentation must include who lives in the home and who provides care for the child.

An examination is performed with attention to any skin lesions. Body charts and photographs assist in documenting the injuries. **A skeletal survey (skull, chest, spine, and limbs) assists in obtaining evidence of prior trauma in children younger than 3 years.** Recent fractures may not be detectable on plain radiographs for 1 to 2 weeks after an injury; if necessary, bone scans demonstrate fractures within 24 to 48 hours of injury. Children with bruising often may be evaluated with a platelet count and coagulation studies to eliminate hematologic disorders as a cause.

Although bruises and lacerations are common abuse indicators, they also are common in nonabused children. **Accidental bruises are usually found over bony areas** (knees, shins, elbows, forehead) and are appropriate for the child's developmental milestones. **Abdomen, face, neck, buttocks, thighs, and inner arm bruises occur less frequently in cases of accidental trauma.** In addition to bleeding disorders, the possibility of other causes of easy bruising such as Ehlers-Danlos syndrome, scurvy, glutaric aciduria, and arteriovenous malformation should be assessed. Some clues to the presence of a bleeding disorder include petechiae at clothing line pressure sites, object pressure sites such as in the pattern seen in infant seat fasteners, or diffuse bruising seen in severe bleeding disorders. If the initial evaluation indicates a need for laboratory testing for bleeding disorders to rule out medical causes of bruising or ecchymosis, initial testing is focused to rule out more common causes like hemophilia, immune (idiopathic) thrombocytopenic purpura (ITP), factor deficiencies, and von Willebrand disease (VWD), and Henoch-Schönlein purpura.

Characteristic child abuse injury patterns include looped cord marks, belt buckle–shaped lesions, multiple bruises in various stages of healing, hand prints, bite marks, and circumferential cord marks around the neck from strangulation. Burn injuries may resemble the insulting object, such as a steam or curling iron. **Intentional hot water immersion usually leaves a sharply demarcated border; the "stocking glove" distribution is a classic pattern.** Cigarette burns are circular and may appear similar to impetigo or insect bites. Patterned injury can also result from folk medicine practices, such as cupping (a heated cup applied to the skin leaves a circular injury) or coin rubbing (leaves linear red marks on the back). A history, physical examination, and a few screening tests can help eliminate these diagnostic considerations.

Skeletal injuries suspicious for abuse include long bone metaphyseal injuries, rib or complex skull fractures, and multiple fractures (especially when seen in various stages of healing). Spiral or oblique long bone fractures can result from unintentional rotating force injuries in ambulatory children. Nursemaid's elbow (radial head subluxation) occurs accidentally when a toddler falls while walking and holding an adult's hand (elbow dislocation occurs as the limb is pulled and twisted). Osteogenesis imperfecta, scurvy, cortical hyperostosis, and Menkes kinky hair disease are rare pediatric conditions with increased risk of bony injury.

CASE CORRELATION

- Child abuse mimics myriad other pediatric conditions. Thus, patients with failure to thrive (Case 10), bruising initially thought to be leukemia (Case 19), the child who appears to have undergone sudden infant death syndrome (Case 21), the pediatric patient with a subdural hematoma (Case 29), or unexplained bone pain such as atypical nursemaid's elbow (Case 36) must have nonaccidental trauma in the differential.

COMPREHENSION QUESTIONS

38.1 A 3-month-old boy is seen by the pediatrician with swelling of his right upper arm without history of trauma. On physical examination the infant has tenderness of the arm without erythema and is noted to have right-sided scalp swelling and multiple small bruises on the torso. The infant is otherwise well appearing and has an interactive smile. Which of the following is the best next step in management?

A. Obtain a radiograph of the right elbow.

B. Order a skeletal survey.

C. Place the right arm in a sling.

D. Order a prothrombin time (PT) and partial thromboplastin time (PTT).

E. Apply traction to the forearm while increasing the degree of pronation.

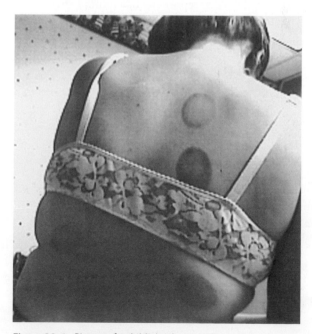

Figure 38–1. Picture of a child's back.

38.2 A 15-year-old adolescent girl has 2 days of nasal congestion and cough. Upon auscultation of her back, you find the lesions noted (Figure 38–1). Which of the following is the most likely etiology for her condition?

A. Cupping

B. Physical abuse

C. Disseminated intravascular coagulation (DIC)

D. Henoch-Schönlein purpura

E. Coining

38.3 A 3-year-old boy presents with a swollen left knee and multiple bruises on the elbows, ankles, and shin. The parents insist that their son is very active and have noted that he "bruises easily" upon minor trauma. They appear to be very concerned by his condition. The child is found to have normal growth and development. The physical examination is consistent with the findings stated earlier. What is the most appropriate next step in evaluation of the patient?

A. Inform Child Protective Services.

B. Order a skeletal survey.

C. Obtain a detailed family history.

D. Order laboratory tests to rule out a bleeding disorder.

E. Consult a pediatric hematologist.

38.4 A 9-month-old girl is fussy, appears to have pain on palpation of the right leg, and has bluish sclerae. Radiographs reveal a right femur fracture. Her parents deny any severe trauma but report she had multiple fractures as a child. Family history is also likely to include which of the following?

A. Blindness

B. Short stature

C. Tall stature

D. Renal disease

E. Aortic aneurysm

ANSWERS

38.1 **B.** This infant has what appears to be multiple injuries without a history of trauma. This is concerning for possible inflicted injury. A skeletal survey must be performed.

38.2 **A.** This adolescent has multiple perfectly circular lesions on her back consistent with cupping; when asked, she gives the history of cupping. Physical abuse injuries likely would not be identical in appearance. Patients with DIC will have significant systemic manifestation, and the pattern of ecchymoses would not be symmetrical. Coining causes ecchymosis in a linear pattern.

38.3 **C.** This presentation is typical for a bleeding diathesis likely hemophilia. In cases with a presentation concerning for physical abuse, it is imperative to get a detailed history including family history to rule out inherited bleeding disorders. The physical examination is consistent with bruises that are not particularly concerning for inflicted trauma. Evaluation with blood tests to rule out a bleeding disorder is indicated.

38.4 **B.** This infant has features of osteogenesis imperfecta, an autosomal dominant genetic disorder most often caused by point mutations of COL1A1 or COL1A2 genes. Features include long bone fractures and vertebral injury with minimal trauma, short stature, deafness, and blue sclerae. Four main types exist: type 1 is mild; type 2 is lethal (*in utero* or shortly thereafter); type 3 is the most severe; and type 4 is moderately severe. The types 5 to 7 do not involve mutations of type 1 collagen.

CLINICAL PEARLS

▶ All cases of suspected child maltreatment must be reported to Child Protective Services and/or law enforcement.

▶ If the history of trauma does not fit a patient's injury pattern, child abuse is suspected.

▶ If a child's development is inconsistent with the injury history, child abuse is suspected.

▶ It is important to rule out accidental and medical causes of bruising and bony injury based on the presentation of the patient.

REFERENCES

Carey JC, Bamshad MJ. Disorders of structural proteins of cartilage. In: Rudolph CD, Rudolph AM, Lister GE, First LR, Gershon AA, eds. *Rudolph's Pediatrics*. 22nd ed. New York, NY: McGraw-Hill; 2011:720-721.

Dubowitz H, Lane WG. Abused and neglected children. In: Kliegman RM, Stanton BF, St. Geme JW, Schor NF, Behrman RE, eds. *Nelson Textbook of Pediatrics*. 19th ed. Philadelphia, PA: WB Saunders; 2011:135-142.

Leventhal JM, Asnes AG. Child maltreatment: neglect to abuse. In: Rudolph CD, Rudolph AM, Lister GE, First LR, Gershon AA, eds. *Rudolph's Pediatrics*. 22nd ed. New York, NY: McGraw-Hill; 2011:137-143.

Marini JC. Osteogenesis imperfecta. In: Kliegman RM, Stanton BF, St. Geme JW, Schor NF, Behrman RE, eds. *Nelson Textbook of Pediatrics*. 19th ed. Philadelphia, PA: WB Saunders; 2011:2437-2440.

Reece RM. Child maltreatment. In: McMillan JA, Feigin RD, DeAngelis CD, Jones MD, eds. *Oski's Pediatrics: Principles and Practice*. 4th ed. Philadelphia, PA: Lippincott Williams & Wilkins; 2006: 174-181.

Reece RM. Child maltreatment. In: McMillan JA, Feigin RD, DeAngelis CD, Jones MD, eds. *Oski's Pediatrics: Principles and Practice*. 4th ed. Philadelphia, PA: Lippincott Williams & Wilkins; 2006: 153-154.

Sponseller PD. Bone, joint and muscle problems (osteogenesis imperfecta). In: McMillan JA, Feigin RD, DeAngelis CD, Jones MD, eds. *Oski's Pediatrics: Principles and Practice*. 4th ed. Philadelphia, PA: Lippincott Williams & Wilkins; 2006:2495.

Wilson P. Injuries. In: Rudolph CD, Rudolph AM, Lister GE, First LR, Gershon AA, eds. *Rudolph's Pediatrics*. 22nd ed. New York, NY: McGraw-Hill; 2011:865-866.

A 3-year-old boy presents to his pediatrician for follow-up. He was seen two days prior with a 4-day history of fever ranging from 102°F (38.9°C) to 104°F (40°C), anorexia, and irritability. He is fully vaccinated and has not traveled outside Houston. His examination at that time was remarkable for bilateral conjunctivitis without discharge, and erythema of the lips, tongue, and pharynx. A rapid strep test was negative. A clean-catch urinalysis showed 2+ leukocytes but no other abnormalities. Because he had no other localizing symptoms, he was started on an oral cephalosporin for presumptive urinary tract infection pending urine culture results. Today he returns with persistent fever and irritability and does not want to walk; his mother attributes it to swelling of his feet. The physical findings noted previously are still present, but now he also has a maculopapular rash over his torso, nonpitting edema of the hands and feet, and a 1.7-cm nonerythematous, nonsuppurative right anterior cervical lymph node. The urine culture and a throat culture from the previous visit show no growth. A complete blood cell count (CBC) shows a white blood cell count of 20,000/mm^3, hemoglobin 10 g/dL, and platelets of 470,000/mm^3. An erythrocyte sedimentation rate (ESR) measures 67 mm/h.

▶ What is the most likely diagnosis?
▶ What is the most common complication associated with the diagnosis?
▶ What further testing is needed?
▶ What is the treatment for this condition?

ANSWERS TO CASE 39:

Kawasaki Disease

Summary: A 3-year-old boy presents with fever and irritability for 6 days (Figure 39–1). Conjunctivitis, unilateral anterior cervical lymphadenopathy, oropharyngeal erythema involving the lips, a maculopapular rash, and edema of the hands and feet are present on examination. Elevated ESR, normocytic anemia, thrombocytosis, and sterile pyuria support the diagnosis.

- **Most likely diagnosis:** Kawasaki disease (KD, also known as mucocutaneous lymph node syndrome).

- **Complication of Kawasaki disease:** Coronary artery dilation with aneurysm formation.

- **Necessary diagnostic test:** Echocardiography is used to identify coronary artery abnormalities, pericarditis, congestive heart failure, and valvular regurgitation.

- **Treatment:** Early anti-inflammatory therapy with high-dose intravenous immunoglobulin (IVIG) and aspirin reduces the risk of coronary complications.

ANALYSIS

Objectives

1. Know the diagnostic criteria for KD.

2. Recognize the need for echocardiography to identify complications.

3. Name the two medications used for treatment of KD.

4. Be familiar with other diagnostic possibilities in the differential diagnosis of KD.

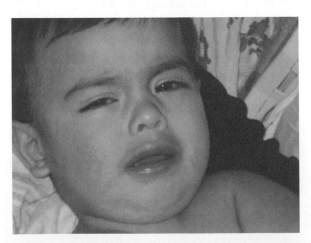

Figure 39–1. A child with Kawasaki disease with conjunctival injection and red fissured lips. (*Reproduced, with permission, from Goldsmith LA, Katz SI, Gilchrest BA, et al. Fitzpatrick's Dermatology in General Medicine. 8th ed. New York, NY: McGraw-Hill Education; 2012. Figure 167-1.*)

Considerations

Diagnosing KD can be difficult in the first few days of illness when only a few classic clinical findings may be present. Ongoing follow-up for fever resolution in any pediatric illness is essential to identify KD because most cases do not have all the findings present simultaneously. Bacterial diseases that share similar features of fever and exanthem include group A streptococcal disease (scarlet fever, toxic-shock syndrome), *Staphylococcus aureus* toxic shock syndrome, Rocky Mountain Spotted fever, and leptospirosis.

Group A streptococcal infection of the pharynx does not have conjunctivitis and the rash of scarlet fever has a "sandpaper" texture with accentuation in flexural creases known as Pastia lines. Viral etiologies of fever, exanthem, and conjunctivitis include measles, varicella, adenovirus, parvovirus B19, roseola, and Epstein-Barr virus (EBV). Measles would be distinguished by an accompanying enanthem (Koplik spots), cough, and coryza. Varicella has a vesicular rash, and adenovirus usually has a purulent conjunctivitis and exudative tonsillitis. EBV will also have exudative tonsillitis. Noninfectious causes of similar symptoms in children are drug hypersensitivity reactions or systemic-onset juvenile idiopathic arthritis (JIA). JIA will not have conjunctival or oropharyngeal findings, the rash is transient, and there is generalized lymphadenopathy. Splenomegaly may be found in EBV and JIA but not in KD.

APPROACH TO:

Kawasaki Disease

DEFINITIONS

POLYMORPHOUS RASH: An exanthem that may take various forms among affected individuals, such as maculopapular, erythema multiforme, morbilliform, or scarlatiniform.

STRAWBERRY TONGUE: Erythema of the tongue with prominent papillae, typically seen only in scarlet fever, KD, and toxic shock syndrome.

THROMBOCYTOSIS: Elevation of the platelet count above $450,000/mm^3$. In KD this usually occurs after the 10th day of illness and may last for a few weeks.

CLINICAL APPROACH

Kawasaki disease is a generalized vasculitis of medium-sized arteries associated with fever and an exanthema. The etiology is unknown but thought to be infectious. The incidence is highest among children of **Asian ancestry,** but it is seen worldwide. It occurs predominantly in **children younger than 5 years of age** (80% of cases). It is the most common cause of acquired heart disease in American children.

The diagnosis of "classic" KD is based on **5 days of fever and at least four physical findings** (Table 39–1). If less than four of the findings are present, the child may have incomplete KD. Incomplete disease occurs most frequently in infants who

Table 39-1 • DIAGNOSTIC CRITERIA FOR KAWASAKI DISEASE

Fever lasting for at least 5 days (or fewer days if defervescence occurs in response to early IVIG therapy) in a child without evidence of other more likely pathology, in addition to the presence of at least four of the following five characteristics:

1. **Bilateral bulbar conjunctivitis**, generally without discharge
2. Oropharyngeal mucosal changes including **pharyngeal erythema, red cracked lips, and strawberry tongue**
3. **Polymorphous generalized erythematous rash** (usually most pronounced in the perineum where there may also be desquamation)
4. **Edema of the hands or feet and erythema of the palms and soles** in the acute phase; periungual desquamation in the subacute phase
5. **Acute nonsuppurative cervical lymphadenopathy** (usually unilateral and measures ≥1.5 cm)

Note: Patients with fever and two of these criteria can be diagnosed with Kawasaki disease when coronary aneurysm or dilatation is recognized by 2D echocardiography or coronary angiography.

are, unfortunately, the group most likely to develop coronary complications. Thus, incomplete disease should be considered when fever is for five or more days and two clinical features along with supportive laboratory data are found. These laboratory tests include an elevated **ESR and C-reactive protein (CRP)**, **normocytic anemia, leukocytosis, thrombocytosis**, hypoalbuminemia, elevated alanine aminotransferase (ALT), and sterile pyuria. **Cerebrospinal fluid pleocytosis and mildly elevated hepatic transaminase levels** are the other most commonly seen laboratory abnormalities. Associated symptoms include painful and frequent urination, meningismus, vomiting, or right upper quadrant pain. Less common physical examination findings that can accompany KD are anterior uveitis, arthritis, pericardial friction rub, gallbladder hydrops, or desquamation in the groin.

Successful treatment depends on **starting high-dose aspirin and IVIG before the 10th day of illness because aneurysms rarely form before then.** Defervescence in the next 2 to 3 days generally occurs with this regimen. Aspirin therapy is later reduced from anti-inflammatory to antithrombotic doses and is discontinued 6 to 8 weeks after disease onset when the ESR normalizes if there are no coronary artery abnormalities. Children with coronary artery disease require prolonged antithrombotic therapy. Echocardiogram should be obtained at time of diagnosis, as well as at 2 weeks and at 6 to 8 weeks.

Without treatment, up to 25% of children may have coronary artery aneurysms and fever lasting 2 weeks. Even with treatment, approximately 2% to 4% of children develop coronary artery abnormalities. Aneurysms can develop at other sites, such as the brachial, axillary, femoral, mesenteric, and renal arteries. Aneurysm risk factors include male gender, fever more than 10 days, age younger than 12 months or older than 8 years, higher baseline neutrophil (>30,000cells/mm^2) and band counts, lower hemoglobin level (<10gm/dL), and platelet count less than 350,000/mm^3. Children with mild coronary artery dilation usually return to their normal state of health within 2 months. Death is rare and is caused by myocardial infarction or, less commonly, aneurysm rupture.

> ## CASE CORRELATION
>
> • The child with Kawasaki typically has a rash, which rarely may be confused with atopic dermatitis (Case 32) but the other diagnostic criteria of adenopathy, fever, oral and ocular changes and extremity findings of Kawasaki typically allow differentiation between these two conditions. The child with Stevens-Johnson syndrome (Case 26) typically presents after an exposure to an inciting agent such as medications (especially antibiotics such as sulfonamides or amoxicillin or anticonvulsants such as phenobarbital), infections (especially *Mycoplasma pneumoniae*) and is more common in patients with HIV disease.

COMPREHENSION QUESTIONS

39.1 An 18-month-old boy is seen in the clinic for evaluation of 4 days of fever, "pink eye," and irritability. Along with the conjunctivitis, he also has a generalized maculopapular rash. The mother reports that there are several sick contacts at his daycare. Which of the following examination findings would prompt you to order an echocardiogram?

    A. A tender 5-mm preauricular lymph node

    B. Shallow ulcers on the gingiva

    C. Red lips, palms, and soles

    D. Hepatosplenomegaly

    E. Bilateral crackles and wheezes

39.2 A 6-year-old girl presents with a history of 4 days of fever, headache, rash, and sore throat. The rash is maculopapular, blanching, with a sandpaper-like texture and located on the cheeks, axillae, and trunk, with streaks of linear confluent petechiae on the axillae and in the antecubital fossa. Tonsillar erythema and exudates are noted along with an erythematous oropharynx and strawberry tongue. The lips and conjunctiva are normal. What is the most appropriate management?

    A. Measles immunoglobulin

    B. Rapid strep test

    C. IVIG and high-dose aspirin

    D. Supportive care with antipyretics

    E. Serum autoantibodies and rheumatology consult

39.3   A 5-month-old irritable infant has 7 days of high fever, an erythematous rash in the diaper region, and swollen, red lips. He has a mild normocytic anemia, a white blood cell count (WBC) of 15,000/mm³ with a predominance of neutrophils and immature forms, and an erythrocyte sedimentation rate (ESR) of 80 mm/h. Urinalysis is normal, but the cerebrospinal fluid shows pleocytosis with a negative Gram stain and negative culture. Blood culture is negative. After 48 hours of ceftriaxone, he continues to have high fever and has developed foot edema. Subsequent management of this child should include which of the following?

A.   Nystatin for the diaper rash

B.   Repeat of the spinal tap

C.   Addition of vancomycin to the antibiotic regimen

D.   Pediatric cardiology consultation for echocardiogram

E.   Continuing current management and following the culture results

39.4   A 7-year-old girl has had 5 days of fever, conjunctivitis, erythema of the oropharynx, and a generalized maculopapular rash. Her lips, lymph nodes, and extremities appear normal. Which of the following laboratory tests would NOT be used to establish a diagnosis?

A.   Complete blood cell count (CBC)

B.   Urinalysis (UA)

C.   C-reactive protein (CRP)

D.   Erythrocyte sedimentation rate (ESR)

E.   Antinuclear antibody (ANA)

ANSWERS

39.1   **C.** Although he has only had 4 days of fever, the erythema of the lips and erythema of the palms and soles are two findings that are not commonly seen in other illnesses. When combined with his other abnormalities, he has four criteria that meet the diagnosis of Kawasaki disease (KD).

39.2   **B.** Rapid strep test should be performed because this patient has findings of scarlet fever, a manifestation of group A streptococcus (GAS) infection of the pharynx. The characteristic oral findings of GAS are strawberry tongue, erythema of the oropharynx, and tonsillar erythema that may also be exudative. The rash is typical of the toxin produced by GAS infection of the pharynx or skin. The absence of conjunctivitis helps exclude measles and she does not meet criteria for KD. Supportive care is indicated for viral pharyngitis. Serum autoantibodies would be indicated if juvenile idiopathic arthritis (JIA) was suspected but it does not present with oropharyngeal abnormalities.

39.3 **D.** This child's presentation is concerning for incomplete KD due to the persistent fever, two physical examination findings (oropharyngeal erythema, foot edema), and abnormal laboratory findings (anemia, cerebrospinal fluid pleocytosis, elevated ESR). Without evidence for another diagnosis, echocardiography is indicated.

39.4 **E.** Laboratory abnormalities found in KD are nonspecific but can be helpful in supporting the possibility as a diagnosis. Leukocytosis, anemia, and/or thrombocytosis would be identified by CBC; sterile pyuria or elevations in CRP and ESR are the other common findings.

CLINICAL PEARLS

▶ The diagnosis of Kawasaki disease (KD) is based on clinical criteria and should be strongly suspected in a young child with a combination of high fever for more than 5 days, oropharyngeal changes, conjunctivitis, extremity changes, rash, and cervical adenopathy.

▶ Children with incomplete disease can develop coronary artery abnormalities.

▶ The most important complication of KD is coronary artery disease. Echocardiography and consultation with a pediatric cardiologist is essential.

▶ Early recognition and initiation of therapy for KD is key to preventing potential coronary complications.

REFERENCES

American Academy of Pediatrics. Kawasaki disease. In: Pickering LK, Baker CJ, Kimberlin DW, Long SS, eds. *Red Book: 2012 Report of the Committee on Infectious Diseases.* 29th ed. Elk Grove Village, IL: American Academy of Pediatrics; 2012:454-459.

Newburger JW, Takahashi M, Gerber MA, et al. Diagnosis, treatment, and long-term management of Kawasaki disease: a statement for health professionals from the Committee on Rheumatic Fever, Endocarditis and Kawasaki Disease, Council on Cardiovascular Disease in the Young, American Heart Association. *Pediatrics.* 2004;114:1708-1733.

Son MB, Newburger JW. Kawasaki disease. In: Rudolph CD, Rudolph AM, Lister GE, First LR, Gershon AA, eds. *Rudolph's Pediatrics.* 22nd ed. New York, NY: McGraw-Hill; 2011:1855-1858.

Son MBF, Newburger JW. Kawasaki disease. In: Kliegman RM, Stanton BF, St. Geme III J, Schor N, Behrman R, eds. *Nelson Textbook of Pediatrics.* 19th ed. Philadelphia, PA: WB Saunders; 2011: 862-867.

An 8-year-old boy presents to your clinic with a 3-day history of a "white coating" in his mouth. He denies having a sore throat, upper respiratory infection symptoms, gastrointestinal distress, change in appetite, or fever. His immunizations are current, he has no significant past medical history, and he has been developing normally per his mother. His weight, however, has fallen from the 25th percentile to the 5th percentile, and he has been hospitalized on three occasions in the last year with pneumonia or dehydration. His family history is remarkable only for maternal hepatitis C infection related to past intravenous (IV) drug use. The patient is afebrile today, but his examination is notable for severe gingivitis, bilateral cervical and axillary lymphadenopathy, exudates on his buccal mucosa, and hepatomegaly.

▶ What is the most likely diagnosis?
▶ What is the next step in evaluation?

ANSWERS TO CASE 40:

Immunodeficiency

Summary: A child with lymphadenopathy, organomegaly, weight loss, recurring infection, and oral lesions consistent with candidiasis.

- **Most likely diagnosis:** Immunodeficiency.

- **Next step in evaluation:** Gather additional history, including birth history, details of hospitalizations, dietary history, and patient and family histories of recurring or atypical infection. Consider testing for human immunodeficiency virus (HIV) type 1 and obtaining a complete blood count and comprehensive metabolic panel to assess cell counts, organ function, and nutritional status.

ANALYSIS

Objectives

1. Differentiate between primary and secondary immunodeficiencies.

2. Understand selected etiologies of pediatric immunodeficiency.

3. Identify and manage pediatric HIV disease.

Considerations

Recurring infections in this patient presenting with oral lesions, weight loss, and lymphadenopathy are concerning for immune system dysfunction. He may have a primary immunodeficiency due to an inheritable defect or an acquired (secondary) immunodeficiency related to HIV infection, malignancy, malnutrition, or other disorder. The maternal history of IV drug use makes pediatric HIV infection a strong likelihood, probably due to vertical transmission. Additional patient and family histories and selected initial laboratory tests will aid in diagnosis and help guide management.

APPROACH TO:

The Child with Immunodeficiency

DEFINITIONS

HIV DNA POLYMERASE CHAIN REACTION (PCR): Recommended assay to diagnose HIV infection in children younger than 18 months; detects HIV DNA in peripheral blood mononuclear cells; sensitivity and specificity greater than 95%; exclusion of HIV with two negative assays after 1 month and 4 months of age, assuming other immunologic studies are negative.

HIV RNA PCR: Assay to quantitate copies of HIV RNA in blood; poor sensitivity in neonates (25%-40%); used to assess response to antiretroviral therapy (ART) in patients diagnosed with HIV; may be detected prior to seroconversion in older children and adults.

HIV ANTIBODY ENZYME-LINKED IMMUNOSORBENT ASSAY (ELISA): Detects HIV immunoglobulin G (IgG); initially detectable 2 weeks to 6 months after exposure; sensitivity and specificity greater than 99%; false-positive rate less than 5 in 100,000 assays; false-negative results may occur after immunization or in hepatic disease, autoimmune disease, or advanced acquired immunodeficiency syndrome (AIDS).

WESTERN BLOT: Direct visualization of antibodies to individual virion proteins; can be used to confirm screening antibody assay; results can be indeterminate and require repeat testing.

CD4$^+$ (T HELPER) CELL: Essential for humoral (B-cell) and cellular (T-cell) immunity; binds to antigens presented by the Class II MHC molecule on the surface of antigen presenting cells, prompting chemokine release and immune activation; rendered dysfunctional in HIV infection.

CLINICAL APPROACH

Evaluation of patients with recurring or atypical infection starts with a comprehensive history and systems review. Clinicians should inquire about perinatal history, growth and development, and past illnesses. **Immunosuppression** is suggested by **failure to thrive (FTT) or atypical or difficult-to-eradicate infections** (recurring otitis refractory to multiple antimicrobials). Family history includes parental health concerns (unexplained weight loss, growth failure, or developmental delay in siblings) and recurring or atypical infection in immediate family members. A focused physical examination should then be performed to identify signs consistent with immunosuppression (wasting, generalized lymphadenopathy, and organomegaly).

Primary (syndromic) **immunodeficiency** is due to a genetic defect, either inherited or related to de novo gene mutation. Most are humoral in origin or characterized by both humoral and cellular dysfunction (severe combined immunodeficiency). Some arise due to congenital malformations that affect proper development of the immune system (thymic dysgenesis in DiGeorge syndrome). Other primary immunodeficiencies include phagocytic cell deficiency (chronic granulomatous disease due to impaired respiratory burst), complement deficiency (autoimmune disease or serious bacterial infection due to C2 deficiency), and neutrophil dysfunction (autosomal-recessive leukocyte adhesion deficiency). Treatment is aimed at compensating for the defective response (IV immune globulin in humoral defects) or, in severe cases, reconstitution of the immune system via bone marrow stem cell transplant.

Patients with **secondary immunodeficiency** have normal immune function at birth, but subsequently develop an illness or metabolic abnormality that disrupts immune cell production or function. Conditions adversely affecting a patient's immune status include HIV infection, diabetes mellitus, sickle cell disease, malnutrition, hepatic disease, autoimmune disease, aging, and stress.

HIV is a global epidemic, with over 35 million people presumably infected worldwide. Unprotected sexual intercourse and needle sharing with IV drug use are known means of transmission. Prior to the mid-1980s, blood transfusion was also a risk factor. In the pediatric population, HIV is typically acquired through vertical transmission. Approximately 75% of pediatric cases diagnosed prior to age 13 involve intrapartum transfer. HIV can also be acquired from infected secretions at delivery and from breast milk. It is important to know the HIV status of the pregnant female, so that ART can be administered during pregnancy to decrease viral replication and diminish the potential for transfer to the neonate. An infected mother has a 25% chance of transmitting the virus to her newborn if no ART is received. With the advent of combined ART and infant prophylaxis with zidovudine, a mother on therapy with an undetectable viral load has less than a 1% chance of transmission. In mothers receiving no ART during pregnancy, infant prophylaxis during the first week of life with three doses of nevirapine added to standard zidovudine therapy reduced transmission rate to 2.2%.

A concerning trend over the past few years is the increase in HIV transmission among adolescents. In 2010, nearly 2300 new HIV cases in the United States were diagnosed in teens. About one in four new infections occur during the ages of 13 to 29 years. Sexual contact was the primary means of transmission in this group, especially among homosexual teens. A comprehensive social history, including sexual orientation and activity, should be obtained at all routine adolescent visits, and counseling regarding safer sex practices should always be provided. For those with identified risk factors (males who have sex with males, high-risk sexual partners, and IV drug use), HIV screening should be offered.

HIV infection gives rise to **dysfunctional CD4 cells** resulting in overall immune system compromise and eventual opportunistic infection. Approximately 75% of pediatric patients who acquire HIV vertically follow a course similar to adults, with an extended period of disease inactivity; a patient will often remain asymptomatic for a decade or more until the CD4 count falls to a critical level. The remainder of patients progress rapidly during the first several months of life. Therefore, early determination of maternal HIV status and measures to decrease transmission are critical (avoiding breast-feeding, aggressive and appropriate neonatal HIV testing, and early antiretroviral therapy).

Verification of HIV infection is made in the patient older than 18 months by performing an HIV antibody ELISA and subsequent Western blot for confirmation. Because of placental transfer of maternal antibodies, **diagnosis in younger patients is made by HIV DNA PCR testing.** Two assays are performed on separate occasions to confirm the diagnosis. Subsequently, HIV RNA activity, CD4 cell count, and clinical findings are used to determine disease status. Centers for Disease Control and Prevention (CDC) classification of HIV status is based on the presence and severity of signs or symptoms and degree of immunosuppression. For example, a patient with *Pneumocystis jiroveci (carinii)* pneumonia (PCP), an AIDS-defining opportunistic infection, is classified "severe" disease (category C). Degree of immunosuppression is based on an age-adjusted CD4 count. For the patient in this case, a normal CD4 count would be more than or equal to 500 or 25%. Severe suppression is denoted by a CD4 count less than 200 or 15%.

Neonates born to HIV-positive women are tested at birth and at selected intervals through approximately 6 months of age. Traditionally, the exposed neonate receives 6 weeks of ART in the form of zidovudine starting in the first few hours of life. Nevirapine may be added to the prophylactic regimen if the mother received no ART during pregnancy. If an infant is diagnosed by two positive DNA PCR tests, then zidovudine monotherapy should be discontinued, and the child referred to a pediatric HIV specialist for combination ART and monitoring. **PCP prophylaxis** in the form of **trimethoprim (TMP)-sulfamethoxazole (SMX)** commences at approximately 6 weeks of age for HIV-positive infants. CD4 levels are followed in quarterly intervals in the patient who becomes HIV positive. HIV RNA activity is followed and typically correlates with disease progression; RNA activity of greater than 100,000 copies/mL has been associated with advanced progression and early death.

Treatment of HIV-positive patients is started early to diminish viral replication before mutation and antiretroviral resistance occur. The **three major classes of antiretrovirals are nucleoside reverse transcriptase inhibitors** (didanosine, stavudine, zidovudine), **nonnucleoside reverse transcriptase inhibitors** (efavirenz, nevirapine), and **protease inhibitors** (indinavir, nelfinavir). A variety of other available medications target different points in the HIV replication cycle (coreceptor binding and integration of retroviral DNA), but are typically used after the above prove ineffective. Combination ART in children has led to a marked decline in child mortality. Common adverse effects for all ARTs include headache, emesis, abdominal pain, and diarrhea. Osteopenia and drug rash can also be seen. Possible other abnormalities include anemia, neutropenia, elevated transaminases, hyperglycemia, and hyperlipidemia.

The current pediatric ART recommendation consists of three drugs: two nucleoside reverse transcriptase inhibitors and either a protease inhibitor or a nonnucleoside reverse transcriptase inhibitor. An existing treatment regimen is altered when toxicity becomes an issue or disease progression occurs. Ultimately, HIV treatment requires a multidisciplinary approach with input from nutritionists, social workers, and pediatric HIV and mental health specialists. In addition to periodic monitoring of viral activity and prophylaxis against opportunistic infection, close monitoring of growth, development, and emotional health is important in pediatric HIV disease management. **Immunizations** should be kept current, with all vaccines administered per the recommended pediatric schedule, excluding live vaccines such as measles, mumps, and rubella (MMR) and varicella for symptomatic HIV-infected children with a CD4 count less than 15%.

CASE CORRELATION

- See also Case 10 (Failure to Thrive) which can present with any chronic medical condition, many of which have immune deficiency as a component. The child with sickle cell disease (Case 13) has an acquired immune deficiency due to splenic auto-infarction and a higher incidence of infection due to encapsulated (pneumococcus) organisms. Patients with frequent pneumonia (Case 14) or as a result to unusual organism and patients who have frequent or unusually severe otitis media (Case 16) may have a primary immune deficiency. The patient with cystic fibrosis (Case 18) has a variety of medical issues such as malnutrition, vitamin deficiency, and frequent pneumonia characteristic of a patient with secondary immune deficiency. Leukemia (Case 19) and neuroblastoma (Case 33) represent secondary immune deficiencies.

COMPREHENSION QUESTIONS

40.1 A 16-year-old boy has a 2-week history of subjective fever, sore throat, and swollen and tender lymph nodes in the neck and groin. He admits to being sexually active, including oral sex, with a male partner over the past month. They do not use condoms. On physical examination, he is afebrile, with cervical and inguinal lymphadenopathy and a nonexudative pharyngitis. HIV ELISA done in the ER was negative. Which of the following is the next best step in your evaluation?

A. Lymph node biopsy

B. HIV RNA PCR

C. CD4 cell count

D. Herpes simplex virus-1 IgG

E. Rapid plasma reagin (RPR)

40.2 A mother notes her 6-week-old son's umbilical cord is still attached. His activity and intake are normal; he has had no illness or fever. Delivery was at term without problems. His examination is notable for a cord without evidence of separation and a shallow, 0.5-cm ulceration at the occiput without discharge or surrounding erythema. The mother declares that the "sore," caused by a scalp probe, has been slowly healing since birth and was deemed unremarkable at his 2-week checkup. Which of the following is consistent with this child's likely diagnosis?

A. Defective humoral response

B. Functional leukocyte adherence glycoproteins

C. Marked neutrophilia

D. Normal wound healing

E. Purulent abscess formation

40.3 A 6-month-old girl is seen after an emergency room visit for decreased intake, emesis, and watery diarrhea for the past 3 days. She was diagnosed yesterday with "stomach flu" and given IV fluids. She is doing better today with improved intake and resolution of her emesis and diarrhea. The father is concerned about her thrush since birth (despite multiple courses of an oral antifungal), and that she has been hospitalized twice for pneumonia over the past 4 months. Her weight has dropped from the 50th percentile on her 4-month visit to the 5th percentile today. She has no findings consistent with dehydration, but she does appear to have some extremity muscle wasting. Her examination is remarkable for buccal mucosal exudates and hyperactive bowel sounds. Vital signs and the remainder of her examination are normal. You suspect severe combined immunodeficiency (SCID). Which of the following is consistent with the diagnosis?

A. Autosomal dominant inheritance

B. Persistent lymphocytosis

C. Defective cellular immunity

D. Normal vaccine immune response

E. No curative therapy

40.4 You are called urgently to examine a term, 2-hour-old newborn with temperature instability, difficulty with feeding, and a suspected seizure. He has atypical facies (wide-set eyes, a prominent nose, and a small mandible), a cleft palate, and a holosystolic murmur. A chest radiograph reveals a boot-shaped heart. Which of the following is consistent with this infant's likely diagnosis?

A. Hypercalcemia

B. Chromosomal duplication

C. Parathyroid hyperplasia

D. Hypophosphatemia

E. Thymic aplasia

ANSWERS

40.1 **B.** This adolescent presents with nonspecific findings of a viral-like illness. Sexual activity, a male partner, and absent barrier protection are risk factors for acquiring HIV. Because an early negative HIV ELISA is possible, HIV RNA PCR to detect replicating virus is a reasonable consideration. CD4 count is premature, routine nodal biopsy may not provide a diagnosis, and herpes or syphilis is not consistent with the clinical scenario. Whether symptomatic or not, selective and judicious testing for sexually transmitted diseases (STDs) is an important consideration in all sexually active adolescents.

40.2 **C.** You suspect leukocyte adhesion deficiency (LAD) as the etiology of this child's problem. LAD is an inheritable disorder of leukocyte chemotaxis and adherence characterized by recurring sinopulmonary, oropharyngeal, and cutaneous infections with delayed wound healing. Neutrophilia is common with white blood cell (WBC) counts typically more than 50,000 cells/mm^3. Severe, life-threatening infection is possible with *Staphylococcus* species, *Enterobacteriaceae*, and *Candida* species. Good skin and oral hygiene are important; broad-spectrum antimicrobials and surgical debridement are early considerations with infection.

40.3 **C.** Severe combined immunodeficiency (SCID) is an autosomal recessive or X-linked disorder of both humoral and cellular immunity. Serum immunoglobulins and T cells are often markedly diminished or absent. Thymic dysgenesis is also seen. Recurring cutaneous, gastrointestinal, or pulmonary infections occur with opportunistic organisms such as cytomegalovirus (CMV) and *Pneumocystis pneumonia* (PCP). Death typically occurs in the first 12 to 24 months of life unless bone marrow transplantation is performed.

40.4 **E.** The child in the question has typical features of DiGeorge syndrome, caused by a 22q11 microdeletion. This syndromic immunodeficiency is characterized by decreased T-cell production and recurring infection. Findings include characteristic facies and velocardiofacial defects, such as ventricular septal defect and tetralogy of Fallot. Thymic or parathyroid dysgenesis can occur, accompanied by hypocalcemia and seizures. Developmental and speech delay are common in older patients.

CLINICAL PEARLS

▶ Primary immunodeficiency is a group of inheritable disorders characterized by weakened immunity and recurring, serious infection early in life.

▶ A variety of illnesses can provoke secondary immunodeficiency; malignancy, malnutrition, hepatic disease, and HIV infection are known to adversely influence both humoral and cellular immunity.

▶ Pediatric HIV disease can be deterred by appropriate testing and treatment of pregnant females and judicious antiretroviral prophylaxis in the exposed neonate. Exposed patients should be closely followed by clinicians and a team approach used in the management of active disease.

▶ Adolescents should be screened for sexual activity and high-risk behaviors at routine health visits, and HIV screening should be offered when history or examination warrants.

REFERENCES

American Academy of Pediatrics. Human immunodeficiency virus infection. In: Pickering LK, ed. *2012 Red Book: Report of the Committee on Infectious Diseases*. 29th ed. Elk Grove Village, IL: American Academy of Pediatrics; 2012:418-439.

Borkowsky W. Acquired immunodeficiency syndrome and human immunodeficiency virus. In: Katz SL, Hotez PJ, Gerson AA, eds. *Krugman's Infectious Diseases of Children*. 11th ed. Philadelphia, PA: Mosby; 2004:1-26.

Buckley RH. Evaluation of suspected immunodeficiency. In: Kliegman RM, Stanton BF, St. Geme JW, Schor NF, Behrman RE, eds. *Nelson Textbook of Pediatrics*. 19th ed. Philadelphia, PA: WB Saunders; 2011:715-722.

CDC. HIV Surveillance Report. 2010. Vol 22. http://www.cdc.gov/hiv/surveillance/resources/reports/2010report/pdf/2010_HIV_Surveillance_Report_vol_22.pdf. Published February 2012. Accessed March 20, 2014.

Church JA. Human immunodeficiency virus infection. In: Osborn LM, DeWitt TG, First LR, Zenel JA, eds. *Pediatrics*. 1st ed. Philadelphia, PA: Elsevier-Mosby; 2005:1132-1139.

Panel on Antiretroviral Therapy and Medical Management of HIV-Infected Children. Guidelines for the use of antiretroviral agents in pediatric HIV infection. http://aidsinfo.nih.gov/contentfiles/lvguidelines/pediatricguidelines.pdf. Accessed March 20, 2014.

Panel on Treatment of HIV-Infected Pregnant Women and Prevention of Perinatal Transmission. Recommendations for use of antiretroviral drugs in pregnant HIV-1-infected women for maternal health and interventions to reduce perinatal HIV transmission in the United States. http://aidsinfo.nih.gov/contentfiles/lvguidelines/PerinatalGL.pdf. Accessed March 20, 2014.

Yogev R, Chadwick EG. Acquired immunodeficiency syndrome (human immunodeficiency virus). In: Kliegman RM, Stanton BF, St. Geme JW, Schor NF, Behrman RE, eds. *Nelson Textbook of Pediatrics*. 19th ed. Philadelphia, PA: WB Saunders; 2011:1157-1177.

A 13-year-old boy presents for routine care. His mother reports that he seems to be much more immature and insecure than her older son was at the same age. His school performance is below average, and this year he has begun to receive special education for language-based classes. On physical examination you note that he is at the 95th percentile for height-age, his extremities are longer than expected, and he is embarrassed by his gynecomastia. His physical examination shows that he has Tanner stage 1 sexual development with small gonads.

▶ What is the most likely diagnosis?
▶ What is the best test to diagnose this condition?

ANSWERS TO CASE 41:

Klinefelter Syndrome

Summary: A tall, immature, and insecure 13-year-old boy with hypogonadism, long limbs, gynecomastia, and developmental delay.

- **Most likely diagnosis:** Klinefelter syndrome, a nondisjunction trisomy of the sex chromosomes affecting approximately 1 in 500 to 800 male infants

- **Best diagnostic test:** Chromosomal analysis

ANALYSIS

Objectives

1. Understand the signs and symptoms of Klinefelter syndrome.

2. Appreciate the variety of causes of childhood intellectual disability (ID).

3. Learn the signs and symptoms of syndromes involving missing or duplicate sex chromosomes.

Considerations

This child's mother has identified his development and behavior to be different from her other children. The school recently identified his need for special education, especially in language-based classes. A thorough history (including all school performance and behavioral problems) and physical examination can provide diagnostic clues. The etiology of his condition impacts his psychosocial outcome, his future medical therapy, and his parents' family planning decisions.

APPROACH TO:

Klinefelter Syndrome

DEFINITIONS

KLINEFELTER SYNDROME: A syndrome comprised of behavioral problems (immaturity, insecurity), developmental delay (speech, language, lower IQ), and physical abnormalities (gynecomastia, hypogonadism, long limbs) caused by an extra X chromosome in males.

INTELLECTUAL DISABILITY (ID): A clinically and socially important impairment of measured intelligence and adaptive behavior that is diagnosed before 18 years of age.

CLINICAL APPROACH

Causes of ID include **preconception and early embryonic disruptions** (teratogens, chromosomal abnormalities, placental dysfunction, congenital central nervous system [CNS] malformations); **fetal brain insults** (infections, toxins); **perinatal difficulties** (prematurity, metabolic disorders, placental problems); **postnatal brain injuries** (infections, trauma, metabolic disorders, toxins, poor nutrition); and miscellaneous **postnatal family difficulties** (poverty, poor caregiver-child interaction, parental mental illness). Children with ID who do not fit into one of these categories are classified as having ID of unknown etiology.

The diagnosis of ID relies upon evaluation of the child's psychosocial skills and a review of school reports, and may require formal IQ testing. A determination of whether formal testing should be performed is based on physical examination findings, developmental and school histories, and concerns of the family and teachers. Males with Klinefelter syndrome often have developmental delay, especially in verbal cognitive areas where they underachieve in reading, spelling, and mathematics; their full IQ may be normal, but their verbal IQ is usually decreased. **Boys with Klinefelter syndrome often go unidentified until puberty because of the subtleness of the clinical findings. The diagnosis should be considered for all boys (regardless of age) who have been identified as having intellectual disability, or psychosocial, school, or adjustment problems.**

Physical findings to be considered in patients with suspected ID include the size of the occiput, unusual hair color or distribution, eye shape and placement, malformed ears or nose, and abnormalities in jaw size, mouth shape, or palate height. The hands and feet may have short metacarpals or metatarsals, overlapping or supernumerary digits, abnormal palmar creases, or nail changes. The skin may have café au lait spots or depigmented nevi, and the genitalia may be abnormally sized or ambiguous. Patients with Klinefelter syndrome typically are tall and thin with long extremities (Figure 41–1). The testes and phallus are often small for age, but this may not become apparent until puberty. As adults, males with Klinefelter syndrome develop gynecomastia, sparse facial hair, and azoospermia. The incidence of breast cancer and some hematologic cancers is elevated in Klinefelter syndrome.

Laboratory testing of a child with ID is based on the clinical findings and developmental milestones. A chromosomal analysis is often included in the evaluation of a child with ID if a genetic or syndromic cause is suspected; for Klinefelter syndrome such an analysis will most often demonstrate one extra X chromosome (47,XXY) but may show additional X chromosomes (48,XXXY) or mosaicism (46,XY/47,XXY). Other ID testing may include urine and serum amino and organic acids, serum levels of ammonia, lead, zinc, and copper, and serum titers for congenital infections. Radiologic evaluation may include cranial computed tomography (CT), magnetic resonance imaging (MRI), or electroencephalogram (EEG).

Management of children with ID includes specialized educational services, early childhood interventions, social services, vocational training, and psychiatric referral. Children with specific syndromes may benefit from diet modification, genetic counselling, and reviewing the natural disease course with the family.

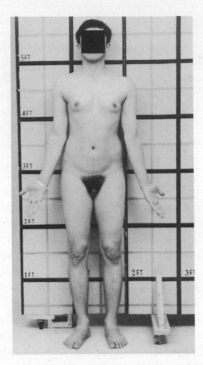

Figure 41–1. Klinefelter syndrome (XXY) in a 20-year-old man. Note relatively increased lower/upper body segment ratio, gynecomastia, small penis, and sparse body hair with a female pubic hair pattern. (*Reproduced, with permission, from Gardner DB, Shoback D.* Greenspan's basic & clinical endocrinology. *9th ed. New York: McGraw-Hill Education, 2011. Figure 12-7.*)

CASE CORRELATION

• See also Case 17 (Cerebral Palsy) which may have intellectual deficiency as part of its presentation.

COMPREHENSION QUESTIONS

41.1 An institutionalized male juvenile delinquent has severe nodulocystic acne, mild pectus excavatum, large teeth, prominent glabella, and relatively long face and fingers. His family says he has poor fine motor skills (such as penmanship), an explosive temper, and a low-normal IQ. What is the most likely diagnosis?

A. Fragile X syndrome

B. Klinefelter syndrome (XXY)

C. Turner syndrome (XO)

D. XXX syndrome

E. XYY male

41.2 A tall, thin 14-year-old adolescent boy has no signs of puberty. He was delayed in his speech development and always has done less well in school than his siblings. He is shy, and teachers report that he is immature. Physical examination reveals breast development and long limbs with a decreased upper segment–lower segment ratio. He has small testes and phallus. What is the most likely diagnosis?

A. Fragile X syndrome

B. Klinefelter syndrome (XXY)

C. Turner syndrome (XO)

D. XXX syndrome

E. XYY male

41.3 A 15-year-old adolescent girl with primary amenorrhea is noted to be well below the fifth percentile for height. She has hypertension, a low posterior hairline, prominent and low-set ears, and excessive nuchal skin. What is the most likely diagnosis?

A. Fragile X syndrome

B. Klinefelter syndrome (XXY)

C. Turner syndrome (XO)

D. XXX syndrome

E. XYY phenotypic female

41.4 A 7-year-old boy with ID was born at home at 26 weeks of gestation to a 28-year-old mother who had received no prenatal care. An evaluation is likely to suggest his ID is related to which of the following?

A. Brain tumor

B. Chromosomal aberration

C. Complications of prematurity

D. Congenital infection with cytomegalovirus

E. Elevated serum lead levels

ANSWERS

41.1 **E.** XYY-affected males often have explosive tempers. Other findings include long and asymmetrical ears, increased length versus breadth for the hands, feet, and cranium, and mild pectus excavatum. By the age of 5 to 6 years, they tend to be taller than their peers and begin displaying aggressive or defiant behavior.

41.2 **B.** With Klinefelter syndrome, testosterone replacement allows for more normal adolescent male development, although azoospermia is the rule; the breast cancer incidence approaches that of women.

41.3 **C.** Turner syndrome also includes widely spaced nipples and broad chest, cubitus valgus (increased carrying angle of arms), edema of the hands and feet in the newborn period, congenital heart disease (coarctation of the aorta or bicuspid aortic valve), horseshoe kidney, short fourth metacarpal and metatarsal, hypothyroidism, and decreased hearing. Intellectual development usually is normal.

41.4 **C.** Prematurity, especially when earlier than 28 weeks of gestation, is associated with complications (such as intraventricular hemorrhage) that can result in developmental delay and low IQ.

CLINICAL PEARLS

▶ Males with Klinefelter syndrome (XXY) have mild mental delay, eunuchoid habitus, gynecomastia, long arms and legs, and hypogonadism.

▶ XYY males have explosive (often antisocial) behavior, weakness with poor fine motor control, accelerated growth in mid-childhood, large teeth, prominent glabella and asymmetrical ears, and severe acne at puberty.

▶ Girls with Turner syndrome (45,XO) have short stature, amenorrhea, excessive nuchal skin, low posterior hairline, broad chests with widely spaced nipples, cubitus valgus, and coarctation of the aorta. Hypertension is common, possibly due to renal abnormalities (horseshoe kidney).

▶ Fragile X syndrome, the most common form of inherited intellectual disability, is seen primarily in boys and can be diagnosed in patients with intellectual disability (particularly boys) who have macrocephaly, long face, high arched palate, large ears, and macroorchidism after puberty.

REFERENCES

Accardo PJ, Accardo JA, Capute AJ. Mental retardation. In: McMillan JA, Feigin RD, DeAngelis CD, Jones MD, eds. *Oski's Pediatrics: Principles and Practice.* 4th ed. Philadelphia, PA: Lippincott Williams & Wilkins; 2006:608-614.

Ali O, Donohoue PA. Hypofunction of the testes. In: Kleigman RM, Stanton BF, St. Geme JW, Schor NF, Behrman RE, eds. *Nelson Textbook of Pediatrics.* 19th ed. Philadelphia, PA: WB Saunders; 2011:1943-1951.

American Academy of Pediatrics: Committee on Genetics. Health supervision for children with fragile X syndrome. *Pediatrics.* 2011;127; 994-1006.

Bacino CA, Lee B. Cytogenetics. In: Kleigman RM, Stanton BF, St. Geme JW, Schor NF, Behrman RE, eds. *Nelson Textbook of Pediatrics.* 19th ed. Philadelphia, PA: WB Saunders; 2011:394-415.

Carey JC. Chromosome disorders. In: Rudolph CD, Rudolph AM, Lister G, First LR, Gershon AA, eds. *Rudolph's Pediatrics.* 22nd ed. New York, NY: McGraw-Hill; 2011:691-697.

Goldson E, Reynolds A. Child development & behavior. In: Hay WW, Levin MJ, Sondheimer JM, Deterding RR. *Current Diagnosis & Treatment: Pediatrics.* 20th ed. New York, NY: McGraw-Hill; 2011:64-103.

Lewanda AF, Boyadjiev SA, Jaabs EW. Dysmorphology: genetic syndromes and associations. In: McMillan JA, Feigin RD, DeAngelis CD, Jones MD, eds. *Oski's Pediatrics: Principles and Practice.* 4th ed. Philadelphia, PA: Lippincott Williams & Wilkins; 2006:2629-2670.

Shapiro BK, Batshaw ML. Intellectual disability. In: Kleigman RM, Stanton BF, St. Geme JW, Schor NF, Behrman RE, eds. *Nelson Textbook of Pediatrics.* 19th ed. Philadelphia, PA: WB Saunders; 2011:122-129.

South ST, Carey JC. Human cytogenetics. In: Rudolph CD, Rudolph AM, Lister G, First LR, Gershon AA, eds. *Rudolph's Pediatrics.* 22nd ed. New York, NY: McGraw-Hill; 2011:688-691.

Stein DS, Blum NJ, Barbaresi WJ. Developmental and behavioral disorders through the life span. *Pediatrics.* 2011;128:364-373.

Tsai AC-H, Manchester DK, Elias ER. Genetics & dysmorphology. In: Hay WW, Levin MJ, Sondheimer JM, Deterding RR. *Current Diagnosis & Treatment: Pediatrics.* 20th ed. New York, NY: McGraw-Hill; 2011:1038-1039.

Vignozzi L, Corona G, Forti G, Jannini EA, Maggi, M. Clinical and therapeutic aspects of Klinefelter's syndrome: sexual function. *Mol Hum Reprod.* 2010;16:418-424.

A 6-year-old boy presents to the emergency department with his mother complaining of abdominal pain and has had several episodes of emesis over the last 3 hours. His mother states that he is extremely tired and has not been acting like himself for the past 2 days. Upon further questioning, you note that despite the patient's recent increase in appetite, he has lost weight. He has been asking for several glasses of water per day and has had new-onset nocturnal enuresis.

His vital signs include a heart rate of 155 beats/min, a respiratory rate of 40 breaths/min, a temperature of 37.5°C (99.5°F), and a blood pressure of 80/50 mm Hg. On examination, the patient is noted to be taking deep, rapid breaths and his capillary refill is prolonged at 4 seconds.

▶ What is the most likely diagnosis?
▶ What is the acute treatment for this condition?
▶ What is the most devastating, acute complication that is often seen with this condition?

ANSWERS TO CASE 42:

Diabetic Ketoacidosis

Summary: A 6-year-old boy with new-onset polyuria, polydipsia, and polyphagia is found to have increased pulse, decreased blood pressure, and increased respiratory rate.

- **Most likely diagnosis:** Diabetic ketoacidosis (DKA)
- **Best management for this condition:** Rehydration with IV fluids and intravenous insulin administration
- **Most devastating, acute complication that is likely to occur:** Cerebral edema

ANALYSIS

Objectives

1. Know the symptoms and laboratory irregularities associated with DKA.

2. Understand the principles of treatment of DKA.

3. Identify the most common complications associated with DKA.

Considerations

The patient has a recent history of polyuria, polydipsia, and polyphagia. He presents with signs consistent with dehydration, including increased pulse, decreased blood pressure, and increased capillary refill time. He also has labored breathing, consistent with Kussmaul respirations. His blood glucose should be checked at the bedside, because the most likely diagnosis is DKA. This condition is a medical emergency, and the first step in treatment should include management of Airway, Breathing, and Circulation. Once this initial evaluation is complete, fluid resuscitation and insulin administration should begin.

APPROACH TO:

Suspected Diabetic Ketoacidosis

DEFINITIONS

DIABETIC KETOACIDOSIS (DKA): A severe insulin deficiency that leads to decreased peripheral glucose utilization. Resultant complications include hypertonic dehydration, ketonuria, and metabolic disturbances including increased serum anion gap, decreased serum bicarbonate, decreased serum pH.

TYPE I DIABETES MELLITUS: An autoimmune insulin deficiency requiring administration of exogenous insulin to prevent ketoacidosis.

TYPE II DIABETES MELLITUS: A tissue-level insulin resistance that can require exogenous insulin administration if severe, but rarely leads to ketoacidosis.

KUSSMAUL RESPIRATIONS: Rapid, deep respirations associated with the compensatory respiratory alkalosis of DKA in response to the body's metabolic acidosis.

CLINICAL APPROACH

Diabetic ketoacidosis is often the presenting sign of type 1 diabetes in children and represents a medical emergency. Patients may complain of nausea and vomiting, fatigue, and severe abdominal pain at presentation. The history is frequently positive for polyuria and polydipsia, which result from serum glucose concentration exceeding the renal threshold for glucose reabsorption, which leads to osmotic diuresis. Consequently, these patients become dehydrated and will increase their caloric intake, while simultaneously losing weight.

Initial assessment of the patient with suspected DKA should include vital signs and a thorough physical examination, including mental status and neurologic evaluation. Vital signs are often indicative of dehydration, with increased pulse and decreased blood pressure. **Respirations are typically rapid and deep (termed Kussmaul respirations) which can eventually lead to fatigue and respiratory failure.** Patients are classically described as having "fruity breath," caused by acetone formation. Laboratory evaluation includes serum glucose, serum electrolytes including blood urea nitrogen (BUN) and creatinine, serum pH, and urinary ketones. Expected serum findings in a patient with DKA include elevated glucose (usually 400-800 mg/dL) and metabolic acidosis (decreased bicarbonate level with increased anion gap). Laboratory work also often reveals hyperkalemia, although total body potassium is invariably low. Hyponatremia is often seen, which is usually dilutional and results from increased serum glucose concentration. The true serum sodium concentration can be calculated by adding 1.6 mEq/L for every 100 mg/dL of serum glucose above the normal range. Because many cases of DKA are precipitated by infection, a complete blood count and cultures (urine and blood) are often obtained.

Because dehydration is usually severe (about 5%-10% in most patients), IV fluids should be administered at presentation. A bolus of 10 mL/kg of isotonic fluids is given prior to treatment with insulin. The remainder of the calculated fluid deficit should be replaced over the ensuing 48 hours. Because most patients are total body hypokalemic and hypophosphatemic, these electrolytes are added to the IV fluids early. Intravenous insulin infusion should also be initiated after the initial bolus at a rate of 0.05 to 0.1 units/kg/h with the infusion titrated based on the patient's hourly glucose concentration. Although the hyperglycemia resolves more quickly than the metabolic acidosis, intravenous insulin therapy is continued until the anion gap has closed. To prevent inadvertent hypoglycemia during the therapy phase, dextrose is added to the IV fluids once serum glucose levels reach 250 to 300 mg/dL. As the patient's hyperglycemia and metabolic acidosis resolve, intravenous insulin therapy can be discontinued and a transition to subcutaneous insulin can be initiated.

Although the treatment phase is benign in most children, the most devastating but fortunately rare complication of DKA is cerebral edema. As many as 20% to 25% of patients who develop cerebral edema will not survive, and those who do often have significant associated morbidities. Signs and symptoms of cerebral edema include severe headache, sudden deterioration of mental status, bradycardia, hypertension, and incontinence. If these signs or symptoms develop, immediate treatment with IV mannitol and hyperventilation should be initiated.

> ## CASE CORRELATION
>
> - See also Case 10 (Failure to Thrive) which can present with any chronic medical condition. Diabetes can be considered a secondary cause of immune deficiency (Case 40) and be heralded by oral or vaginal candidiasis.

COMPREHENSION QUESTIONS

42.1 A 16-year-old girl has enuresis, frequent urination, a white vaginal discharge, and a dark rash around her neck. Her weight is more than the 95th percentile for her age. Her serum glucose level is 250 mg/dL, and her urinalysis is positive for 2+ glucose but is otherwise negative. Which of the following is the most likely diagnosis?

A. Chemical vaginitis

B. Chlamydia cervicitis

C. Psoriasis

D. Type II diabetes

E. Urinary tract infection (UTI)

42.2 Six months after being diagnosed with what appears to be insulin-dependent diabetes, a 5-year-old boy has a significant decrease in his insulin requirement. Which of the following the most likely explanation?

A. His diagnosis of insulin-dependent diabetes was incorrect.

B. He had a chronic infection that is now under control.

C. He has followed his diabetes diet so well that he requires less insulin.

D. He is demonstrating the Somogyi phenomenon.

E. He has entered the "honeymoon phase" of his diabetes.

42.3 Upon presentation to the emergency department, a 6-year-old girl is found to have a serum glucose concentration of 650 mg/dL, pH of 7.2, bicarbonate of 13 mEq/L, and a potassium of 6.5 mEq/L. What is the first step in treatment?

A. Administer a normal saline bolus.

B. Administer a potassium binder.

C. Administer subcutaneous insulin.

D. Administer intravenous insulin.

E. Administer bicarbonate.

42.4 Thirty-six hours after initiation of treatment with insulin for DKA, a 4-year-old girl's serum glucose level is 230 mEq/L. Further laboratory work reveals a bicarbonate level of 16 mEq/L. She is currently receiving 0.1 units/kg/h of regular insulin as well as normal saline. What is the next step in treatment?

A. Continue current therapy.

B. Continue intravenous insulin therapy and change IVF to D5 0.45% normal saline.

C. Stop intravenous insulin therapy and allow the patient to begin subcutaneous insulin administration.

D. Continue intravenous insulin therapy and administer bicarbonate.

E. Stop intravenous insulin therapy and administer bicarbonate.

ANSWERS

42.1 **D.** The description is of an obese adolescent girl with candida vaginitis (white vaginal discharge) and acanthosis nigricans (the nuchal dark rash), which is consistent with type II diabetes. This condition is far more common in overweight children, especially those with a family history of the condition. Although each of these conditions alone could be caused by other diagnoses, the constellation is concerning for diabetes mellitus.

42.2 **E.** Up to 75% of newly diagnosed diabetics have a progressive decrease in the daily insulin requirement in the months after their diabetes diagnosis; a few patients temporarily require no insulin. This "honeymoon" period usually lasts a few months, and then an insulin requirement returns. A strict adherence to diabetic diet will not increase endogenous insulin production and the disease does not resolve with treatment.

42.3 **A.** The first step in treatment of DKA is intravenous fluid resuscitation which is done prior to the administration of any insulin. Although many patients have hyperkalemia on initial laboratory work due to their acidosis, they are often intracellularly depleted of potassium. Administering a potassium binder would further decrease her total-body potassium and could result in cardiac arrhythmias. Because insulin and correction of acidosis drives potassium intracellularly, administering insulin without supplementing the patient's potassium in IVF could also result in hypokalemia.

42.4 **B.** Although the patient's serum glucose is decreasing, her metabolic acidosis has not yet resolved and will require continued intravenous insulin therapy and IVF for treatment. The patient should not be converted to subcutaneous insulin until her glucose has normalized, her bicarbonate level is greater than 18 mEq/L, and her serum pH is greater than 7.3. Because of the risk of causing hypoglycemia with continued insulin therapy, dextrose should be added to her fluids. Bicarbonate therapy has not been shown to be effective in the treatment of metabolic acidosis associated with DKA and can actually be harmful.

CLINICAL PEARLS

▶ Although patients in DKA frequently have high potassium on initial laboratory tests, they are almost invariably intracellularly depleted. This will become evident once treatment with insulin is initiated.

▶ Hyponatremia may be because of the dilutional effects of increased serum glucose. To evaluate for the true value of sodium, add 1.6 mEq/L to the measured sodium value for each 100 mg/dL glucose which is elevated above the normal range.

▶ Correction of hyperglycemia occurs more quickly than metabolic acidosis. Intravenous infusion of insulin should continue until acidosis resolves and the anion gap closes.

▶ The most common complication of DKA is cerebral edema, which has high morbidity and mortality rates. Any child diagnosed with ketoacidosis who also exhibits signs of neurologic dysfunction should be evaluated for cerebral edema so that treatment can be initiated quickly.

REFERENCES

Alemzadeh R, Ali O. Diabetes mellitus. In: Kleigman RM, Stanton BF, St. Geme JW, Schor NF, Behrman RE, eds. *Nelson Textbook of Pediatrics.* 19th ed. Philadelphia, PA: WB Saunders; 2011:1068-1997.

Chase HP, Eisenbarth GS. Diabetes mellitus. In: Hay WW, Levin MJ, Sondheimer JM, Deterding RR, eds. *Current Diagnosis & Treatment: Pediatrics.* 20th ed. New York, NY: McGraw-Hill; 2011:984-991.

Cook DW, Plotnick L. Management of diabetic ketoacidosis in children and adolescents. *Pediatr Rev.* 2008;29:430-437.

Cooke DW. Type 2 diabetes mellitus. In: McMillan JA, Feigin RD, DeAngelis CD, Jones MD, eds. *Oski's Pediatrics: Principles and Practice.* 4th ed. Philadelphia, PA: Lippincott Williams & Wilkins; 2006:2115-2122.

Olivieri L, Chasm R. Diabetic ketoacidosis in the pediatric emergency department. *Emerg Med Clin N Am.* 2013;31:755-773.

Plotnick LP. Type 1 (insulin-dependent) diabetes mellitus. In: McMillan JA, Feigin RD, DeAngelis CD, Jones MD, eds. *Oski's Pediatrics: Principles and Practice.* 4th ed. Philadelphia, PA: Lippincott Williams & Wilkins; 2006:2103-2115.

Rosenbloom AL. Diabetes mellitus. In: Rudolph CD, Rudolph AM, Lister G, First LR, Gershon AA, eds. *Rudolph's Pediatrics.* 22nd ed. New York, NY: McGraw-Hill; 2011:2104-2125.

Tebben PJ, Schwenk WF. Diabetic ketoacidosis. In: McInerny TK, Adam HM, Campbell DE, Kamat DM, Kelleher KJ, Hoekelman RA, eds. *AAP Textbook of Pediatric Care.* https://www.pediatriccareonline.org/pco/ub/view/AAP-Textbook-of-Pediatric-Care/394342/0/chapter_342:_diabetic_ketoacidosis. Accessed April 14, 2014.

A 6-year-old boy is seen by his pediatrician for his yearly well-child visit. His mother is concerned about his weight gain since his last visit. She reports that he has added about 15 lb, but she has not noticed a major growth spurt. She admits frequent and daily eating of fast food. Further questions reveals that he often snores while sleeping and that he sometimes seems to gasp for air at night. At school, he is hyperactive and is having trouble keeping up his grades, often falling asleep in class. On physical examination, his weight is in the 95th percentile for his age (up from the 75th percentile on his last visit), and his body mass index has increased from 25 to 35. His physical examination is normal other than his oropharynx demonstrating bilateral tonsillar hypertrophy.

▶ What is the most likely diagnosis?
▶ What is the next step in the evaluation?
▶ What is the recommended first line management for this condition?

ANSWERS TO CASE 43:

Obstructive Sleep Apnea Syndrome

Summary: A 6-year-old obese boy with nighttime symptoms of snoring and gasping for air as well as daytime symptoms of hyperactivity, poor grades, and excessive daytime sleepiness.

- **Most likely diagnosis:** Obstructive sleep apnea syndrome (OSAS).

- **Next step:** Obtain an overnight polysomnogram (PSG) also known as a sleep study.

- **Best initial management:** Referral to an ENT (otolaryngologist) for evaluation and possible adenotonsillectomy (AT).

ANALYSIS

Objectives

1. Recognize the nighttime and daytime symptoms of OSAS.

2. Understand comorbid conditions of untreated OSAS.

3. Understand the diagnostic approach and management of patients with OSAS.

Considerations

This 6-year-old-boy exhibits classic nighttime and some daytime symptoms of OSAS. His comorbid obesity and hypertrophic tonsils are risk factors and key diagnostic clues for OSAS. Initial steps of management include ordering a nocturnal PSG, which will evaluate fully physiologic parameters during sleep and will help to diagnose the disorder. Should this testing suggest OSAS, his pediatrician should refer him to an otolaryngologist for evaluation of his tonsils and adenoids. If these structures are enlarged, an AT could relieve the obstructive component of his syndrome. While most patient do well after AT, some patients may have persistent OSAS. Appropriate weight management is appropriate for all obese children which will further reduce symptoms and a variety of health-related risks.

APPROACH TO:

Obstructive Sleep Apnea

DEFINITIONS

OBSTRUCTIVE SLEEP APNEA SYNDROME (OSAS): A breathing disorder in sleep with prolonged partial or complete obstruction of the upper airway during sleep, with resultant oxygen desaturation and hypercapnia.

PRIMARY SNORING: Snoring without associated respiratory disturbances such as apnea or hypopnea, hypoxemia, hypercapnia, or arousal from sleep.

POLYSOMNOGRAPHY (PSG): A comprehensive recording of the biophysiological changes that occur during sleep. The PSG monitors many body functions during sleep including brain (electroencephalogram [EEG]), eye movements (electrooculography [EOG]), muscle activity or skeletal muscle activation (electromyography [EMG]) and heart rhythm (electrocardiography [ECG]). Testing allows for the quantification of the severity of OSAS via the apnea-hypopnea index (AHI).

CLINICAL APPROACH

OSAS is a common health problem encountered by primary care physicians. The prevalence has been reported to range between 1% and 5% with the peak prevalence occurring between the ages of 2 to 8 years and without gender differences. Risk factors for this condition include obesity, anatomical factors (adenotonsillar hypertrophy, retro/micrognathia, tongue size), and increased upper airway collapsibility (altered neurological upper airway reflexes, hypotonia, upper airway inflammation). Obesity is an independent risk factor, especially in older children with OSAS. If left untreated, OSAS carries long-term morbidity such as behavioral, cognitive, cardiovascular, and growth problems. Neuropsychological and cognitive problems include attention deficit hyperactivity disorder (ADHD) or ADHD symptoms, hypersomnolence, somatization, depression, aggression, and abnormal social behaviors. Failure to thrive is seen in severe cases of OSAS.

Cardiovascular abnormalities such as left and right ventricular hypertrophy and elevated systolic and diastolic blooding pressures are associated with OSAS. Several studies suggest patients with OSAS have autonomic dysfunction such as increased heart rate variability, increased sympathetic vascular reactivity, and decreased cerebral blood flow. Some patients with OSAS have evidence of systemic inflammation (increased C-reactive protein and peripheral inflammatory markers). Thus, the increased sympathetic activity and upregulation of the inflammatory pathways may explain the increased cardiovascular risk in patients with OSAS.

The evaluation of OSAS starts with a history and physical examination, although both have a poor positive predictive value of 65% and 45%, respectively. One challenge of gathering a good history is that the symptoms of OSAS depend on parental observation and report. Snoring is a commonly reported symptom, but not all snoring is associated with OSAS. Primary snoring happens in individuals who do not have any associated ventilatory problems or sleep disturbances. A high level of suspicion from the clinician is required to pursue the diagnosis. Nighttime symptoms include snoring, excessive sweating, restless sleep, mouth breathing, apneas, gasping, labored or paradoxical breathing, and hyperextension of neck during sleep. Daytime symptoms include difficulty concentrating, behavioral and mood problems, morning headaches, excessive daytime sleepiness, and failure to thrive. The physical examination should include evaluation of growth parameters (obesity or failure to thrive), head and neck structures (enlarged tonsils/adenoids, excessive pharyngeal tissues, narrowed oropharynx, septal deviation, hypertrophic nasal turbinate, abnormal facial structures), and the cardiopulmonary system (hypertension, pulmonary hypertension, cor pulmonale, and right-sided heart failure).

When OSAS is suspected based on the history and physical examination, the next step is an overnight PSG. Nocturnal PSG is the current gold standard recommended by the American Academy of Pediatrics (AAP) because it can provide evidence of upper airways obstruction and differentiate obstructive apnea from central apnea. It can also record epileptic episodes in children with neurological disorders via EEG monitoring. Positive findings on the PSG trigger referral to an otolaryngologist for evaluation of the upper airway.

The most common cause of OSAS is adenotonsillar hypertrophy. Thus, AT typically is the primary treatment per AAP recommendations. Other treatment options include adenoidectomy, partial tonsillectomy, and nasal CPAP. A postoperative PSG is recommended to evaluate for complete resolution of OSAS symptoms. Most of the children with OSAS improve after AT, but some children have incomplete or no resolution in their symptoms. Risk factors for persistence of OSAS postoperatively include childhood obesity, worse baseline severity of OSAS, children older than 7 years, and children with asthma. Additional risk factors are based on underlying illnesses such as craniofacial anomalies, Down syndrome, and neuromuscular disease.

Nasal CPAP has been found to be an effective treatment of both clinical symptoms and PSG evidence of OSAS in young children. However, compliance is a major problem and, therefore, is not the recommended first-line treatment. Nasal CPAP use is reserved for children who have had poor response to surgery or are not surgical candidates.

Other therapies less commonly utilized include intranasal steroids and montelukast for mild OSAS. Maxillary expansion has been used to treat OSAS, but is relatively expensive.

COMPREHENSION QUESTIONS

43.1 A 3-year-old girl has been snoring and having excessive nighttime sweating as well as restless sleep. Which of the following symptoms would be most helpful in confirming your suspicion for obstructive sleep apnea syndrome (OSAS)?

A. Palpitations

B. Morning headaches

C. Urinary incontinence

D. Fevers

E. Skin rashes

43.2 A mother was concerned about OSAS in her 8-year-old child who snores and has attentional problems. Of the following, which is the most important independent risk factor associated with OSAS in older children?

A. Obesity

B. Being a twin

C. Prematurity

D. Congenital heart disease

E. Cerebral palsy

43.3 A father brings his 10-year-old son to his pediatrician concerned that he may have OSAS. The father was recently diagnosed with OSAS, but admits that his symptoms are a little different from his son's. What symptom is more commonly seen with adults with OSAS than in children with OSAS?

A. Excessive daytime sleepiness

B. Obesity

C. Nighttime sweating

D. Attention problems

E. Snoring

43.4 What does the American Academy of Pediatrics recommend as the gold standard for diagnosis of OSAS in children?

A. Apnea test

B. History and physical examination

C. Electroencephalography

D. Nocturnal polysomnogram

E. Nocturnal pulse oximetry

43.5 A 5-year-old-boy snores during sleep. On examination, he is found to have enlarged adenoids. After a diagnosis of OSAS has been made by PSG, what is the next step in management?

A. Prescribe CPAP.

B. Instruct patient to use intranasal steroids.

C. Perform rapid maxillary expansion.

D. Start montelukast orally.

E. Refer to otolaryngology for consideration of adenotonsillectomy.

ANSWERS

43.1 **B.** Nighttime symptoms are more easily recognizable, but daytime symptoms include morning headaches, difficulty concentrating, behavior and mood problems, excessive daytime sleepiness, and failure to thrive.

43.2 **A.** Obesity has become one of the most significant risk factors for OSAS in older children. Furthermore, obesity is also a risk for failure of adenotonsillectomy procedure to cure OSAS. For preschool-age children, the predominant remedial problem is adenotonsillar hypertrophy.

43.3 **A.** In contrast to adults, excessive daytime sleepiness does not seem to be as prominent in pediatric OSAS. Nonetheless, children with OSAS have been shown to have more daytime sleepiness than normal controls.

43.4 **D.** Gold standard for diagnosing OSAS in children according to the AAP is a nocturnal polysomnogram, which can quantify the severity of OSAS. History and physical examination alone have poor positive predictive values and can sometimes be misleading.

43.5 **E.** The first step in treatment of OSAS is a referral to an otolaryngologist for evaluation of adenotonsillectomy. Adenoidectomy alone and partial tonsillectomy allow for the regrowth of lymphoid tissue and recurrence of OSAS. Nasal CPAP is not well tolerated. Rapid maxillary expansion is not proven to be beneficial. Intranasal steroids and montelukast might help only for mild OSAS.

CLINICAL PEARLS

▶ Obstructive sleep apnea syndrome (OSAS) is common in children and is not readily distinguished from primary snoring by history and physical examination alone.

▶ The American Academy of Pediatrics recommends an overnight polysomnogram (PSG) as the gold standard to diagnose OSAS because it can provide an assessment of its severity.

▶ Untreated OSAS can lead to comorbidities such as behavioral, cognitive, cardiovascular, and growth problems.

▶ Adenotonsillectomy by an otolaryngologist is the first-line treatment of OSAS in most cases.

REFERENCES

Fitzgerald NM, Fitzgerald DA. Managing snoring and obstructive sleep apnea in childhood. *J Paediatr Child Health*. 2013;49:800-806.

Marcus CL, Brooks LJ, Draper KA. American Academy of Pediatrics. Diagnosis and management of childhood obstructive sleep apnea syndrome. *Pediatrics*. 2012;130:e714-e755.

Owens, JA. Sleep medicine. In: Kliegman RM, Stanton BF, St. Geme III JW, Schor NF, and Behrman RE, eds. *Nelson Textbook of Pediatrics*. 19th ed. Philadelphia, PA: Elsevier; 2011:46-55.

Tan HL, Gozal D, Kheirandish-Gozal L. Obstructive sleep apnea in children: a critical update. *Nat Sci Sleep*. 2013;5:109-123.

The parents of a healthy 8-year-old boy are concerned that he is the shortest child in his class. His height and weight growth curves are shown in Figure 44–1. He was a full-term infant, has experienced no significant medical problems, and is developmentally appropriate. Other than being small, his examination is normal. His upper and lower body segment measurements demonstrate normal body proportions. His father is 6 ft 4 in (193 cm) tall; he began pubertal development at 13 years of age. His mother is 5 ft 11 in (180 cm) tall; she had her first menstrual cycle at the age of 14 years.

▶ What is the most likely diagnosis?
▶ What is the best diagnostic test?
▶ What is the best therapy?

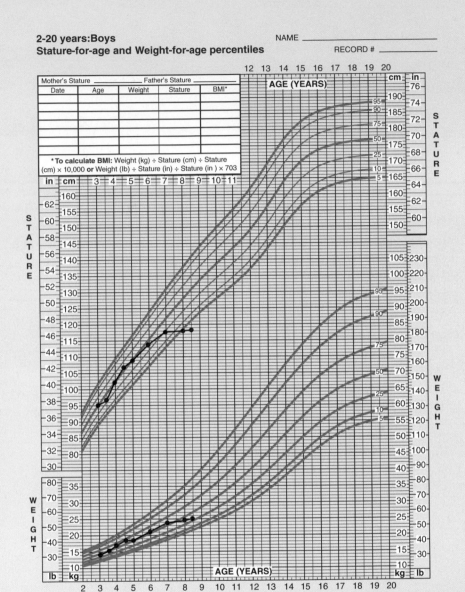

2-20 years:Boys
Stature-for-age and Weight-for-age percentiles

NAME _____

RECORD # _____

Figure 44–1. Childhood growth curve. (*Reproduced from the Centers for Disease Control and Prevention.*) Available at http://www.cdc.gov/growthcharts/clinical_charts.htm. Accessed on April 19, 2012.

ANSWERS TO CASE 44:
Growth Hormone Deficiency

Summary: An 8-year-old boy with no significant medical history and a normal examination presents with failure to grow.

- **Most likely diagnosis:** Growth hormone (GH) deficiency.

- **Best diagnostic test:** Screening tests might include a complete blood count (CBC) and erythrocyte sedimentation rate (ESR); electrolytes and general health chemistry panel; urinalysis; serum for thyroid function studies, insulin-like growth factor-1 (IGF-1), and insulin-like growth factor–binding protein-3 (IGF-BP3); bone age radiograph; and, if this were a girl, possibly chromosomal karyotype.

- **Best therapy:** Replace GH via injection.

ANALYSIS

Objectives

1. Understand the common causes of growth delay in children.

2. Appreciate the evaluation strategies for the various forms of growth failure.

3. Learn treatment options for common causes of childhood growth delay.

Considerations

This patient has essentially stopped growing (or is growing at a rate less than expected). He has no medical problems and a normal examination. His parents are tall, and their pubertal development was not delayed. An evaluation to determine the reason for his growth failure is appropriate.

APPROACH TO:
Growth Hormone Deficiency

DEFINITIONS

BONE AGE: Childhood bone development occurs in a predictable sequence. Left wrist radiographs on children older than 2 years (or the knee in those younger) are compared to published "normals" to determine how old the bones appear compared to chronologic age, thus providing an estimate of the remaining growth potential of the bones.

CONSTITUTIONAL GROWTH DELAY: A condition in which a healthy child's growth is slower than expected but for whom one or more parents demonstrated a pubertal development delay and ultimately normal adult height. In this case, the "bone age" equals the "height age."

FAMILIAL SHORT STATURE: A condition in which a short child is born to short parents who had normal timing of their pubertal development.

GROWTH VELOCITY: The increase in measured height or length over time as compared to standardized growth curves.

HEIGHT AGE: The age at which a child's measured height is at the 50th percentile.

IDIOPATHIC SHORT STATURE: A condition in which a short stature diagnosis cannot be reached.

CLINICAL APPROACH

Many parents become concerned if their child is noticeably shorter than their child's peers. Many conditions can result in short stature; a growth and social history (to identify psychosocial growth failure), physical examination, and selected screening tests usually help to identify the problem's etiology.

The growth velocity of a child is assessed by obtaining height and weight measurements over time and plotting them on standardized growth charts. Deviations from the normal on a growth chart are often the first clue a problem with growth exists. **In the first year of life, children grow at a rate of approximately 23 to 28 cm per year.** This rate **drops to approximately 7.5 to 13 cm per year for children aged 1 to 3 years.** Until puberty, they grow approximately 4.5 to 7 cm per year. **At puberty, growth increases to 8 to 9 cm per year for girls and to 10 to 11 cm per year for boys.** By approximately 24 months of age, most children settle into a percentile growth channel, remaining there for the remainder of their childhood. Significant deviations from these expectations alert the clinician to potential growth problems (ie, "fall off their curve").

Constitutional growth delay is a common cause of short stature. These children have no history or examination abnormalities. In contrast to children with GH deficiency, children with constitutional delay have a **growth rate that is normal.** Their family history is positive, however, for one or more parents with pubertal development delays ("late bloomers") who developed normal adult height. A short child in a family with a classic history of "late bloomers" often requires no laboratory or radiographic evaluation. Sometimes a bone age is helpful to reassure the patient and family that much bone growth remains and normal height will be achieved. For some of these children, testosterone injections will hasten pubertal changes (which eventually will begin on their own without treatment); consultation with a pediatric endocrinologist can be helpful.

The child born to short parents often is short **(familial short stature).** The growth curve shows growth parallel to a growth line at or just below the third to fifth percentile. Laboratory and radiographic testing usually are not necessary; a **bone age equals the chronologic age,** indicating no "extra" growth potential. An estimate of a child's ultimate height potential is calculated using the parents' heights. A boy's final height can be predicted as follows: (Father's height in cm + [Mother's height in cm + 13])/2. A girl's final height can be predicted as follows: (Mother's height in cm + [Father's height in cm + 13])/2. Reassurance is indicated for children with familial short stature.

Growth hormone (GH) deficiency occurs in approximately 1 in 4000 school-age children. These children demonstrate a **growth rate that is slow, usually falling away from the normal growth curve** (in contrast to constitutional delay where growth parallels the third to fifth percentile curves). On examination these children often appear younger than their stated age and frequently appear chubby (weight age > height age). **Bone ages are delayed,** indicating catch-up growth potential. Random sampling of GH level is of little diagnostic value because secretion is pulsatile and difficult to interpret. GH screening tests include serum IGF-1 or somatomedin C and IGF-BP3. Confirmation often requires GH stimulation testing and interpretation by a pediatric endocrinologist. Replacement therapy involves recombinant GH injections several times per week until the child reaches full adult height.

Clues that growth failure may be caused by an underlying condition not already mentioned include **poor appetite, weight loss, abdominal pain or diarrhea, unexplained fevers, headaches or vomiting, weight gain out of proportion to height, or dysmorphic features.** Screening tests might include a CBC (anemia), ESR (chronic inflammatory diseases), electrolytes (acidosis or renal abnormalities), general health chemistry panel (hepatitis, liver dysfunction), urinalysis (infection, renal disease), thyroid function tests (hypothyroidism), IGF-1, and IGF-BP3 (GH deficiency), and, for girls, possibly chromosomal analysis (Turner syndrome). Children with growth failure who do not fall into another, more appropriate category are classified as having idiopathic short stature.

CASE CORRELATION

- See also Case 10 (Failure to Thrive) which can present with growth failure.

COMPREHENSION QUESTIONS

44.1 An 8-year-old boy has short stature. He has no significant past medical history and his physical examination is normal. The growth curve shows growth parallel to a growth line at the fifth percentile. His father is 5 ft 4 in (163 cm), and his mother is 5 ft 1 in (155 cm). Radiograph of the left wrist shows a bone age equal to the chronological age. Which of the following is the most appropriate next step?

A. Reassure the parents that the child has normal prepubertal development.

B. Order thyroid function tests.

C. Order chromosomal analysis.

D. Refer to pediatric endocrinology for evaluation.

E. Obtain further radiographic imaging.

44.2 A 16-year-old boy complains that he is the shortest boy in his class. He has a normal past medical history, and although always a bit small for age, he has really noticed that he has fallen behind his peers in the last 2 years. He is Tanner stage 3 and is at the 5th percentile for height. His father began puberty at the age of 16 and completed his growth at the age of 19; he is now 6 ft 2 in (188 cm) tall. His mother began her pubertal development at the age of 10 and had her first menstrual period at the age of 13; her height is 5 ft 4 in (163 cm). Which of the following is the single most appropriate first intervention?

   A. Chromosomal analysis

   B. Liver function studies

   C. Measurement of bone age

   D. Measurement of somatomedin C

   E. Pediatric endocrinology referral

44.3 You are seeing 10-year-old girl for evaluation of short stature. Which of the following are important to the workup?

   A. History and physical including examination of growth chart

   B. Parental height, growth pattern, and timing of puberty

   C. Birth weight and length

   D. Assessment for underlying systemic disease

   E. All of the above

44.4 A 10-year-old girl is 4 ft 10 in (147 cm) tall. Her father is 5 ft 10 in (178 cm) tall, and her mother is 5 ft 5 in (165 cm) tall. Over the past 3 years she has dropped from the 25th percentile for height to the 5th percentile. Her weight has remained stable. Radiographs show bone age is delayed. Which of the following is the most appropriate next step in her management?

   A. Send patient to the emergency department for CT evaluation of the brain.

   B. Obtain growth hormone level.

   C. Obtain IGF-1 level.

   D. Start growth hormone injections.

   E. Provide reassurance to parents.

ANSWERS

44.1 **A.** This child likely has familial short stature because both his parents are short. Bone age does not show catch-up potential in this case. Additional imaging or laboratory evaluations would not be necessary in this case because this child has no other symptoms aside from short stature. Reassurance is the most appropriate choice.

44.2 **C.** This boy likely has constitutional growth delay, similar to that of his father. Bone age would be delayed, indicating potential growth. He eventually will enter puberty, but the psychosocial ramifications of remaining shorter and appearing more immature than his peers may warrant treatment. Monthly testosterone injections "jump start" the pubertal process without altering final growth potential; a pediatric endocrinologist might be required to assist.

44.3 **E.** All of the above should be investigated. The differential diagnosis for growth delay is broad (Table 44–1). A careful history and physical examination is the most important initial step. Any signs or symptoms of chronic disease would then warrant further evaluation. If a child's growth chart is unavailable, questions about a child's clothing or shoe size changes may provide valuable information. Obtaining history about parental growth pattern and their onset of puberty also provides important diagnostic clues to the child's etiology of short stature.

44.4 **C.** This child has evidence of possible growth hormone deficiency. Obtaining an IGF-1 level would be the most appropriate initial choice. Growth hormone deficiency is not an emergent condition but the earlier the diagnosis is made the sooner appropriate treatment can be initiated. Obtaining a growth hormone level would not be diagnostically helpful because its secretion is pulsatile. Referral to a pediatric endocrinologist would be warranted if initial screening tests confirm the suspected growth hormone deficiency.

Table 44–1 • CAUSES OF SHORT STATURE

Organ system disease
- Renal: renal tubular acidosis, electrolyte abnormalities
- Hematologic: anemia
- Rheumatologic: chronic inflammatory disease
- Gastrointestinal: hepatitis, liver dysfunction, inflammatory bowel disease (IBD), poor nutrition, malabsorption
- Cardiac: heart failure
- Pulmonary: asthma, cystic fibrosis
- Endocrinologic: growth hormone deficiency, hypothyroidism, glucocorticoid excess
- Skeletal disorders

Intrauterine growth restriction (IUGR)/Small for Gestational Age (SGA)

Genetic disorders
- Turner syndrome, Prader-Willi syndrome, Noonan syndrome
- Inborn errors of metabolism

Psychological/psychosocial
- Anorexia nervosa, depression, abuse/deprivation

Constitutional growth delay

Familial short stature

Medication use

CLINICAL PEARLS

▶ Constitutional growth delay is a condition in which a healthy child's growth is slower than expected and for whom at least one parent demonstrated a pubertal development delay but normal adult height ("late bloomers"). Growth parallels the third or fifth percentile growth curve; bone age is delayed.

▶ Familial short stature is a condition in which a short child is born to short parents who had normal timing of their pubertal development. Growth parallels the third or fifth percentile growth curve; bone age is normal.

▶ Idiopathic short stature includes children with short stature for whom a more appropriate diagnosis cannot be found.

▶ Growth hormone (GH) deficiency is a condition in which inadequate GH secretion results in growth failure, delayed bone age, and catch-up growth upon GH replacement.

REFERENCES

Ali O, Donohoue PA. Hypergonadotropic hypogonadism in the male (primary hypogonadism). In: Kleigman RM, Stanton BF, St. Geme JW, Schor NF, Behrman RE, eds. *Nelson Textbook of Pediatrics*. 19th ed. Philadelphia, PA: WB Saunders; 2011:1944-1948.

Moshang T, Grimberg A. Neuroendocrine disorders. In: McMillan JA, Feigin RD, DeAngelis CD, Jones MD, eds. *Oski's Pediatrics: Principles and Practice*. 4th ed. Philadelphia, PA: Lippincott Williams & Wilkins; 2006:2097-2103.

Parks JS, Felner EI. Hypopituitarism. In: Kleigman RM, Stanton BF, St. Geme JW, Schor NF, Behrman RE, eds. *Nelson Textbook of Pediatrics*. 19th ed. Philadelphia, PA: WB Saunders; 2011:1876-1881.

Plotnick LP, Miller RS. Growth, growth hormone, and pituitary disorders. In: McMillan JA, Feigin RD, DeAngelis CD, Jones MD, eds. *Oski's Pediatrics: Principles and Practice*. 4th ed. Philadelphia, PA: Lippincott Williams & Wilkins; 2006:2084-2092.

Reiter EO. Disorders of the anterior pituitary gland. In: Rudolph CD, Rudolph AM, Lister G, First LR, Gershon AA, eds. *Rudolph's Pediatrics*. 22nd ed. New York, NY: McGraw-Hill; 2011:2009-2012.

Reiter EO. Growth and growth impairment. In: Rudolph CD, Rudolph AM, Lister G, First LR, Gershon AA, eds. *Rudolph's Pediatrics*. 22nd ed. New York, NY: McGraw-Hill; 2011:2012-2017.

Thilo EH, Rosenberg AA. Disturbances of growth. In: Hay WW, Levin MJ, Sondheimer JM, Deterding RR. *Current Diagnosis & Treatment: Pediatrics*. 20th ed. New York, NY: McGraw-Hill; 2011:944-951.

Parents bring their 5-year-old daughter to your clinic because she has developed breast and pubic hair over the previous 3 months. Physical examination reveals a girl whose height and weight are above the 95th percentile, Tanner stage II breast and pubic hair development, oily skin, and facial acne.

▶ What is the most likely diagnosis?
▶ What is the best next step in the evaluation?

ANSWERS TO CASE 45:

Precocious Puberty

Summary: A 5-year-old girl has breast and pubic hair development, tall stature, and facial acne.

- **Most likely diagnosis:** Idiopathic central precocious puberty.

- **Next step in the evaluation:** Inquire about birth history, illnesses, hospitalizations, medications, siblings' health status, and family history of early puberty and diseases. Serum follicle-stimulating hormone (FSH) and luteinizing hormone (LH) levels and bone age radiographs are helpful.

ANALYSIS

Objectives

1. Understand the underlying causes of precocious puberty.

2. Describe laboratory and radiologic tests that are helpful in determining the etiology of precocious puberty.

3. Establish the treatment and follow-up necessary for a child with precocious puberty.

Considerations

This 5-year-old girl has precocious puberty signs (breast and pubic hair development and tall stature). She may have true (central) precocious puberty or precocious (noncentral) pseudopuberty. A central nervous system (CNS) cause of true precocious puberty must be ruled in girls younger than 6 to 8 years, and a CNS cause must be ruled out in boys at any age below or up to 9 years.

Of note, timing of puberty events approximates a normal distribution with a strong genetic component. Racial variation exists. For example African American children start puberty earlier on average than Caucasian children. Onset of puberty is likely multifactoral. A trend toward earlier start of puberty among today's children, as compared to previous generations, has been noted.

APPROACH TO:

Precocious Puberty

DEFINITIONS

DELAYED PUBERTY: No signs of puberty in girls by the age of 13 years or in boys by the age of 14 years. May be caused by gonadal failure, chromosomal abnormalities (Turner syndrome, Klinefelter syndrome), hypopituitarism, chronic disease, or malnutrition.

PRECOCIOUS PUBERTY: Onset of secondary sexual development before the age of 8 years in girls and 9 years in boys (2.5-3 standard deviations below the mean of 10.5 years in girls and 11.5 years in boys). Categorized as central or noncentral.

TRUE (CENTRAL) PRECOCIOUS PUBERTY: Gonadotropin dependent. Hypothalamic-pituitary-gonadal activation leading to secondary sex characteristics.

PRECOCIOUS (NONCENTRAL) PSEUDOPUBERTY: Gonadotropin independent. No hypothalamic-pituitary-gonadal activation. Hormones usually are either exogenous (birth control pills, estrogen, testosterone cream) or from adrenal/ovarian tumors.

INCOMPLETE PRECOCIOUS PUBERTY: Early breast development (typically in girls ages 1-4 years), no pubic/axillary hair development or linear growth acceleration (premature thelarche), or early activation of adrenal androgens (typically in girls ages 6-8 years), with gradually increasing pubic/axillary hair development and body odor (premature adrenarche).

CLINICAL APPROACH

More common in girls, true precocious puberty stems from secretion of hypothalamic GnRH with normal-appearing, but early, progression of pubertal events. Sexual precocity is **idiopathic in more than 90% of girls,** whereas a **structural CNS abnormality is present in 25% to 75% of boys.**

Girls with precocious pseudopuberty have an independent source of estrogens causing their pubertal changes. An exogenous source of estrogen (birth control pills, hormone replacement) or an **estrogen-producing tumor of the ovary or adrenal gland** must be considered. **CNS lesions** causing precocious puberty without neurologic symptoms are rarely malignant and seldom require neurosurgical intervention.

A detailed history offers important clues regarding the onset of puberty. Three main patterns of precocious pubertal progression can be identified, particularly in girls. Most girls who are younger than 6 years at onset have rapidly progressing sexual precocity, characterized by early physical and osseous maturation with a loss of ultimate height potential. Girls older than 6 years typically have a slowly progressing variant with parallel advancement of osseous maturation and linear growth and preserved height potential. In a small percentage of girls, a spontaneous regression or unsustained central precocious puberty at a young age is seen, with normal pubertal development at an expected age.

A neurologic history may identify past hydrocephalus, head trauma, meningoencephalitis, or the presence of headaches, visual problems, or behavioral changes. The type, sequence, and age at which pubertal changes were first noticed (breast and pubic/axillary hair development, external genitalia maturation, menarche) give valuable information regarding the etiology of the problem. Important questions include the following:

- Has the child been rapidly outgrowing shoes and clothes (evidence of linear growth acceleration)?

- Has the child's appetite increased?

- Has the child developed body odor?

- Was the child possibly exposed to an exogenous source of sex steroids (oral contraceptives, hormone replacement, anabolic steroids)?

- At what ages did parents and siblings undergo puberty?

- Can a known or suspected family history of congenital adrenal hyperplasia be identified?

Physical examination offers further important information. Serial height measurements are critical for determining the child's growth velocity. The skin should be examined for café-au-lait spots (neurofibromatosis, tuberous sclerosis), oiliness, and acne. The presence of axillary hair and body odor, the amount of breast tissue, whether the nipples and areolae are enlarging and thinning, and the amount, location, and character of pubic hair are documented (Tanner staging, Figures 45–1 and 45–2). The abdomen is palpated for masses.

Boys are examined for enlargement of the penis and testes (>2.5 cm in precocious puberty) and thinning of the scrotum (prepubertal scrotum is thick and nonvascular). If the testes are different in size and consistency, a unilateral mass is considered. Testicular transillumination may be helpful in differentiating a mass which is solid versus cystic (hydroceles usually transilluminate). In girls, the clitoris, labia, and vaginal orifice are examined to identify vaginal secretions, maturation of the labia minora, and vaginal mucosa estrogenization (dull, gray-pink, and ruggated rather than shiny, smooth, and red). A neurologic examination also is performed.

In precocious puberty, serum sex hormone concentrations usually are appropriate for the observed stage of puberty, but inappropriate for the child's chronologic age. Serum estradiol concentration is elevated in girls, and serum testosterone level is elevated in boys with precocious puberty. Because LH and FSH levels fluctuate, single samples often are inadequate. An immunometric assay for LH is more sensitive than the radioimmunoassay when using random blood samples; with this test, serum LH is undetectable in prepubertal children, but is detectable in 50% to 70% of girls (and an even higher percentage of boys) with central precocious puberty. A gonadotropin-releasing hormone (GnRH) stimulation test, measuring response time and peak values of LH and FSH after intravenous administration of GnRH, is a helpful diagnostic tool.

Bone age radiographs are advanced beyond chronologic age in precocious puberty. Organic CNS causes of central sexual precocity are ruled out by computed tomography (CT) or magnetic resonance imaging (MRI), particularly in girls younger than 6 years and in all boys. Pelvic ultrasonography is indicated if gonadotropin-independent causes of precocious puberty (ovarian tumors/cysts, adrenal tumors) are suspected based on examination.

The goal of treating precocious puberty is to prevent premature closure of the epiphyses, allowing the child to reach full adult growth potential. Gonadotropin-releasing hormone agonists are used for the treatment of central precocious puberty. These analogues desensitize the gonadotropic cells of the pituitary to the stimulatory effect of GnRH produced by the hypothalamus. Nearly all boys and most girls with rapidly progressive precocious puberty are candidates for treatment.

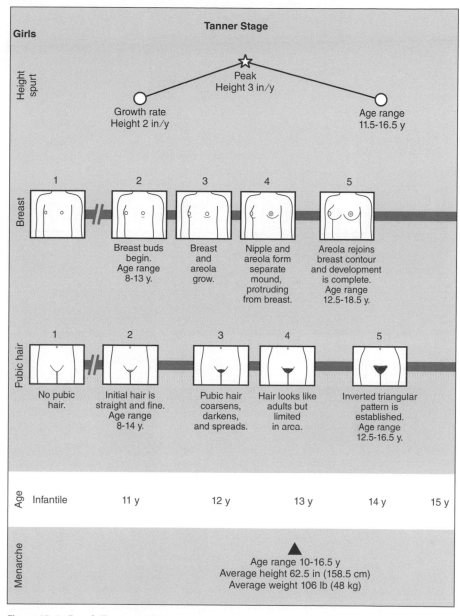

Figure 45–1. Female Tanner staging.

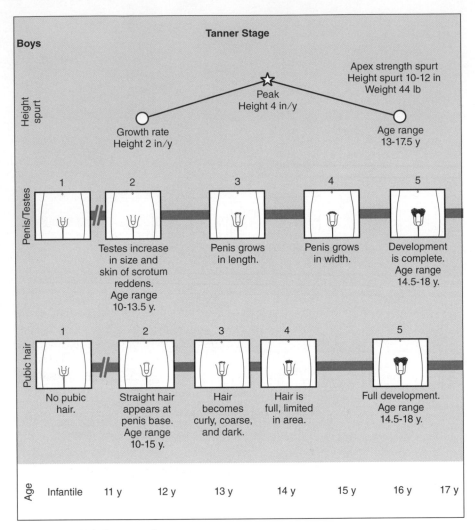

Figure 45–2. Male Tanner staging.

Girls with slowly progressive puberty do not seem to benefit from GnRH agonist therapy in adult height prognosis. A pediatric endocrinologist should evaluate children considered for GnRH agonist treatment.

> ## CASE CORRELATION
> - See also Case 5 (Ambiguous Genitalia) for a description of congenital adrenal hyperplasia in the newborn period.

COMPREHENSION QUESTIONS

45.1 A 5-year-old girl has bilateral breast development that was first noticed 6 months ago. She takes no medications, and no source of exogenous estrogen is present in the home. Family history is unremarkable. Physical examination reveals a girl who is at the 50th percentile for height and weight, with normal blood pressure, normal skin without oiliness, Tanner stage II breasts, soft abdomen without palpable masses, no body odor, no pubic/axillary hair, and mild estrogenization of the vagina. Which of the following is the most likely explanation for the child's breast development?

A. Adrenal tumor

B. Central precocious puberty

C. Congenital adrenal hyperplasia

D. Premature adrenarche

E. Premature thelarche

45.2 A 7-year-old girl presents to your office with her mother noting pubic hair growth over the last month. The girl also has started to develop breast buds. Growth and development are normal. Maternal history is remarkable for pubarche at age 11 years. Past medical history and family history are otherwise unremarkable. Your physical examination reveals genitalia and breast Tanner stage 3. Which of the following laboratory findings is most likely to be found?

A. Decreased estradiol, luteinizing hormone (LH) detectable, normal bone age for age

B. Decreased estradiol, LH undetectable, normal bone age for age

C. Elevated estradiol, LH detectable, advanced bone age for age

D. Elevated estradiol, LH detectable, normal bone age for age

E. Elevated estradiol, LH undetectable, advanced bone age for age

45.3 A 2-year-old boy presents to the office with his father due to concerns over the appearance of his son's genitals. He reports that over the last 2 months he has noticed his penis has gotten longer, frequent erections, and what appears to be a few dark strands of hair. On examination, you confirm that the phallus is long for stated age, pubic hair that is curly, and testicles that are less than 2.5 cm. His father denies any past medical history for his son and even states that he had imaging of his head during an ER visit for a fall 2 weeks prior which was normal. When you question the father about his onset of puberty, he claims to have noticed changes at 14 years old. He denies any other family history of illness. The child lives with his mother and father. Medications in the home include maternal intake of daily multivitamins and paternal gel for decreased libido. Which of the following statements is likely an explanation for this child's presentation?

A. Noncentral precocious puberty hypothalamic-pituitary-gonadal axis early activation

B. Noncentral precocious puberty from exogenous source of sex hormone

C. Central precocious puberty hypothalamic-pituitary-gonadal axis early activation

D. Central precocious puberty from exogenous source of sex hormone

E. Incomplete precocious puberty based on history and early thelarche

45.4 You are giving a lecture to medical students about the treatment of precocious puberty and its importance in preserving height. You discuss certain population segments where treatment would be most indicated and beneficial. Which of the following patient populations would benefit most from GnRH agonist therapy?

A. Younger children with rapidly progressing noncentral precocious puberty

B. Younger children with rapidly progressing central precocious puberty

C. Older children with rapidly progressing noncentral precocious puberty

D. Older children with rapidly progressing central precocious puberty

E. Younger boys with slowly progressing central precocious puberty

ANSWERS

45.1 **E.** All this child's findings are estrogen related and represent premature thelarche, a form of incomplete precocious puberty. She has no virilization. Postulated premature thelarche causes include ovarian cysts and transient gonadotropin secretion. No treatment is necessary. Bone age would be normal.

45.2 **C.** The child likely has precious puberty. With true precocious puberty hormonal levels mirror the physical appearance of the child (increased estrogen and detectable LH) because a premature activation of the hypothalamic pituitary gonadal axis has occurred. The bone age would also reflect these changes and appear older on wrist x-ray than her chronologic age.

45.3 **B.** Noncentral precocious is due to exogenous sources of sex hormones. This may be from a tumor or from the use of medications. In addition, the testicle size is greater than 2.5 cm in central precocious puberty. This question highlights a black box warning regarding the use of topical testosterone. Multiple case reports of males using testosterone gel and direct skin exposure resulting in virilization of close contacts including children have been noted. This virilization usually regresses after exposure to testosterone is withdrawn.

45.4 **B.** GnRH agonists are beneficial in patients with precocious puberty that is rapidly progressing. The younger the onset of precocious puberty, the greater the loss to final height a child will experience. Once the epiphyseal plates close, no additional growth potential exists. GnRH agonist shows no benefit in noncentral precocious puberty because the pathology involves an excess of exogenous sex hormone not affected by the hypothalamic-pituitary-gonadal axis.

CLINICAL PEARLS

▶ True precocious puberty is the onset of secondary sexual characteristics before the age of 8 years in girls and 9 years in boys. It stems from the secretion of hypothalamic gonadotropin-releasing hormone and is more common in girls.

▶ Precocious puberty is idiopathic in more than 90% of girls, and a structural central nervous system abnormality is noted in 25% to 75% of boys.

▶ When compared to norms, the serum estradiol level is elevated in girls and the testosterone level is elevated in boys with precocious puberty. Bone age radiographs are advanced beyond chronologic age.

▶ The goal of treating precocious puberty is to prevent premature closure of the epiphyses, allowing the child to reach full adult growth potential.

REFERENCES

Bhowmick SK, Ricke T, Rettig KR. Sexual precocity in a 16-month-old boy induced by indirect topical exposure to testosterone. *Clin Pediatr (Phila)*. 2007;46(6):540-543.

Boepple PA, Crowley WF Jr. Precocious puberty. In: Adashi EY, Rock JA, Rosenwaks Z, eds. *Reproductive Endocrinology, Surgery, and Technology*. Vol 1. Philadelphia, PA: Lippincott-Raven; 1996:989.

Garibaldi L, Chemaitilly W. Disorders of pubertal development. In: Kliegman RM, Stanton BF, St. Geme JW, Schor NF, Behrman RE, eds. *Nelson Textbook of Pediatrics*. 19th ed. Philadelphia, PA: WB Saunders; 2011:1886-1894.

Plotnick LP, Long DN. Puberty and gonadal disorders. In: McMillan JA, Feigin RD, DeAngelis CD, Jones MD, eds. *Oski's Pediatrics: Principles and Practice*. 4th ed. Philadelphia, PA: Lippincott Williams & Wilkins; 2006:2079-2084.

Rosen DS. Physiologic growth and development during adolescence. *Pediatr Rev*. 2004;25:194-200. doi: 10.1542/pir.25-6-194.

Styne DM, Cuttler L. Normal pubertal development. In: Rudolph CD, Rudolph AM, Lister GE, First R, Gershon AA, eds. *Rudolph's Pediatrics*. 22nd ed. New York, NY: McGraw-Hill; 2011:2074-2077.

White PC. Congenital adrenal hyperplasia and related disorders. In: Kliegman RM, Stanton BF, St. Geme JW, Schor NF, Behrman RE, eds. *Nelson Textbook of Pediatrics*. 19th ed. Philadelphia, PA: WB Saunders; 2011:1930-1939.

A mother reports that her 4-year-old daughter complains of sore throat and difficulty swallowing for 3 days. She has been irritable and does not want to move her neck. Her appetite and intake have decreased, and she has vomited twice overnight. She exhibits no symptoms of upper respiratory tract infection (URI). She is otherwise healthy with up-to-date immunizations. Her physical examination is remarkable for fever to 102°F (38.9°C), bilateral tonsillar exudates, and an erythematous posterior oropharynx with right posterior pharyngeal wall swelling.

▶ What is the most likely diagnosis?
▶ What is the most appropriate next step in the evaluation?

ANSWERS TO CASE 46:

Retropharyngeal Abscess

Summary: An ill-appearing toddler with sore throat, odynophagia, fever, and an abnormal oropharyngeal examination.

- **Most likely diagnosis:** Retropharyngeal abscess.

- **Next step in evaluation:** Laboratory testing might include group A β-hemolytic streptococcus (GAS) immunoassay and culture. Radiologic evaluation might include lateral cervical x-ray and computed tomography (CT) or magnetic resonance imaging (MRI) to elucidate location and extent of infection.

ANALYSIS

Objectives

1. Discuss the diagnosis and treatment of retropharyngeal abscess.

2. Differentiate between various forms of neck abscess.

3. Discuss neck conditions presenting similarly to retropharyngeal abscess.

Considerations

History and examination for this toddler with odynophagia, fever, and posterior pharyngeal swelling is consistent with retropharyngeal abscess. Because a variety of head and neck lesions can present similarly, the diagnostic challenge lies in determining whether a bacterial infection is present, the extent of infection, whether the potential exists for spread to surrounding vital structures, and the need for urgent surgical intervention.

APPROACH TO:

Retropharyngeal Abscess

DEFINITIONS

RETROPHARYNGEAL SPACE: Located posterior to the esophagus and extending inferiorly into the superior mediastinum; bordered by layers of the deep cervical fascia; contains lymphatics draining the middle ears, sinuses, and nasopharynx.

PARAPHARYNGEAL (LATERAL) SPACE: Located lateral to the pharynx and bordered by muscles of the styloid process; comprises anterior and posterior compartments containing lymph nodes, cranial nerves, and carotid sheaths; infections in the lateral space can originate from the oropharynx, middle ears, and teeth.

PERITONSILLAR SPACE: Located superior and lateral to the tonsillar capsule and bordered by pharyngeal musculature; infection in the peritonsillar space typically is an extension of acute or recurrent tonsillitis.

EPIGLOTTITIS: Infection of the cartilaginous structure that protects the airway during swallowing; often characterized by a toxic-appearing child with drooling and fever; bacterial etiology historically *Haemophilus influenzae* type B (HiB) before widespread use of the HiB vaccine; most cases now involve *Streptococcus pyogenes*, *Streptococcus pneumoniae*, or *Staphylococcus aureus*; emergent airway obstruction is possible, and treatment involves intravenous antibiotics.

RAPID STREP IMMUNOASSAY: Detects GAS antigen by latex agglutination or enzyme-linked immunosorbent assay; high specificity and variable sensitivity with false-negative results possible.

MONOSPOT: Latex agglutination of heterophile antibodies to erythrocytes in Epstein-Barr virus (EBV) infection; high specificity and sensitivity in patients older than 3 years; infection may be confirmed by EBV immunoglobulin (Ig)M antibody if heterophile is negative.

STRIDOR: Abnormal, musical breathing because of large airway obstruction.

DYSPHAGIA: Difficulty swallowing.

ODYNOPHAGIA: Pain on swallowing.

TRISMUS: Inability to open the mouth secondary to pain or inflammation or mass effect involving facial neuromusculature.

CLINICAL APPROACH

Categorization of deep neck infections is based on a combination of **examination findings** and **neck imaging.** Multiple compartments exist within the neck, bordered by musculature and fascia and containing various neurovascular structures (cranial nerves and carotid arteries); infections can easily spread along these fascial planes. The type and extent of infection ultimately determine whether a patient requires surgery and could be at risk for infection of nearby vital structures, including the mediastinum.

Some age predilections are noted in neck abscess. **The typical pediatric patient with retropharyngeal abscess, for example, is a toddler younger than 4 years,** coinciding with the time when retropharyngeal lymph nodes are prominent (which atrophy by puberty) and when the majority of URI and otitis cases are seen. **Peritonsillar abscess** can be seen at any age, but **prevalence is greater in the adolescents or young adults.** Of all abscess types, **peritonsillar abscess is the most common type in the pediatric population.**

Infections of the various neck spaces may present similarly. Fever, irritability, toxicity, and decreased oral intake are common, with patients usually complaining of sore throat, dysphagia, odynophagia, or trismus (with trismus noted more frequently in peritonsillar or parapharyngeal infection). Drooling, increased work of breathing, or frank stridor may be seen with oropharyngeal infection or edema. Torticollis, neck pain (particularly on neck extension), or limited neck mobility in the context of a patient with sore throat and fever, is suspicious for retropharyngeal infection; on examination, posterior oropharyngeal wall edema or bulge may be seen. Neck lymphadenopathy is noted more often in patients with peritonsillar or parapharyngeal abscess. Peritonsillar or soft palatal swelling is more prominent with peritonsillar abscess.

Imaging in the patient with suspected neck abscess starts with a **lateral cervical x-ray.** Radiographic evidence for retropharyngeal abscess on a lateral film includes widening of the retropharyngeal space. Findings on a lateral film in a patient with sore throat and fever may lead to an alternative diagnosis such as epiglottitis which presents with epiglottic edema and **classic "thumb sign."** Cervical CT imaging offers a more precise radiologic diagnosis in deep neck abscess, and is an excellent study for determining whether a patient has only cellulitis and edema surrounding a neck space, or hypodensity and rim enhancement consistent with an abscess. It also delineates whether there has been extension to contiguous structures. An MRI is an alternative when there is a concern for infection involving a compartment with neurovascular elements and more accurate visualization is desired.

Specific neck space infections have specific origins and complications, dependent upon lymphatic channels, fascial planes, and nearby vital structures. An infection in one compartment often can spread to another. Generally, a neck abscess results when there is contiguous spread of bacteria in a patient with pharyngitis, odontogenic infection, otitis, mastoiditis, sinusitis, or other head and neck infection. Parapharyngeal space abscess stems from the teeth, ears, and pharynx, and may ultimately impact neurovascular elements in the lateral space, specifically by erosion or mass effect involving the carotid artery sheath. **Lymph chains draining the sinuses, nasopharynx, and oropharynx can seed the retropharyngeal space, with potential for spread to the mediastinum,** where impact on cardiorespiratory function (upper airway obstruction, aspiration pneumonia following abscess rupture), or mediastinitis could develop.

Bacterial etiologies for neck abscess include *Streptococcus pyogenes* (GAS), *Staphylococcus* sp, *Haemophilus influenzae*, *Peptostreptococcus* sp, *Bacteroides* sp, and *Fusobacterium* sp. Polymicrobial infection is typically seen, often reflective of the organisms most commonly found in infections involving the oropharynx, ear, or sinuses.

Viral etiologies include EBV, cytomegalovirus, adenovirus, and rhinovirus and may present similarly to bacterial infection. Viruses can present with oropharyngeal exudate and swelling or neck masses in the form of lymphadenopathy. A viral process usually can be differentiated from a more concerning bacterial process by ancillary testing previously described and observing symptomatology more frequently seen in viremia. For example, an exudative pharyngitis with neck findings, rhinorrhea, and cough is more consistent with viral infection.

Standard therapies include intravenous penicillins, advanced-generation cephalosporins, or carbapenems. Clindamycin or metronidazole is added if anaerobes are suspected and broad coverage is desired. Clindamycin often is a good choice for monotherapy in the patient with penicillin allergy. Broad-spectrum antibiotics are started in the patient with neck abscess, with treatment modification if an organism is identified from oropharyngeal or surgical samples.

Ultimately, pediatricians and surgeons determine whether to pursue a "watchful waiting" approach with a patient receiving antibiotics, or to proceed quickly with needle aspiration or incision and drainage. The severity of clinical presentation and imaging studies, extent of infection, current impact on surrounding structures, and expectations for progression often drive this decision. **Emergent surgical drainage may be required in the patient with respiratory distress (concerning for abscess-related airway obstruction), or with rapid, progressive deterioration (toxicity, persistent high fever) despite intravenous antibiotics.**

Other abnormalities, unrelated to deep neck infection can present with sore throat, odynophagia, or swelling and pain of the oropharynx and neck. They include anatomic variants such as thyroglossal duct cyst or second branchial cleft cyst. Arising from vestigial structures, these cysts can become secondarily infected and develop overlying tenderness and erythema that might be confused with deeper infection. Thyroiditis and sialadenitis also present with fairly localized neck findings. Depending on location, one also should consider thyroid nodule, goiter, or salivary gland tumor, particularly in the case of an initially nontender mass that grows slowly.

COMPREHENSION QUESTIONS

46.1 A mother notices a lump on her 5-year-old son's neck. He complains about pain in the region and difficulty swallowing. Appetite and intake are normal. On examination, he is afebrile with a 3 × 3-cm area of mild erythema, fluctuance, and tenderness of the central anterior neck. The mass moves superiorly when he opens his mouth. His oropharynx is clear. Which of the following symptoms was most likely present during the preceding week?

A. Diarrhea

B. Abdominal pain

C. Dizziness

D. Urinary frequency

E. Cough

46.2 A 9-year-old girl complains of sore throat and anterior neck pain of 1-day duration, and nasal congestion and cough over the past 3 days. There has been no nausea or change in appetite. She describes "lumps growing in her neck" over the past day. Her past medical history is unremarkable. She is afebrile with a clear posterior oropharynx and a supple neck. She has four firm, fixed, and minimally tender submandibular masses without overlying skin changes; the largest mass is 1 cm in diameter. Which of the following is the most likely explanation for these findings?

A. Lymphadenopathy

B. Peritonsillar abscess

C. Retropharyngeal abscess

D. Sialadenitis

E. Streptococcal pharyngitis

46.3 A father states that his 7-year-old daughter has a 1-week history of mouth and neck pain. She describes pain on chewing and swallowing. Slight swelling around her right, lower jaw was first noted yesterday. She has been afebrile and exhibits no upper respiratory tract infection (URI) symptoms. Her examination reveals a temperature of 100.2°F (37.9°C) with swelling, tenderness, and warmth overlying the right, posterior mandible without fluctuance or skin changes. Scattered, bilateral neck lymphadenopathy is appreciated. Her posterior oropharynx is minimally erythematous, with marked swelling and tenderness of the gum surrounding the posterior molars of the right mandible. Which of the following is the most appropriate next step?

A. Admit her immediately to the hospital for intravenous antibiotics.

B. Commence a broad-spectrum antibiotic and advise her to see a dentist as soon as possible.

C. Obtain an immediate surgery consult.

D. Order a cervical CT and obtain ear, nose, and throat (ENT) consultation today.

E. Perform a rapid strep immunoassay in your clinic.

46.4 A previously healthy 4-year-old boy has been febrile for a day. He does not want to drink and vomited this morning. There have been no URI symptoms or diarrhea. On examination, he is sleepy, but arousable, and has a temperature of 102.8°F (39.3°C). His posterior oropharynx is markedly erythematous with enlarged, symmetrical, and cryptic tonsils that are laden with exudate. Shoddy cervical lymphadenopathy is noted. He moves his head vigorously in an effort to thwart your examination. Which of the following is the next best step in your evaluation?

A. Lumbar puncture

B. Cervical CT

C. Tonsillar needle aspiration

D. Rapid streptococcal testing

E. Complete blood count

ANSWERS

46.1 **E.** Thyroglossal duct cysts, arising from the embryonic thyroglossal tract, are typically midline, often move on tongue protrusion, and often are noted after an URI. Treatment is usually surgical excision, sometimes after neck CT imaging to ascertain cyst and thyroid anatomy. About half can become infected.

46.2 **A.** This patient has viral URI symptoms, most likely causing reactive lymphadenopathy. Supportive care such as analgesics would be a reasonable treatment recommendation. Rapid streptococcal testing usually is not warranted for classic URI symptoms; streptococcal pharyngitis more commonly presents with sore throat (typically exudative pharyngitis), headache, nausea, and/or fever. Signs of viremia and her neck examination do not suggest sial-adenitis or neck abscess.

46.3 **B.** Tooth abscess is her most likely diagnosis, as evidenced by obvious gingival inflammation and other signs of ongoing infection in the area, despite the absence of frank pus from an evident cavity. Potential causative organisms include *Streptococcus mutans* and *Fusobacterium nucleatum*. Therapy includes an antibiotic (amoxicillin or clindamycin) and referral to her dentist within the next 24 hours. Deep neck infection is unlikely; imaging and IV antibiotics are not warranted at this time.

46.4 **D.** This child has a fairly classic examination for streptococcal tonsillitis. The potential for a retropharyngeal or peritonsillar process is diminished by the lack of tonsillar asymmetry, soft palatal changes, and nuchal rigidity. A rapid streptococcal immunoassay would be a good initial test; a swab for culture may be sent as well. Standard therapy would include oral or intramuscular penicillin in the nonallergic patient and an analgesic/antipyretic. If the strep-tococcal immunoassay is negative, some treat patients whose history and examination are consistent with streptococcal infection while awaiting cul-ture results.

CLINICAL PEARLS

▶ Infections involving specific compartments of the neck have specific complications, such as the potential for mediastinitis in the patient with retropharyngeal abscess.

▶ Multiple bacterial and viral etiologies, including GAS and EBV, are possible in the patient with constitutional symptoms and neck findings. Extension of these infections into cervical compartments may endanger surrounding vital structures.

▶ Treatment of deep neck infection involves intravenous antibiotics and possible surgical intervention, depending on the severity of presentation and radiographic extent of infection.

▶ Various head and neck abnormalities (infected thyroglossal duct cyst or extensive reactive lymphadenopathy) may mimic deep neck infection.

REFERENCES

Goldstein NA, Hammersclag MR. Peritonsillar, retropharyngeal, and parapharyngeal abscesses. In: Feigin RD, Cherry JD, Demmler-Harrison GJ, Kaplan SL, eds. *Textbook of Pediatric Infectious Disease*. 6th ed. Philadelphia, PA: Saunders; 2009:177-181.

Inkelis SH. Disorders of the pharynx. In: Osborn LM, DeWitt TG, First LR, Zenel JA, eds. *Pediatrics*. Philadelphia, PA: Elsevier Mosby; 2005:460-470.

Milczuk H. Disorders of the neck and salivary glands. In: Osborn LM, DeWitt TG, First LA, Zenel JA, eds. *Pediatrics*. Philadelphia, PA: Elsevier Mosby; 2005:471-479.

Pappas DE, Hendley JO. Retropharyngeal abscess, lateral pharyngeal (parapharyngeal) abscess, and peritonsillar cellulitis/abscess. In: Kliegman RM, Stanton BF, St. Geme JW, Schor NF, Behrman RE, eds. *Nelson Textbook of Pediatrics*. 19th ed. Philadelphia, PA: WB Saunders; 2011:1440-1442.

Weed HG, Forest LA. Deep neck infection. In: Flint PW, Haughey BH, Lund VJ, Niparko JK, Robbins KT, Thomas JR, Richardson MA, eds. *Cummings Otolaryngology: Head and Neck Surgery*. 5th ed. Philadelphia, PA: Elsevier-Mosby; 2010:201-208.

A 13-year-old boy presents with left knee pain of 1 month's duration. His mother says that she has noticed him limping for the past 3 days. The pain is described as dull and aching. He denies any history of trauma or paresthesias. The pain is exacerbated with exertion and relieved by rest. The pain does not awaken the patient at night nor does it radiate. On physical examination, his blood pressure is 100/70 mm Hg, heart rate 105 beats/min, the height at the 50th percentile for age, and the weight greater than the 90th percentile for age. The knee does not appear red, warm, or swollen and has no obvious deformities. While supine, his left leg is slightly externally rotated at rest as compared to the right. He has no tenderness to palpation of the left knee. Passive motion is limited by intense pain. On gait, he limps to avoid bearing weight on the left leg with downward pelvic tilt toward the right when he steps on his left leg.

▶ What is the most likely diagnosis?
▶ What are complications that can occur due to this condition?
▶ What is the best management for this condition?

ANSWERS TO CASE 47:

Slipped Capital Femoral Epiphysis

Summary: A 13-year-old obese boy complains of left knee pain and is found to be limping on examination. He has an antalgic and Trendelenburg gait.

- **Most likely diagnosis:** Slipped capital femoral epiphysis (SCFE).

- **Complications that can occur:** Osteonecrosis and chondrolysis.

- **Best management for this condition:** Consult orthopedic surgery for in situ pinning.

ANALYSIS

Objectives

1. Know the differential diagnosis of knee pain with limp in a child.

2. Understand the clinical presentation of SCFE.

3. Understand that identification of SCFE requires a high degree of suspicion. Management includes immediate institution of non–weight-bearing status on the suspected extremity and evaluation by orthopedic surgery.

4. Know the most common complications of SCFE.

Considerations

Slipped capital femoral epiphysis (SCFE) is a disorder involving the displacement of the femoral head. The condition occurs most commonly in early adolescence with an incidence varying from 1 in 100,000 children to 8 in 100,000. The condition occurs more frequently in boys and in African American children. The peak age for presentation is 11 to 13 years for girls and 13 to 15 years for boys. Roughly 65% of affected individuals are above the 90th percentile for their weight for age. The condition occurs on the contralateral side in 20% to 25% of affected children.

This patient demonstrates the typical presentation of SCFE: *overweight adolescent boy who presents with knee pain and limp.* SCFE can present as groin, hip, or knee pain. In many cases where the patient presents with knee pain, the diagnosis may be delayed due to normal knee examination and knee radiographs. Knee pain can occur because of hip pathology, especially in children. To prevent a delay in SCFE diagnosis and possible transformation of a stable to an unstable condition, a thorough examination of the hips in children complaining of knee pain is warranted. A diagnostic clue on physical examination is external rotation during hip flexion.

APPROACH TO:
Slipped Capital Femoral Epiphysis

DEFINITIONS

SLIPPED CAPITAL FEMORAL EPIPHYSIS (SCFE): A displacement of the femoral neck from the femoral head. This condition can be divided into a "stable SCFE" characterized by an ability to bear weight *or* no displacement of the femoral epiphysis. An "unstable SCFE" is characterized as an inability to bear weight *or* displacement of the femoral epiphysis.

OSTEONECROSIS: Also known as avascular necrosis is a complication of SCFE.

CHONDROLYSIS: A breakdown of the femoroacetabular joint cartilage with no clear etiology, but more commonly seen in unstable slips.

ANTALGIC GAIT: The gait cycle can be broken down into two components: the stance phase and the swing phase. In conditions where it is painful to bear weight on the affected leg, the body adapts an antalgic gait, characterized by a short stance phase (the time the foot is touching the ground).

TRENDELENBURG GAIT: Downward pelvic tilt when stepping on the affected leg from gluteal muscle weakness on the affected side.

DEVELOPMENTAL DYSPLASIA OF THE HIP (DDH): A condition of abnormal development of the hip joint. Multiple causes may lead to DDH. An underlying risk factor for the multiple causes is conditions that limit mobility of the hip joint whether in utero or after birth. These conditions include breech presentation, oligohydramnios, and large-for-gestational age infants. Because screening of the hip mobility begins at birth, DDH is usually diagnosed in the newborn period. Screening consists of provocative physical examination maneuvers to test for hip joint laxity, namely the Ortolani and Barlow test.

LEGG-CALVE-PERTHES DISEASE (LCPD): An idiopathic avascular necrosis of the femoral head. LCPD typically presents as thigh or knee pain with limp in a child. Similar to SCFE, the limp can be an antalgic with a Trendelenburg gait. The age of onset ranges between 3 and 12 years of age. Although the clinical presentation is similar to SCFE, radiographs of the hip in anteroposterior (AP) and frog leg views help differentiate the etiology. LCPD will show joint space widening due to loss (necrosis) of the femoral head height. With suspected LCPD, the patient should be made non–weight bearing and have immediate orthopedic evaluation. The goal of treatment is to prevent further necrosis and to promote bone remodeling by maintaining the femoral head within the acetabulum. These goals are best accomplished by casting the affected leg in an abducted and internally rotated fashion.

CLINICAL APPROACH

Slipped capital femoral epiphysis is characterized as displacement through the growth plate of the femoral neck from the femoral head. It classically appears on a radiograph as an ice-cream scoop slipping off a cone, which represents the displacement of the shaft from the femoral epiphysis (Figure 47–1). Note that it is actually anterior superior displacement of femoral epiphysis that in plain radiographs appears as posterior inferior displacement of the femoral epiphysis (ice-cream scoop slipping). The relationship between the femoral head and acetabulum is maintained.

On physical examination this condition is characterized by an antalgic and Trendelenburg gait. The diagnosis is confirmed by clinical presentation and plain films of the hip: AP and lateral (which may include the frog-leg view). Imaging of both

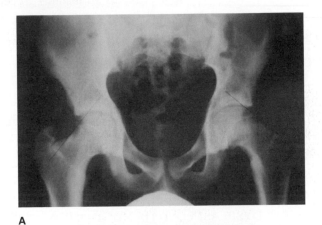

A

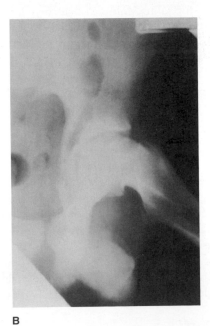

B

Figure 47–1. X-ray picture of slipped capital femoral epiphysis. (*Reproduced, with permission, from Skinner HB, McMahon PJ. Current Diagnosis & Treatment in Orthopedics. 5th ed. New York: McGraw-Hill Education, 2013. Figure 10-14.*)

hips is indicated due to the high frequency of bilateral involvement. If strong clinical suspicion for SCFE exists despite normal plain radiograph, magnetic resource imaging (MRI) can be used to detect early SCFE. Early MRI findings include haziness between the interface of the femoral epiphysis and metaphysis, widening of the joint angle, and effusion. These findings can later progress to displacement of the femoral metaphysis from the epiphysis. The degree of displacement is characterized by mild, moderate, and severe categorizations.

The onset of SCFE is most commonly seen during early adolescence. During puberty, physiologic widening of the growth plate is seen which increases the risk of mechanical forces to cause shear stress. Mechanical load (obesity) and endocrine issues (eg, hypothyroidism and renal osteodystrophy) may play a role. Identification of endocrinopathies should be sought especially in the child with an atypical presentation and who is less than 10th percentile in height and/or less than 50th percentile in weight.

The differential diagnosis of an adolescent patient with a limp and Trendelenburg gait includes DDH and LCPD. Physical examination and radiographs can help distinguish the etiology. Helpful features that differentiate DDH from SCFE include the lack of pain being a chief complaint in DDH, earlier onset of DDH (typically presents when the child first begins walking around 2 years of age), and toe walking in DDH on the affected side to compensate for the shortened leg length.

When SCFE is suspected, the patient should immediately be made non–weight bearing (crutches, wheelchair, or stretcher). Then, imaging to confirm the diagnosis can begin. These precautions help prevent worsening of an unstable SCFE or transforming a stable to an unstable SCFE. After confirmation by radiographs, the patient will require immediate orthopedic surgery evaluation to determine the timeframe for surgical pinning of the femoral head. The overall goal of treatment is stabilization of the femoral head and neck. Uniquely, in patients with a *displaced* SCFE, reduction is NOT performed during pinning of the femoral head. Reduction increases the risk of vascular compromise and subsequent avascular necrosis of the femoral head.

Because in up to 30% to 60% of cases, SCFE eventually occurs on the contralateral hip; some surgeons elect to simultaneously perform bilateral femoral pinning as prophylaxis.

CASE CORRELATION

- Other conditions that may present with a limp, abnormal gait, or leg pain include rickets (Case 12), sickle cell disease (Case 13), and leukemia (Case 19).

COMPREHENSION QUESTIONS

47.1 A 7-year-old boy is seen in the pediatrician's office because his mother has noticed him limping for the past few days. She has given him acetaminophen with only mild relief of pain. His temperature is 101°F (38°C), HR 120 beats/min, BP 100/70 mm Hg, and his weight is at the 97th percentile for age. On examination, his right knee is red, warm, and swollen. Range of motion testing is limited because the patient is guarding and begins crying. What of the following is the best next step in management?

A.   Send the patient for an x-ray of his knee and hip joint and ask them to return the same day.

B.   Provide reassurance. The mainstay of therapy is *rest, ice, compression, and elevation*.

C.   Immediately admit the patient to the hospital for IV antibiotics.

D.   Obtain an erythrocyte sedimentation rate (ESR) and C-reactive protein (CRP) and ensure early follow-up the following day.

E.   Send a referral to orthopedic surgery.

47.2 A 2-year-old boy is seen by the pediatrician for a 1-week history of limping. His father says he slipped and fell after playing outside the previous week. On physical examination, his left thigh is swollen and he has an antalgic gait. You notice bruises on his buttocks and inner thighs. His father comments that he is very active and always gets bumps and bruises. The patient's past medical history is significant for two previous ER visits for fractures. Which of the following would be the best diagnostic test for this patient's condition?

A.   Skeletal survey

B.   Anteroposterior (AP) and frog-legged radiographs of the hip

C.   Complete blood count (CBC), coagulation studies, von Willebrand factor activity, serum factor 8 and 9 level

D.   Ultrasound of the hip joint

E.   Observation and reassurance

47.3 A new 16-year-old patient is seen by the pediatrician before beginning her school year; her family has just moved into town. Her past medical history is significant recent hospitalization for slipped capital femoral epiphysis (SCFE) 6 months prior where she underwent internal pinning of her left hip. Her growth curve shows declining growth velocity from 50th percentile several years ago to the 15th percentile currently. Her weight is in the 85th percentile. Her mother notes that she often is tired and sleeps until noon every day, but attributes it to being a teenager on summer vacation. Her physical examination is within normal limits. Upon questioning she reports no trouble falling or staying asleep and goes to bed around 10 PM nightly. Which of the following is the best next step in management?

A. Repeat magnetic resource imaging (MRI) of the left hip.

B. Thyroid function studies.

C. Noncontrast computed tomography (CT) of the head.

D. Provide reassurance.

E. Start the patient on an antidepressant.

47.4 An 11-year-old boy is seen in the physician's office complaining of right hip pain when he walks. On physical examination, he has an antalgic gait, pain on passive range of motion of his right hip, and external rotation during hip flexion. What of the following is the next best step in management?

A. Place the patient in non–weight-bearing status and obtain bilateral hip films.

B. Send a referral to orthopedic surgery.

C. Obtain synovial fluid by arthrocentesis of the right hip joint.

D. Recommend nonsteroidal anti-inflammatory drugs (NSAIDs) and follow-up in 2 weeks.

E. Obtain bilateral knee films.

ANSWERS

47.1 **C.** The patient likely has septic arthritis of his right knee and needs immediate hospital admission for intravenous antibiotics. His evaluation would include complete blood count, an ESR, a CRP, and blood cultures. In addition, he requires a joint aspiration for Gram stain and culture. Immediate inpatient or emergency center orthopedic surgery evaluation for the possibility of surgical drainage and wash out of his knee joint is appropriate. Septic joint is an emergency because the joint can be destroyed within hours. Depending on his hospital course, the patient may require long-term IV antibiotics or may be transitioned to oral therapy. SCFE, developmental dysplasia of the hip (DDH), or Legg-Calve-Perthes do not present with fever. Moreover, erythema and warmth are not typical features of any of these latter conditions.

47.2 **A.** This patient requires an immediate evaluation for nonaccidental trauma (NAT). After a thorough history and physical examination, the best diagnostic tool for NAT is a skeletal survey. Such patients typically are admitted to the hospital, and a skeletal survey will be done to evaluate for active or healing fractures. Child protective services should also be contacted. Important features that support NAT are delay in seeking medical care, inconsistent or vague history, and physical examination findings that appear as bruises in the shape of an object (hand, spatula), burns in the shape of the end of a cigarette, and bruising behind the ear, neck, trunk, or inner thighs.

47.3 **B.** Given her older age of onset and her short stature, this patient has atypical SCFE. A patient who presents with atypical SCFE deserves an evaluation for an underlying etiology. Given this adolescent's findings of fatigue and excessive sleeping, hypothyroidism is the most likely cause. The best diagnostic test would be thyroid function studies. Depression can also result in a complaint of excessive sleeping. An evaluation for depression, rather than simply initiating antidepressant therapy, is appropriate.

47.4 **A.** This patient has characteristic clinical symptomatology of SCFE: a male in early adolescence who demonstrates a gait characterized by pain during weight bearing and a key diagnostic clue on physical examination of external rotation of the hip during hip flexion. Prior to obtaining radiographs in the patient with suspected SCFE, the patient is immediately made non–weight bearing to prevent further displacement.

CLINICAL PEARLS

▶ The typical presentation of SCFE is an *overweight adolescent boy who presents with knee pain and limp.*

▶ Films of both hips are indicated if one suspects SCFE due to the high rate of bilateral involvement.

▶ The mainstay of therapy for SCFE is immediate immobilization and surgical pinning of the femoral head.

REFERENCES

Boos SC, Endom EE. Physical abuse in children: diagnostic evaluation and management. In: Wiley JF, ed. *UpToDate.* http://www.uptodate.com/home/index.html. Accessed May 20, 2014.

Clark MD. Approach to the child with a limp. In: Wiley JF, ed. *UpToDate.* http://www.uptodate.com/home/index.html. Accessed May 20, 2014.

Kienstra A, Macias C. Evaluation and management of slipped capital femoral epiphysis. In: Wiley JF, ed. *UpToDate.* http://www.uptodate.com/home/index.html. Accessed May 20, 2014.

Krogstad P. Bacterial arthritis: clinical features and diagnosis in infants and children. In: Torchia MM, ed. *UpToDate.* http://www.uptodate.com/home/index.html. Accessed May 20, 2014.

Podeszwa D. Slipped capital femoral epiphysis. In: Rudolph CD, Rudolph AM, Lister GE, First LR, Gershon AA, eds. *Rudolph's Pediatrics.* 22nd ed. New York, NY: McGraw-Hill; 2011:855-856.

Sponseller PD. Bone, joint, and muscle problems. In: McMillan JA, Feigin RD, DeAngelis CD, Jones MD, eds. *Oski's Pediatrics: Principles and Practice*. 4th ed. Philadelphia, PA: Lippincott Williams & Wilkins; 2006:2471-2476.

Wudbhav N, Sankar B, Horn D, Wells L, Dormans JP. Developmental dysplasia of the hip. In: Kliegman RM, Stanton BF, St. Geme JW, Schor NF, Behrman RE, eds. *Nelson Textbook of Pediatrics*. 19th ed. Philadelphia, PA: WB Saunders; 2011: 2356-2360.

Wudbhav N, Sankar B, Horn D, Wells L, Dourmans JP. Legg-Calve-Perthes disease. In: Kliegman RM, Stanton BF, St. Geme JW, Schor NF, Behrman RE, eds. *Nelson Textbook of Pediatrics*. 19th ed. Philadelphia, PA: WB Saunders; 2011:2361-2363.

Wudbhav N, Sankar B, Horn D, Wells L, Dourmans JP. Slipped capital femoral epiphysis. In: Kliegman RM, Stanton BF, St. Geme JW, Schor NF, Behrman RE, eds. *Nelson Textbook of Pediatrics*. 19th ed. Philadelphia, PA: WB Saunders; 2011:2363-2365.

CASE 48

A 10-year-old boy is accompanied by his parents to the pediatrician's office with complaints of headache and decreased activity for the previous week. The patient reports bilateral throbbing frontal pain that is associated with nausea. The headaches last for 1 to 3 hours and occur throughout the day. He has had one episode of vomiting the previous afternoon. The headaches do not wake him from sleep, but he does report that bright lights bother him. The headaches have been severe enough to force him to miss school 3 days In the previous week. His past medical history is positive for similar episodes of headaches when he was 5 years old. He denies seeing flashing lights, having vision changes, or weakness prior to or associated with the headache. His mother reports she has a similar history of headaches.

▶ What is the next step in the management of this patient?
▶ What is the most likely diagnosis?
▶ What is the best management?

ANSWERS TO CASE 48:

Migraine Without Aura

Summary: A 10-year-old boy with a recurrent history of bilateral throbbing frontal headaches lasting for hours associated with vomiting and photophobia.

- **Next step in evaluation:** Gather more information, including birth, past medical, family, social, and developmental histories. Perform thorough physical examination, with particular attention to neurologic examination.

- **Most likely diagnosis:** Primary headache, most likely migraine without aura.

- **Best management:** Nonsteroidal anti-inflammatory drugs (NSAIDs) to treat acute headache, antiemetics to help with nausea, and biobehavioral therapy to identify triggers and perform biofeedback-assisted relaxation therapy.

ANALYSIS

Objectives

1. Identify primary versus secondary headache.

2. Identify and understand common signs for serious disease for a patient with headache.

3. Understand diagnosis and management of migraines and tension headaches.

4. Understand workup and evaluation of secondary headaches.

Considerations

This 10-year-old's presentation does not identify any concerns for a secondary headache (intracranial lesion, infection, etc). His symptoms, recurrent nature, and presence of positive family history are highly suggestive for the diagnosis of migraine. When a patient presents with complaints of headache, it is important to be able to identify signs or symptoms suggestive of a more serious headache or secondary headache (where the headache is a symptoms of an underlying cause). This requires detailed history taking and a thorough physical and neurologic examination.

Areas of concern for secondary headache are as follows:

- Headache is more severe, frequent or is new/different from previous episodes.

- Nocturnal/morning headaches with emesis or headache awakens patient from sleep.

- Neurologic signs or symptoms other than headache are present.

- Sudden onset of explosive headache.

- Headache worsens with coughing, straining, or exertion.

- Absence of family history of migraines.

- Systemic symptoms such as fever, hypertension, etc are present.

APPROACH TO:
Headache in Children

DEFINITIONS

PRIMARY HEADACHE: A usually benign headache disorder that is recurrent and episodic in nature and cannot be attributed to another disorder. Examples include migraines and tension headaches.

SECONDARY HEADACHE: Headache that is a symptom of an underlying cause. Examples include increased intracranial pressure, infection, trauma, bleeding, tumors, and medication overuse.

MIGRAINE: Primary headache disorder characterized by moderate to severe, episodic focal headaches often associated with nausea, vomiting, photophobia, or phonophobia. This condition usually has a strong hereditary component, can cause disability, and may be associated with an aura. The pain can last from 1 to 72 hours.

AURA: Neurologic warning that a migraine may occur. Usually lasts 5 to 60 minutes and the headache begins during or within an hour of the aura. Auras may be visual, sensory, or dysphasic.

STATUS MIGRAINOSUS: Migraine lasting more than 72 hours.

TENSION HEADACHE: Primary headache disorder characterized by mild to moderate diffuse headache with pain described as being tight, pressure, or band-like. Often has associated muscle pain and tension in neck and shoulders. Pain can last for 1 hour to several days.

CLINICAL APPROACH

Headache is a common complaint in pediatrics. The history and physical examination are the most important tools in evaluating a patient with headaches. The goals of the history and physical examination are first to identify whether the patient is experiencing any signs or symptoms for serious, emergent pathology (as described previously) and then to determine whether the headache is primary or secondary.

Primary headaches are common, benign, recurrent, and episodic headache disorders such as tension headaches and migraines. Secondary headaches are headaches that are a symptom of an underlying cause. Secondary headaches may be due to infection (such as meningitis, sinusitis, acute viral illness), trauma, tumors, intracranial hemorrhage, increased intracranial pressure, analgesic medication overuse, carbon monoxide poisoning, caffeine or alcohol withdrawal, or lead toxicity. Secondary headaches often require further laboratory and imaging evaluation.

Tension headaches are mild to moderate band-like, tightening headaches that are not localized. They may be episodic or chronic, and the duration can vary from 1 hour to several days. They typically are not associated with nausea, vomiting, photophobia, phonophobia, or auras. They are not affected by activity and are often associated with muscle pain of the shoulders and neck. Treatment involves behavioral therapy (identifying stressors, relaxation techniques) and analgesia with NSAIDs and acetaminophen.

Migraines commonly begin in children aged 5 to 15 years. Causes of migraines are multifactorial; however, they are associated with a strong genetic predisposition. Migraines can be triggered by stress, illness, fatigue, dehydration, and poor sleep. Unlike adults in whom migraine headaches are usually unilateral, children can present with unilateral or bilateral migraine headaches. Children may also have associated symptoms of nausea and vomiting, abdominal pain, and decrease in activity or appetite. Sleep often relieves the migraine symptoms.

Migraines without aura are the most common form of migraines in adults and children (Table 48–1). Migraine headaches can have a large impact on a patient's quality of life. Debilitating migraines can cause prolonged absences or poor performance in school, anxiety, and social withdrawal. The diagnosis of migraine headaches does not require workup with laboratory testing or imaging. Imaging may be warranted in the presence of signs or symptoms of more serious disease or in the absence of family history of migraine headaches.

Treatment of migraines includes acute, preventive, and behavioral therapy. The goal of abortive or acute therapy is to stop the headache and help the patient to return to their baseline function as quickly as possible. The treatment of choice and first step in therapy is NSAIDs. If the headache does not remit with NSAIDs, triptans may be used. FDA-approved medications for childhood migraines include rizatriptan (for ages 6-17 years) and almotriptan (for adolescents). Antiemetics also are useful to combat the migraine-associated nausea. Preventive therapy is recommended for patients who experience frequent (two to three episodes per month) and disabling migraines. Medications used for preventive therapy include topiramate, valproic acid, β-blockers, tricyclic antidepressants, and cyproheptadine. Biobehavioral therapy (identifying migraine triggers, learning to avoid them, and

Table 48–1 • DIAGNOSTIC CRITERIA FOR MIGRAINE

The diagnostic criteria for migraines without aura require at least five attacks that:
1. Last 1-72 hours (untreated or unsuccessfully treated)
2. Have two or more of the following characteristics:
   a. Unilateral or bilateral frontal or temporal pain
   b. Pulsing or throbbing in nature
   c. Moderate to severe pain
   d. Aggravated or causes avoidance of routine physical activity
3. Have at least one of the following:
   a. Nausea or vomiting
   b. Photophobia or phonophobia
4. Is not due to another disorder

Modified, with permission, from Headache Classification Subcommittee of the International Headache Society. The International Classification of Headache Disorders. 2nd ed. Cephalgia 2004;24(suppl 1):9-160.

utilizing behavioral techniques such as relaxation and biofeedback therapy) can be helpful in the treatment of migraines and tension headaches. Proper hydration, regular meals, adequate sleep, and caffeine avoidance are important lifestyle factors that may decrease migraine frequency.

CASE CORRELATION

- Myriad other conditions may present with headaches. Failure to thrive (Case 10) and headache may suggest a chronic condition such as brain tumor. Acute onset of headache, especially if associated with acute neurologic symptoms in the patient with sickle cell disease (Case 13) may represent stroke. The younger child with developing neurologic symptoms and headache may be a victim of lead toxicity (Case 25). Bacterial meningitis (Case 27) may present with acute headache along with other symptoms such as fever for organism such as pneumococcus or with more chronic headache if associated with organisms such as tuberculosis. A child with head injury (accidental or inflicted) may have a headache associated with subdural hematoma (Case 29).

COMPREHENSION QUESTIONS

48.1 A 3-year-old boy is brought to the emergency room for vomiting, decreased oral intake, and lethargy. The parents report that for the previous week he has been vomiting, crying, and irritable every morning after awakening from his sleep. They report he holds his head while complaining of pain and that he seems to be bothered by lights and loud sounds. He was seen by his pediatrician earlier in the week and diagnosed with gastroenteritis. Despite being prescribed antiemetics, the vomiting has not resolved. The family denies fevers, trauma, or diarrhea. After completing a thorough physical examination, which of the following is the most appropriate diagnostic test?

A. Serum electrolytes

B. Plain radiograph of the skull

C. Magnetic resonance imaging (MRI) of the brain

D. Lumbar puncture

E. Complete blood count with differential

48.2 An obese 15-year-old girl complains of daily headaches for the previous 5 days. She describes the headaches as being throbbing in quality, diffuse, and 9/10 in severity. She reports nausea and notes blurry vision and ringing in her ears the previous few days. The pain worsens when she sneezes or coughs. She has had no relief with over-the-counter medications; sleep does not improve her symptoms. Her vital signs include temperature 99.1°F (37.3°C), BP 152/91 mm Hg systolic and diastolic, respectively, HR 90 beats/min, and RR 12 breaths/min. Physical examination reveals papilledema. Which of the following is the most likely diagnosis?

A. Subdural hemorrhage

B. Pseudotumor cerebri

C. Migraine headache

D. Meningitis

E. Tension headache

48.3 A 9-year-old boy with a past medical history significant for migraines is seen by the pediatrician during a particularly debilitating episode. He has missed a week of school and has not been able to resume his normal activities due to pain. The mother reports she has been giving him acetaminophen for pain without improvement. Which of the following medications would be the next step in treating his migraine?

A. Morphine

B. Rizatriptan

C. Cyproheptadine

D. Ibuprofen

E. Phenobarbital

48.4 A 16-year-old girl is diagnosed with tension headaches. She is a very ambitious and high-achieving student. She has final examinations due in the upcoming week and she is very anxious. She takes naproxen for the headaches with some relief. The patient and her parents ask about possible lifestyle modifications that may reduce her headache frequency. Which of the following would be the LEAST useful recommendation?

A. Limit your caffeine intake to less than three servings per week.

B. Avoid skipping meals during the day.

C. Turn off and remove your laptop from your bedroom at night.

D. Drink at least eight cups of water per day.

E. Avoid aerobic exercise as it would make her more tired.

ANSWERS

48.1 **C.** Imaging the brain would be the next diagnostic test of choice because the patient is demonstrating signs and symptoms of serious pathology (history with early morning vomiting and headaches awakening him from sleep). In this case, a secondary headache due to increased intracranial pressure is of concern. At present the cause of the intracranial pressure is unknown. Thus, MRI is imaging of choice because it can evaluate for structural abnormalities, masses, infection, inflammation, and ischemia. Computerized tomography (CT) of the head may be considered in cases concerning for fracture or hemorrhages.

48.2 **B.** Pseudotumor cerebri is an idiopathic condition characterized by increased intracranial pressure resulting in a secondary headache. Symptoms include daily headaches, nausea/vomiting, diplopia, tinnitus, blurry vision, and transient blindness. It is often seen in obese female adolescents. Physical examination can show papilledema and cranial nerve III, IV, or VI palsies. Imaging such as CT or MRI is normal, but lumbar puncture will show increased opening pressure (>25 mm Hg). Other causes of increased intracranial pressure include hydrocephalus, tumor, edema, and hemorrhage.

48.3 **D.** NSAIDS are the first line for abortive therapy for migraines. Rizatriptan is a second-line therapy used for abortive therapy if NSAIDS do not work. In this case, the patient has tried acetaminophen only. Therefore, ibuprofen would be treatment of choice. Cyproheptadine is used in prophylactic therapy. Opioids and barbiturates are not recommended for initial migraine therapy.

48.4 **E.** Lifestyle interventions in managing primary headaches can be remembered by the mnemonic SMART: regular and adequate SLEEP (avoiding computer use/television use immediately prior to bedtime), regular and nutritious MEALS and hydration, ACTIVITY with regular but not excessive aerobic exercise, RELAXATION and stress reduction, and TRIGGER avoidance (stress, sleep deprivation, caffeine).

CLINICAL PEARLS

▶ A thorough history and physical examination is the most important diagnostic tool in the evaluation of a headache.

▶ Secondary headaches are headaches due to an underlying cause.

▶ Signs and symptoms of serious pathology for headaches include headache that is more severe, frequent or is new/different from previous episodes; nocturnal/morning headaches with emesis or headache that awakens patient from sleep; neurologic signs or symptoms are present; sudden onset of explosive headache; headache worsens with coughing, straining, or exertion; no family history of migraines; presence of systemic symptoms.

▶ Migraines treatment includes abortive therapy with NSAIDs as first choice and then triptans if these fail. Preventive therapy includes topiramate, valproic acid, β-blockers, tricyclic antidepressants, cyproheptadine (especially in young children), and biobehavioral therapy.

▶ MRI is imaging of choice to evaluate for secondary headache, unless hemorrhage or fracture is suspected based on history and physical in which case CT is recommended.

REFERENCES

Blume, HK. Pediatric headache: a review. *Pediatr Rev*. 2012;33:562-575.

El-Chammas K, Keyes J, Thompson N, Vijayakumar J, Becher D, Jackson JL. Pharmacologic treatment of pediatric headaches: a metanalysis. *JAMA Pediatrics*. 2013;167:250-258.

Hershey AD. Headaches. In: Kleigman RM, Stanton BF, St. Geme JW, Schor NF, Behrman RE, eds. *Nelson Textbook of Pediatrics*. 19th ed. Philadelphia, PA: WB Saunders; 2011:2039-2046.

Hershey AD. Headache. In: McInerny TK, Adam HM, Campbell DE, Kamat DM, Kelleher KJ, eds. *American Academy of Pediatrics Textbook of Pediatric Care*. Elk Grove Village, IL: American Academy of Pediatrics; 2009:1550-1556.

Prensky AL. Headache. In: McMillan JA, Feigin RD, DeAngelis CD, Jones MD, eds. *Oski's Pediatrics: Principles and Practice*. 4th ed. Philadelphia, PA: Lippincott Williams & Wilkins; 2006:2389-2395.

CASE 49

A 13-year-old boy presents to the emergency room by ambulance from a city park. An elderly couple noted his bizarre behavior and called 911. He arrives disoriented and complaining of double vision. He is noted by the triage nurse to have flushed skin and excessive salivation. His parents soon arrive, and report that he has been more argumentative over the past month, with occasional erratic behavior and nonsensical speech. They question whether he may be hallucinating at times, because he occasionally reports seeing odd shapes and colors. He has been spending less time at home, hanging out with a new set of "unsavory" friends, and asking for more allowance money of late. Also, his grades have dropped significantly over the previous semester. His mother declares no known recent or recurring illness, and he was given a "clean bill of health" by his family doctor 3 months prior. On physical examination, he has normal vital signs, except for slight tachycardia to 110 beats/min with an occasionally irregular rhythm. He is disoriented and exhibits horizontal nystagmus.

▶ What is the most likely diagnosis?
▶ What are potential complications related to the diagnosis?
▶ What important diagnostic tests should be considered?

ANSWERS TO CASE 49:
Adolescent Substance Use Disorder

Summary: A disoriented teenager with double vision, flushed skin, and excessive salivation, along with concerning behavioral, school performance, and peer group changes.

- **Most likely diagnosis:** Adolescent substance use disorder in the form of inhalant use ("huffing").

- **Potential complications:** Inhalant use can lead to sudden death from dysrhythmias. Chronic use is associated with neurotoxic sequelae.

- **Important diagnostic tests:** An electrocardiogram (ECG) should be obtained to assess for possible dysrhythmia, along with a basic metabolic panel (BMP) to ascertain any electrolyte abnormalities. A urine drug screen (UDS) should be considered, given the possibility of concomitant drug abuse.

ANALYSIS

Objectives

1. Understand the definition and modifiers of substance use disorder.

2. Appreciate the importance of fully assessing for possible drug use/abuse when encountering significant adolescent dysfunction.

3. Know the signs of substance abuse in adolescents, and the major physiologic (somatic) and behavioral consequences attributable to their long-term use.

4. Understand the dynamics behind select drugs used by adolescents.

Considerations

An adolescent with disorientation, hallucinations, and recent decline in school performance strongly suggests substance use until proven otherwise. The most likely substance in this scenario is an inhalant, because its use is historically more common among younger teens. Although alcohol is the most commonly abused substance among adolescents overall, it rarely manifests with hallucinations. Inhalants initially present with an excitatory phase, including euphoria, delusions, slurred speech, and hallucinations. Acute cardiotoxicity via dysrythmogenesis is the most common cause of death from inhalant use, and thought due to increased myocardial sensitization. Chronic effects from inhalant abuse include cardiomyopathy, leukoencephalopathy, cerebellar degeneration, and neuropathy. Possible electrolyte abnormality and acid-base imbalance are important considerations during the evaluation of intoxication, particularly with toluene-based products.

| APPROACH TO: |
| Adolescent Substance Use Disorder |

DEFINITIONS

SUBSTANCE USE DISORDER: A maladaptive pattern of substance use leading to clinically significant impairment or distress manifested by two or more positive answers to 11 diagnostic questions (see the section Defining Substance Use Disorder later); this DSM-V disorder replaces the previous diagnoses of substance abuse and substance dependence.

URINE DRUG SCREEN (UDS): Typically, an immunoassay that, when quantified by a spectrophotometer, can detect most of the commonly abused mood-altering substances with the exception of solvents/inhalants and bath salts; the usual assay screens for alcohol, amphetamines, barbiturates, benzodiazepines, cocaine, codeine, heroin, hydromorphone, methadone, morphine, phencyclidine (PCP), propoxyphene, and tetrahydrocannabinol (THC).

CLINICAL APPROACH

The transition from childhood to adolescence is a critical developmental period that involves pubertal maturation, establishment of identity, changing relationships, and an increase in risky behaviors, such as substance use. Although the transition from becoming a nonuser to a user of some drugs may be considered developmentally normative behavior, some adolescents progress to a more regular pattern of substance use with associated consequences. Initially, most adolescents use mood-altering substances intermittently or experimentally. The sequence of progression in substance use generally begins with use of alcohol and tobacco, followed by marijuana and then other illicit drugs. This sequence of use is best described by the "gateway hypothesis": the use of less harmful drugs can lead to the future risk of using more dangerous *hard* drugs.

Ongoing monitoring of legal and illicit drug use by children in the United States suggests that adolescents have been and will likely continue using substances at alarming rates. The best data on adolescent substance abuse come from the Monitoring the Future (MTF) study, which surveys roughly 50,000 students in the 8th, 10th, and 12th grades. In 2013, when asked about any drug usage in the previous 12 months, nearly 40% of high school seniors reported marijuana use, 20% reported use of other illegal drugs, and 43% reported consumption of at least one alcoholic drink during their senior year.

The prevalence of substance use and associated risky behaviors vary by age, gender, ethnicity, and other socioeconomic factors. With the exception of inhalants, younger teenagers report less drug use than do older teens. Teenage boys have higher rates of drug use than teen girls. African American youth have significantly lower rates of illicit drug use than Caucasian youth for all drug categories. Hispanic youth rates fall between, except for 12th grade Hispanics, who report the highest rate of crack cocaine, injected heroin, and crystal methamphetamine use.

Over the past decade, lysergic acid diethylamide (LSD) and methamphetamine use has decreased, whereas cocaine and ecstasy use has risen. Numbers are likely underestimated, though, because the survey only targets those who are in school, and excludes drop-outs, the homeless and incarcerated; illicit drug use is typically higher in these three groups.

DEFINING SUBSTANCE USE DISORDER

With the introduction of the *Diagnostic and Statistical Manual of Mental Disorders, Fifth Edition (DSM-V)* in 2013, a new definition, encompassing substance use, abuse, and dependence, was introduced to reclassify these similar, but different, diagnoses. *Substance use disorder* combines their previous diagnostic criteria, strengthening their ability to classify substance use and abuse onto a scale. Two or three symptoms indicate a mild substance use disorder; four or five a moderate disorder; and six or more a severe disorder. *DSM-V* defines the disorder as "[a] maladaptive pattern of substance use leading to clinically significant impairment or distress," as manifested by two or more of the following occurring within a 12-month period:

1. Craving or a strong desire or urge to use a specific substance.

2. Recurrent substance use resulting in a failure to fulfill major role obligations (poor school performance, suspensions, expulsions).

3. Recurrent substance use in situations in which it is physically hazardous (driving an automobile).

4. Continued substance use despite having persistent or recurrent social or interpersonal problems.

5. Tolerance to the substance (a need for markedly increased amounts of the substance to achieve intoxication and/or markedly diminished effect with continued use of the same amount of the substance).

6. Withdrawal from the substance (the characteristic withdrawal syndrome for the substance, or the same [or a closely related] substance is taken to relieve or avoid withdrawal symptoms).

7. The substance is often taken in larger amounts or over a longer period than was intended.

8. There is a persistent desire to cut down and control substance use.

9. A great deal of time is spent in activities necessary to obtain the substance, use the substance, or recover from its effects.

10. Important social or recreational activities are given up or reduced because of substance use.

11. The substance use is continued despite knowledge of having a persistent or recurrent physical or psychological problem that is likely to have been caused or exacerbated by the substance.

These criteria are somewhat limited in practice with adolescents, due to differing patterns of use, developmental implications, and other age-related consequences. As yet, criteria for diagnostic use have not been developed for adolescents, though most clinicians will refer them for substance abuse treatment based on the previously listed points.

COMMONLY ABUSED DRUGS

Alcohol

When compared to adults, adolescent alcohol use is more likely to be episodic and heavy ("binge drinking"), making its use particularly dangerous. Such binge-drinking adolescents are at a higher risk of alcohol poisoning (suppression of the gag reflex and respiratory drive), high-risk sexual behaviors, academic problems, and more injuries than nonbinge drinking peers. Alcohol use is the primary contributor to the leading causes of death among adolescents (motor vehicle accidents, homicide, suicide). Acute ingestion can result in erosive gastritis, manifested by epigastric pain, anorexia, vomiting, and hematochezia and pancreatitis (mid-epigastric pain and vomiting). Alcohol overdose should be suspected in an adolescent who is disoriented, lethargic, comatose, or who smells of alcohol. An alcohol (EtOH) blood level greater than 0.2 g/dL puts the adolescent at risk of death. A level greater than 0.5 g/dL is usually associated with a fatal outcome. In alcohol poisoning, if obtundation appears out of proportion to the reported blood alcohol level, head trauma, hypoglycemia, or other drug ingestion, it should be considered as a possible confounding factor.

Marijuana

Marijuana's active ingredient is delta-9-tetrahydrocannabinol (THC). In addition to traditional inhalation of marijuana smoke, THC can also be ingested in a number of pharmaceutical food products, homemade recipes, or through electronic cigarettes (hashish or hashish oil). Lacing with other illicit substances is common.

Marijuana effects include euphoria, elation, and decreased social inhibition. Unwanted side effects include decreased reaction time, impaired attention and concentration, and short-term memory loss. Physiologic signs of cannabis intoxication include tachycardia, increased blood pressure, increased respiratory rate, conjunctival injection, dry mouth, and increased appetite. "Amotivational syndrome" has been described in long-term marijuana users, especially adolescents, characterized by inattention to environmental stimuli and impaired goal-directed thinking and behavior. Chronic use by males results in dose-related suppression of plasma testosterone levels and spermatogenesis. A similar pubertal suppression has been described in females.

Cocaine and Amphetamines

Cocaine and amphetamines are central nervous system stimulants that increase dopamine levels by preventing reuptake. Cocaine may elicit euphoria, increased motor activity, decreased fatigability, and mental alertness. Chronic use of intranasal cocaine is associated with loss of smell, nosebleeds, and chronic rhinorrhea. When mixed with alcohol, cocaine is metabolized by the liver to produce cocaethylene, a substance that is significantly more cardio- and hepatotoxic than alcohol or cocaine alone.

Amphetamines are stimulants with a high potential for abuse. Increased diagnosis of attention deficit hyperactivity disorder (ADHD) has made schedule II treatment with stimulants (Ritalin, Adderall) more common. These medications have become a significant drug of abuse among children and adolescents. Illicit methamphetamine is produced in illegal laboratories and is popular among adolescents and young adults because of its potency and ease of absorption.

Amphetamines and cocaine are associated with increased physical activity, rapid and/or irregular heart rate, increased blood pressure, and decreased appetite. Binge effects result in the development of psychotic ideation with the potential for sudden violence. Cerebrovascular damage, psychosis, severe receding of the gums with tooth decay (smoking crack), arrhythmias, and infection with HIV and hepatitis B and C can result from long-term use. Adolescents presenting with chest pain and cardiac signs (brady- or tachyarrhythmias, pathologic rhythms) should be evaluated for possible drug ingestion; ECG and cardiac isoenzymes may be warranted.

Acute agitation and delusional behaviors can be treated with haloperidol and may be diminished by administering a sedating dose of lorazepam or diazepam. Cooling blankets may be used for reactive hyperthermia. Marked reactive hypertension or dysrhythmia may need treatment with a cardiovascular agent (β-blocker) until the intoxication resolves. As in teens with other drug use, comprehensive cognitive-behavioral interventions have been shown to be an effective treatment modality.

Hallucinogens

Members of this group are both naturally occurring and synthetically derived, and include classic hallucinogens (LSD, psilocybin [magic mushrooms]), and designer hallucinogens (3,4-methylenedioxy-N-methylamphetamine [MDMA] and related amphetamine derivatives, PCP, ketamine). All produce alterations in perception, thought, or mood. When taken in high doses, dextromethorphan can produce effects similar to those of PCP and ketamine. Among adolescents, LSD and MDMA are the two most commonly used hallucinogenic substances.

LSD is a potent psychoactive compound resulting in psychedelic effects mediated through the serotonergic system as a serotonin type 2 agonist. Sympathomimetic effects include mydriasis, tachycardia, hypertension, and hyperreflexia. Overdoses have been associated with respiratory arrest, severe hyperthermia, and coagulopathy.

MDMA (X, E, Ecstasy) has "desired" effects of euphoria, a heightened sensual awareness, and somatic hypersensitivity, whereas anxiety, panic attacks, and psychosis are the adverse psychiatric outcomes. Somatic symptoms of ingestion include nausea, jaw clenching, teeth grinding (bruxism), and blurred vision. Repeated MDMA use results in neurotoxic injury to serotonin axon terminals, causing long-term cognitive sequelae from reductions in both the number of serotonin transporters in the brain and levels of serotonin metabolites in the cerebrospinal fluid. Reported impairments include memory loss, diminished learning ability, sleep disturbances, and depression. Acute overdose can cause hyperthermia and multiorgan system failure. Treatment is primarily supportive.

Table 49–1 • COMMON INHALANTS OF ABUSE	
Toluene (gasoline and paint thinners)	Impaired cognition Gait disturbance Loss of coordination Liver and kidney damage
Amyl or butyl nitrite ("poppers")	Sudden death due to cardiorespiratory arrest/failure Immune suppression Methemoglobinemia
Benzene (gasoline)	Bone marrow suppression Impaired immunologic function Increased risk of leukemia Reproductive system toxicity
Butane, propane (lighter fluid, hair and paint sprays)	Sudden death due to cardiorespiratory arrest/failure Risk for burn injuries
Freon (refrigerant, aerosol propellant)	Sudden death due to cardiorespiratory arrest/failure Liver damage
Methylene chloride (paint thinners, degreasers)	Reduction of oxygen-carrying capacity of blood Myocardial dysregulation (arrhythmias)
Hexane, nitrous oxide ("laughing gas")	Hypoxia Limb spasms and sensory loss Blackouts due to hypotension

Inhalants

Inhalants produce immediate effects similar to alcohol: euphoria, slurred speech, and decreased coordination (Table 49–1). Its use is popular among younger adolescents. Common products include volatile solvents (paint thinners, glue), aerosols (spray paint, hair spray), and gases (propane tanks, lighter fluid). Paint "huffers" often present with residual perioral or fingertip paint from inhalation. Because of the increased solvent content in metallic-colored paints, gold and silver spray paints are particularly popular. Initial stages of acute inhalant use are characterized by euphoria, excitation, exhilaration, dizziness, hallucinations, excess salivation, sneezing, flushed skin, and bizarre behavior. More concerning signs of inhalant intoxication are disorientation, double vision, nystagmus, bizarre dreams, epileptiform activity, arrhythmias, and unconsciousness.

Chronic use causes difficulty coordinating movement, gait disorders, muscle tremors, and spasticity due to neurotoxic effects of inhalants, hypoxia, or both. Other toxicity includes pulmonary hypertension, restrictive lung defects or reduced diffusion capacity, hematuria, tubular acidosis, and possibly cerebral and cerebellar atrophy. Death from solvent abuse occurs most commonly from cardiac dysrhythmias.

Treatment is supportive and directed toward control of dysrhythmias and stabilization of respirations and circulation. Withdrawal symptoms do not usually occur.

Bath Salts

"Bath salts" are newly popular drugs that act as a central nervous system stimulant by inhibiting norepinephrine-dopaminergic reuptake. Their primary effects are similar to those of other stimulants like PCP, ecstasy, cocaine, and amphetamines. Although dozens of active ingredients have been isolated, the most common is 4-methylene-dioxypyrovalerone (MDPV). Legal until early 2012, "bath salts" consumption and distribution was widespread and difficult to follow. Common symptoms include euphoria, dilated pupils, loss of inhibition, involuntary muscle movement, tachycardia, and hypertension. Less common side effects of MDPV such as paranoia, panic attacks, and violent behavior are seen. Overdoses can potentially be severe and lethal. Routine drug screens do not detect MDPV in urine; gas chromatography is required.

ADOLESCENT DRUG USE PREVENTION, EVALUATION, AND TREATMENT

Early detection of drug use with regular screening at the health care provider's office is key to diminishing preventable morbidity and mortality in the adolescent population. Early onset of drug use correlates to more severe substance use in later life. Thus, early diagnosis and intervention at routine health screenings is an important component of the well-child examination. Several self-reported screening questionnaires (HEADSS, CRAFFT) provide a format for direct questioning of school performance, family relationships, peer activities, and other possible risk factors for substance use (Boxes 49–1 and 49–2). In addition, a family history of drug addiction or abuse should raise the level of concern about potential drug abuse.

A routine UDS is not recommended in the evaluation of an adolescent suspected of drug use. A UDS may be beneficial when other psychiatric symptoms are present to rule out dual diagnoses. A significant change in school performance or other daily behaviors is noted, and frequent or serious accidents occur (atypical motor vehicular accidents). It may also be helpful as a monitoring procedure during a recovery program. Screening and diagnostic testing in an older, competent adolescent may be carried out, with few exceptions, only with the patient's consent. Parental permission is not sufficient for involuntary screening in these patients. Consent may be waived when the patient's competency is questionable or when findings from the interview and physical examination strongly suggest the patient is at high risk for serious harm from substance use. A UDS usually fails to detect alcohol, is subject to false-positive results, and is notoriously easy for a savvy teenager to falsify. Furthermore, because they measure only "instantaneous use," a UDS may provide a false sense of reassurance if results are negative. The most common

---

Box 49–1 • HEADSS Examination

- *H*ome: safety, stability, support, responsibilities, privileges
- *E*ducation: achievement, skills, strengths, plans, employment
- *A*ctivities: pastimes, sports, religion, civic and community involvement
- *D*rugs: tobacco, alcohol, and other drug use by patient, friends, and family
- *S*exuality: satisfaction with body and self, concerns about sexuality, sexual activity, sexual identity
- *S*uicidality: depressive symptoms, anxiety, mood disorder, thinking problems

Box 49–2 • CRAFFT Examination

- Have you ever ridden in a **c**ar driven by someone (including yourself) who was high or had been using alcohol or drugs?
- Do you ever use alcohol or drugs to **r**elax, feel better about yourself, or fit in?
- Do you ever use alcohol or drugs while you are **a**lone?
- Do you ever **f**orget things you did while using alcohol or drugs?
- Do your **f**amily or **f**riends ever tell you that you should cut down on your drinking or drug use?
- Have you ever gotten into **t**rouble while you were using alcohol or drugs?

Note: Two or more positive responses usually indicate a serious problem.

reason for false-negative results is infrequent use, but results can be "falsified" when the sample is diluted or the adolescent substitutes "clean" urine. False positives also are possible, though infrequent, with select medication use.

Staging substance abuse provides the clinician with a means of monitoring progress and providing an objective means of conveying treatment goals (Table 49–2). Group counseling, individualized counseling, and multifamily educational intervention have been found to be effective interventions for teens with substance use disorders. Outpatient management is often the first line of treatment for teens identified as meeting Stage 4 or Stage 5 criteria. Candidates for inpatient treatment have significant comorbid psychiatric illness; are experiencing withdrawal; have suicidal ideation, runaway behavior, behavior that threatens the lives of their family and/or friends; or have not responded to intensive outpatient treatment.

PSYCHIATRIC COMORBIDITIES

Psychiatric disorders often are comorbidities substance use, especially depression, anxiety, and bipolar disorder. ADHD, eating disorders, conduct disorder, and various personality disorders also have been described. Certain substances are commonly associated with specific comorbid psychiatric diagnoses: amphetamines with eating disorders; cocaine with depression; marijuana with amotivational syndrome; and alcohol use with affective disorder, anxiety disorder, and mania.

CASE CORRELATION

- The child with intentional or nonintentional ingestion may present in myriad ways; this diagnosis should be on the differential for many pediatric conditions. Asthma (Case 20) can be triggered by any pulmonary irritant, tobacco being one of the most common. The substance abusing adolescent often participates in high-risk activities, thus having a higher rate of accidents which may present as a subdural hematoma (Case 29), headache (Case 48), and exposure to acquired immune deficiency (Case 40) such as HIV. The younger child who is exposed to exogenous testosterone, such as accidental exposure to parental testosterone replacement, may have precocious puberty (Case 45) as a finding. Young infants who are born to or in homes with substance abusing caretakers are at higher risk of sudden infant death syndrome (Case 21) and child abuse (Case 38).

Table 49–2 • STAGES OF DRUG ABUSE IN ADOLESCENTS		
Stage 1	No Drug Use	• No health risks from direct use of illicit substances; still subject to risk from use of drugs by friends (riding with an impaired driver, victim in a fight with an intoxicated individual). • Primary focus is on promoting safety, praising, and encouraging abstinence.
Stage 2	Experimentation	• May try various drugs, typically out of curiosity or to "fit in with friends." • At risk from the health effects associated with illicit drug use (cardiac, neurologic, metabolic). • Some adolescents revert to Stage 1, after experiencing unpleasant side effects. • Primary focus is on reviewing risks of drug use, emphasizing safety, encouraging and normalizing abstinence, and rehearsing refusal skills.
Stage 3	Regular Use: Seeking the Euphoria	• Use of other drugs increases (stimulant, LSD, sedative). • Behavioral changes may or may not be present. • Increased frequency of use. • Possible use alone. • Continues to experiment with drugs, if available, but does not make a concerted effort to obtain them. • Use typically occurs on weekends. • Primary focus is on assessing and reviewing risk factors associated with progression, emphasizing safety, encouraging and normalizing abstinence, and rehearsing refusal skills.
Stage 4	Regular Use: Drug Seeking Preoccupation	• Daily use of drugs, coupled with loss of control. • Multiple consequences and risk taking in order to obtain drugs or hide drug use. • Estrangement from family and nonuser friends. • Types of drugs used continue to expand. • Behavioral changes are typically apparent. • Primary focus is per prior stage, but affected adolescents now need careful follow-up; some will meet the criteria for moderate to severe substance use disorder; referral to a drug use specialist is warranted.
Stage 5	Problem Use/Dependence	• Uses drugs to feel "normal." • Polysubstance use/cross-addiction common. • Feels guilt, withdrawal, shame, and remorse. • Comorbid depression often present. • Physical and mental deterioration possible. • Self-destruction/suicidality may occur. • Requires a comprehensive evaluation and will need intensive treatment; most at this stage will meet criteria for moderate to severe substance use disorder, and some may require inpatient treatment.

COMPREHENSION QUESTIONS

49.1 A 14-year-old boy has ataxia. He is brought to the local emergency department, where he appears euphoric, emotionally labile, and a bit disoriented. He has nystagmus and hypersalivation. Many notice his abusive language. Which of the following agents is most likely responsible for his condition?

A. Alcohol

B. Amphetamines

C. Barbiturates

D. Cocaine

E. Phencyclidine (PCP)

49.2 Parents bring their 16-year-old daughter for a "well-child" checkup. She looks normal on examination. As part of your routine care you order a urinalysis. The father pulls you aside and asks you to secretly run a urine drug screen (UDS) on his daughter. Which of the following is the most appropriate course of action?

A. Explore the reasons for the request with the parents and the adolescent, and perform a UDS with the adolescent's permission if the history warrants.

B. Perform the UDS as requested, but have the family and girl return for the results.

C. Perform the UDS in the manner requested.

D. Refer the adolescent to a psychiatrist for further evaluation.

E. Tell the family to bring the adolescent back for a UDS when she is exhibiting signs or symptoms of intoxication, such as euphoria or ataxia.

49.3 A previously healthy adolescent boy has a 3-month history of increasing headaches, blurred vision, and personality changes. Previously he admitted to marijuana experimentation more than a year ago. On examination he is a healthy, athletic-appearing 17 year old with decreased extraocular range of motion and left eye visual acuity. Which of the following is the best next step in his management?

A. Ophthalmology referral

B. Glucose measurement

C. Neuroimaging

D. Trial of methysergide (Sansert) for migraine

E. Urine drug screen

49.4 A 15-year-old boy was found smoking weed by a teacher patrolling an outdoor patio at his school. Parents are unaware of drug use, but did note he has
been acting "dazed and confused" at times, and that his hygiene has worsened
over the past few months. Which one of the following would NOT be used
as an assessment of substance use disorder in this teenager?

A. Problems with law enforcement

B. Desire to cut down smoking marijuana

C. Driving while using marijuana

D. No longer attending soccer practice to smoke with friends

E. Craving of marijuana use while at school

ANSWERS

49.1 **E.** PCP is associated with hyperactivity, hallucinations, abusive language, and
nystagmus.

49.2 **A.** The adolescent's permission should be obtained before drug testing.
Testing "secretly" in this situation destroys the doctor-patient relationship.

49.3 **C.** Despite previous drug experimentation, his current neurologic symptoms
and physical findings make drug use a less likely etiology. Urgent evaluation
for possible brain tumor is warranted.

49.4 **A.** "Problems with law enforcement" was eliminated from drug abuse criteria
when reformatting *DSM-IV* criteria into the current model. Substance use
disorder requires 2 or more criteria of 11 for diagnosis in *DSM-V*. Previous
criteria were combined for abuse and dependence, with the exception of "drug
craving," a new addition, and "problems with law enforcement," eliminated
due to cultural considerations.

CLINICAL PEARLS

▶ Cigarettes and alcohol are the most commonly used drugs in adolescence.

▶ Marijuana is the most common illicit drug used in adolescence.

▶ Substance abuse behaviors include drug dealing, prostitution, unprotected
sex, depression, suicide attempt, school delinquency or failure, burglary,
and physical violence.

▶ Children at risk for drug use include those with significant behavior problems, learning difficulties, and impaired family functioning.

REFERENCES

American Academy of Pediatrics, Committee on Substance Abuse. Testing for drugs of abuse in children and adolescents. *Pediatrics.*1996;98:305-307.

Bukstein OG, Horner MS. Management of the adolescent with substance use disorders and comorbid psychopathology. *Child Adolesc Psychiatr Clin N Am.* July 2010;19(3):609-623.

Heyman RB. Adolescent substance abuse and other high-risk behaviors. In: McMillan JA, Feigin RD, DeAngelis CD, Jones MD, eds. *Oski's Pediatrics: Principles and Practice.* 4th ed. Philadelphia, PA: Lippincott Williams & Wilkins; 2006:578-584.

Knight JR, Mears CJ. Committee on Substance Abuse, American Academy of Pediatrics; Council on School Health, American Academy of Pediatrics. Testing for drugs of abuse in children and adolescents: addendum—testing in schools and at home. *Pediatrics.* 2007;119:627.

Lloyd DJ, O'Malley PM, Bachman JG, Schulenberg JE, Miech RA . Overview, key findings on adolescent drug use. *Monitoring the Future National Survey Results on Drug Use. 1975–2013.* Ann Arbor, MI: Institute for Social Research, The University of Michigan; 2014.

Stager MM. Substance abuse. In: Kleigman RM, Stanton BF, St. Geme JW, Schor NF, Behrman RE, eds. *Nelson Textbook of Pediatrics.* 19th ed. Philadelphia, PA: WB Saunders; 2011:671-1149.

A mother brings her 12-year-old daughter to the clinic to establish care and to get immunizations for school. The mother reports that because of lack of insurance she has not had a regular pediatrician for her children for the previous 8 years. She reports the girl to be in generally good health other than recurrent bouts of otitis media. The mother is concerned that she and her other two daughters began their growth spurts and their menstrual cycles by age 11 years, but this child "hasn't got her period." The child reports that she is doing well in school except for mathematics and she requires help with attention and planning in school activities. On physical examination, she is at the 5th percentile for height and the 90th percentile for weight. She is afebrile, heart rate 90 beats/min, respiratory rate 16 breaths/min, and BP 117/92 mm Hg. Her chest is broad her femoral pulses diminished.

▶ What is the most likely diagnosis?
▶ What are the most appropriate diagnostic tests to order?
▶ What is the best management for this condition?

ANSWERS TO CASE 50:

Turner Syndrome

Summary: A 12-year-old girl has short stature, hypertension, and amenorrhea.

- **Most likely diagnosis:** Turner syndrome
- **Diagnostic tests to order:** Chromosome analysis to confirm the diagnosis and echocardiogram to evaluate for coarctation
- **Best management:** Monitor for cardiac and renal abnormalities, growth hormone for short stature, and laboratory work to check for hypothyroidism and dyslipidemia

ANALYSIS

Objectives

1. Understand the genetic basis of Turner syndrome.

2. Know the clinical manifestations of Turner syndrome.

3. Select appropriate diagnostic tests and treatments for a patient with Turner syndrome.

Considerations

The patient has several of the common clinical abnormalities found in individuals with Turner syndrome. While no single, "classic" presentation of Turner syndrome is seen, girls often are diagnosed later in childhood due to short stature or primary amenorrhea. Findings that prompt earlier diagnosis include webbed neck, lymphedema, cubitus valgus, and low posterior hairline.

APPROACH TO:

Turner Syndrome

DEFINITIONS

MOSAICISM: Varying chromosomal makeup in a single individual due to the presence of different cell lines (45X and 45XX).

CUBITUS VALGUS: Physical finding in which the angle between the shaft of the ulna and humerus is increased greater than 15% in females.

CLINICAL APPROACH

Girls with Turner syndrome have a single X chromosome with absence of all or part of the second sex chromosome (45 X). Mosaicism can be seen and can ameliorate expression of some of the clinical findings. Turner syndrome generally is not inherited but rather is caused by nondisjunction. The prevalence of Turner syndrome is between 1 in 2000 to 5000 live female births. The majority of 45X embryos are aborted during the first trimester. With high-resolution prenatal ultrasound, a fetus with severe lymphedema or hydrops fetalis can be identified. Current research suggests that a homeobox gene (SHOX) located on the short arm of the X chromosome is primarily responsible for short stature and skeletal issues.

Girls with Turner syndrome have a wide variety of clinical abnormalities that necessitate comprehensive care. When Turner syndrome is suspected, a karyotype is performed to confirm the diagnosis. If the diagnosis is suspected during a prenatal ultrasound, chorionic villi sampling or amniocentesis can harvest fetal cells for karyotyping. Neonates with Turner syndrome are often noted to have lymphedema which creates swollen hands and feet. Other clinical features in the newborn period include webbed neck, low set ears, low hairline, broad chest with wide spaced nipples, drooping eyes, and a higher incidence of hip dysplasia. Renal ultrasound is performed to identify renal anomalies. At the time of diagnosis, a team consisting of cardiology, genetics, and endocrinology is established to evaluate and manage the disorder.

CARDIOLOGY

Coarctation of the aorta is the most serious cardiac condition to identify. On physical examination, differences in upper and lower body pulse intensity or blood pressure differences are evaluated. Less commonly seen defects include aortic root dilation, bicuspid aortic valve, mitral valve prolapse, and hypoplastic left heart syndrome. Overall, patients with monosomy X are more likely to have these structural abnormalities. Surveillance of these heart problems by a pediatric cardiologist is warranted; periodic echocardiograms or cardiac MRI may be warranted.

ENDOCRINOLOGY

Autoimmune disorders such as Hashimoto thyroiditis, celiac disease, and inflammatory bowel disease are more prevalent in girls with Turner syndrome. Hypothyroidism and glucose intolerance are common; thyroid function tests and serum glucoses are tested routinely. Short stature is universally present; treatment by a pediatric endocrinologist with growth hormone is considered. Many girls with Turner syndrome (especially those with monosomy X) have absent pubertal development and have "streak" ovaries that do not ovulate. To promote the development of secondary sex characteristics (pubic hair, breast development), estrogens can be initiated in these girls early in their teen years. Mosaic Turner syndrome patients are more likely to have appropriate start of puberty and can become pregnant.

OTHER SERVICES

Girls with Turner syndrome have structural anomalies in the ear which leads to frequent otitis media and effusion, and then to progressive sensorineural hearing loss severe enough to require hearing aids in some cases. Thus, a regular assessment of hearing is required. Strabismus is frequently seen in young girls with Turner syndrome. Amblyopia is possible; evaluation as well as treatment by an ophthalmologist is imperative. Other ocular abnormalities include congenital glaucoma and anterior chamber deformities. Plastic surgery can be considered for girls for whom defects of the neck, face, and ears are particularly troublesome. Dental malocclusion is often seen and requires the services of a pediatric orthodontist. Congenital hip dysplasia requires the services of a pediatric orthopedist. In addition, scoliosis, kyphosis, and lordosis are more commonly seen and are monitored by the primary care provider. Other, less commonly seen findings include pigmented nevi, osteoporosis, inflammatory bowel disease, neuroblastoma, and liver disease.

Girls with Turner syndrome have normal intelligence but can have difficulty in school. Developmental delay and learning difficulties, including problems with special perception and mathematics, can occur. Attention deficit disorders and challenges with social interaction are seen; regular visits to the primary care provider can identify these challenges and appropriate interventions initiated.

CASE CORRELATION

- See also Case 10 (Failure to Thrive) which might be considered in the young girl who is shorter than her peers. Case 45 (Preciocious Puberty) has a thorough description of the normal cascade of pubertal changes as a reference base. Case 22 (Ventricular Septal Defect) is an example of a noncyanotic heart lesion; Table 22–1 lists other noncyanotic heart lesions including a thorough review of coarctation of the aorta which is classically described as being seen with Turner syndrome. Growth hormone deficiency (Case 44) should be considered not as a diagnostic possibility for a girl with short stature, but also as a treatment for those diagnosed with Turner syndrome to improve their final adult height.

COMPREHENSION QUESTIONS

50.1 An infant girl is noted to have a webbed neck, low hairline, and edematous hands and feet. What of the following tests should be performed to confirm the diagnosis?

   A. Echocardiography

   B. Complete blood count (CBC) with differential

   C. Karyotype

   D. Brain ultrasound

   E. Electrocardiography (ECG)

50.2 Which of the following anomalies is most commonly seen on echocardiogram in a patient with Turner syndrome?

A. Transposition of the great arteries

B. Ventricular septal defect

C. Truncus arteriosus

D. Coarctation of the aorta

E. Patent ductus arteriosus

50.3 A term, appropriate for gestational-age infant girl is found to have neck webbing and edematous feet. A karyotype was performed and results show normal 46 XX chromosomes. What other diagnosis must be considered?

A. Fetal alcohol syndrome

B. Noonan syndrome

C. Down syndrome

D. Beckwith-Wiedemann syndrome

E. Trisomy 18

50.4 Which of the following statements about a girl with Turner syndrome is true?

A. By adolescence they are social advanced as compared to their peers.

B. Hyperthyroidism commonly occurs by the third decade of life.

C. Intelligence is normal and difficulty in school is rarely seen.

D. Pigmented nevi are commonly seen, but transformation to melanoma is rare.

E. Infants with proven Turner syndrome but with normal blood pressures and pulses do not require cardiac evaluation.

ANSWERS

50.1 **C.** The physical findings described in this child are concerning for Turner syndrome. The criterion standard to make the diagnosis is chromosome evaluation to identify the missing X chromosome (XO karyotype). If Turner syndrome is suspected/confirmed, evaluation for coarctation of the aorta by physical examination (femoral pulses will be weaker than upper extremity pulses) and echocardiogram is required. The complete blood count, brain ultrasound, and ECG will not confirm the diagnosis of Turner syndrome.

50.2 **D.** Coarctation of the aorta is the most common cardiac lesion associated with Turner syndrome. This condition consists of narrowing of the aorta and can occur in various locations based on the proximity to the ductus arteriosus. Approximately 5% of girls with Turner syndrome have preductal stenosis, which makes the blood flow to lower half of the body dependent on the ductus remaining open; this can be a life-threatening condition if the ductus closes. Coarctation can be asymptomatic and treated conservatively or be repaired through cardiac catheterization with stent placement or surgical resection. The other lesions listed do not have a high predilection for girls with Turner syndrome.

50.3 **B.** Noonan syndrome has similar features to Turner syndrome and was initially thought to be a variant of Turner syndrome. Noonan syndrome is seen in both genders, and both syndromes present with lymphedema at birth and with neck webbing. Both conditions result in short stature and developmental delay. Noonan syndrome patients have a normal karyotype. Patients with fetal alcohol syndrome have normal karyotype with distinct facial features including wide set eyes, microcephaly, and smooth philtrum. Patients with Down syndrome have an extra chromosome 21 but normal XX (female) or XY (male) on their karyotype. Beckwith-Wiedemann syndrome patients are macrosomic, macroglossic, and often hypoglycemic at birth; they have a higher incidence of Wilms tumor. Features of trisomy 18 include severe mental retardation, microcephaly, microphthalmia, micrognathia, clenched fingers and toes, malformed ears, high incidence of ventricular septal defect, omphalocele, cryptorchidism, and thyroid hypoplasia.

50.4 **D.** Infants with Turner syndrome require a cardiac evaluation for aortic root abnormalities even if the concern for significant coarctation is reduced by normal blood pressures and pulses on clinical examination. Hypothyroidism commonly develops in girls with Turner syndrome, mostly after their fourth year of life. Overall, the intelligence of girls with Turner syndrome is normal, but often are socially delayed compared to their peers and frequently have difficulty in school with attention deficit disorder and specific learning difficulties. Pigmented nevi are commonly seen (especially in adolescents), can be disfiguring and irritated by clothing, but are at low risk of malignant transformation.

CLINICAL PEARLS

▶ Prenatal diagnosis of Turner syndrome is suspected in the female fetus with nuchal cysts and severe lymphedema.

▶ The newborn female with edema of hands and feet, unusual shape of ears, low posterior hairline, short fourth metacarpals, and webbed neck may have Turner syndrome.

▶ The adolescent girl with unexpected short stature and primary amenorrhea should be evaluated for features of Turner syndrome; chromosome evaluation is indicated if features such as cubitus valgus, webbed neck, low hairline, or reduced lower extremity pulses are found.

▶ The most common cardiac defect associated with Turner syndrome is coarctation of the aorta.

REFERENCES

American Academy of Pediatrics. Health supervision for children with Turner syndrome. *Pediatrics*. 2003;111:692-702.

Bondy CA. Turner Syndrome Consensus Study Group. Care of girls and women with Turner syndrome: a guideline of the Turner Syndrome Study Group. *J Clin Endocrinol Metab*. 2007;92:10 25.

Cacino CA, Lee B. Turner syndrome. In: Kleigman RM, Stanton BF, St. Geme JW, Schor NF, Behrman RE, eds. *Nelson Textbook of Pediatrics*. 19th ed. Philadelphia, PA: WB Saunders; 2011:409-410.

Carey JC. Sex chromosome abnormalities. In: Rudolph CD, Rudolph AM, Lister G, First LR, Gershon AA, eds. *Rudolph's Pediatrics*. 22nd ed. New York, NY: McGraw-Hill; 2011:696-697.

Grumbach MM. Syndromes of gonadal dysgenesis and variants. In: Rudolph CD, Rudolph AM, Lister G, First LR, Gershon AA, eds. *Rudolph's Pediatrics*. 22nd ed. New York, NY: McGraw-Hill; 2011:2068-2069.

Kansra AR, Donohoue PA. Turner syndrome. In: Kleigman RM, Stanton BF, St. Geme JW, Schor NF, Behrman RE, eds. *Nelson Textbook of Pediatrics*. 19th ed. Philadelphia, PA: WB Saunders; 2011:1951-1954.

Lewanda AF, Boyadjiev SA, Jabs EW. Turner syndrome. In: McMillan JA, Feigin RD, DeAngelis CD, Jones MD, eds. *Oski's Pediatrics: Principles and Practice*. 4th ed. Philadelphia, PA: Lippincott Williams & Wilkins; 2006:2635-2636.

A 15-year-old girl is seen in the pediatrician's office with a 1-week history of intermittent fever, ranging from 100.2°F (37.9°C) to 100.8°F (38.2°C) and a rash. The rash itches slightly and is located on her cheeks and over the nose (Figure 51–1). It appeared when she started playing soccer with her school team; she and her mother initially believed it was a sunburn but it has not resolved. The girl also reports 2 weeks of malaise and 8 out of 10 pain in both of her metacarpophalangeal (MCP) joints. The joint pain is usually in the morning and the MCPs feel very stiff for about 30 minutes; the discomfort resolves with ibuprofen. One month ago she had bilateral knee pain that spontaneously subsided after 2 weeks. She denies any otalgia, sore throat, cough, abdominal pain, or vaginal discharge but reports she has right-sided chest pain with deep inspiration. On examination, you note a blood pressure of 150/90 mm Hg and heart rate of 90 beats/min. She has two small painless ulcerations on the buccal mucosa, hepatomegaly, splenomegaly, and mild swelling of the bilateral MCP joints. A chest radiograph shows a small right pleural effusion. A complete blood count (CBC) shows a white blood cell count of 2,500/mm³, hemoglobin of 9 mg/dL, and platelets of 80,000/mm³. Her direct Coombs test is positive. Urinalysis shows trace blood and 4+ protein; on microscopy she has red blood cell casts. Hepatitis serologies and HIV enzyme-linked immunosorbent assay (ELISA) are negative; the rapid plasma reagin (RPR) test is reactive with a titer of 1:1 but the *Treponema* pallidum particle agglutination (TP-PA) is negative.

► What is the most likely diagnosis?
► What are the diagnostic criteria for this condition?
► What are the possible complications of this condition?

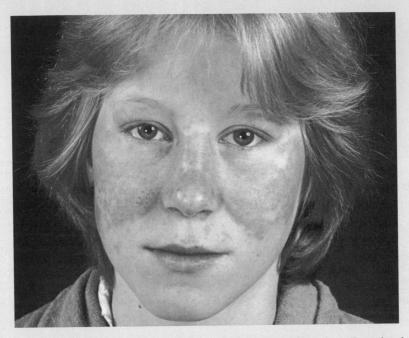

Figure 51–1. Erythematous macules over the malar region in a "butterfly" pattern. (*Reproduced, with permission, from Wolff K, Johnson RA, Saavedra AP. Fitzpatrick's Color Atlas and Synopsis of Clinical Dermatology. 7th ed. New York: McGraw-Hill Education, 2013. Figure 14-33.*)

ANSWERS TO CASE 51:
Systemic Lupus Erythematosus

Summary: A 15-year-old girl has an acute history of fever, facial rash, malaise, and bilateral migratory arthralgias. Physical examination reveals an adolescent who is hypertensive with erythematous macules over the malar aspect of the face, ulcerations on the buccal mucosa, swelling of the MCP joints bilaterally, and hepatosplenomegaly. Chest radiography reveals a pleural effusion that, combined with her symptoms, indicates pleuritis. Laboratory examination shows proteinuria and a CBC with leukopenia, hemolytic anemia, and thrombocytopenia.

- **Most likely diagnosis:** Systemic lupus erythematosus (SLE).

- **Diagnostic criteria:** This patient has 8 of the possible 11 criteria required for the diagnosis of SLE (Table 51-1). To establish the diagnosis, a patient must demonstrate 4 of the 11 features of SLE, which includes malar rash, discoid rash, photosensitivity, oral or nasal ulcers, nonerosive arthritis, serositis, renal disease, neurologic dysfunction, hematologic abnormalities, abnormal antibodies, and a positive antinuclear antibody (ANA).

- **Possible complications:** Cutaneous involvement can result in scarring, alopecia, and Raynaud phenomena. Nephritis in SLE causes hypertension and can result in renal failure, a common cause of mortality in the disease. Central nervous system (CNS) involvement and infection are the other frequent causes of mortality; immunosuppression can result from the disease or most often, from the medications needed to control it. Cardiac and pulmonary involvement increase morbidity.

Table 51-1 • REVISED AMERICAN COLLEGE OF RHEUMATOLOGY (ACR) CRITERIA FOR SYSTEMIC LUPUS ERYTHEMATOSUS (SLE)
Serositis
Oral ulcers
Arthritis
Photosensitivity
Blood Disorders
Renal involvement
Antinuclear antibodies
Immunological disorders (dsDNA, anti-Smith, anti-phospholipid antibodies)
Neurological disorder
Malar Rash
Discord Rash

The American College of Rheumatology (ACR) criteria for SLE revised in 2012 can be summarized by the mnemonic: "SOAP BRAIN MD."

ANALYSIS

Objectives

1. Know the diagnostic criteria for SLE.

2. Distinguish SLE from the other types of pediatric rheumatologic disease.

3. Recognize the complications of SLE.

Considerations

Lupus is a difficult condition to diagnose and requires investigation for a constellation of symptoms that cannot be due to other more common conditions. An extensive workup is often required. The differential diagnosis for a patient who presents with symptoms suggestive of SLE includes juvenile idiopathic arthritis (JIA), dermatomyositis, reactive and postinfectious arthritis, other forms of acute glomerulonephritis and proteinuria, systemic infection, thrombotic thrombocytopenic purpura (TTP), and malignancy.

APPROACH TO:
Systemic Lupus Erythematosus

DEFINITIONS

ARTHRALGIA: Any pain which affects a joint

ARTHRITIS: Swelling or effusion of a joint along with two of the following: limited range of motion, tenderness or pain on motion, and increased heat in one or more joints.

SYSTEMIC LUPUS ERYTHEMATOSUS (SLE): A multisystem disease in which widespread inflammatory involvement of the connective tissues occurs along with an immune-complex vasculitis.

CLINICAL APPROACH

Systemic lupus erythematosus usually **occurs in children after 5 years of age and is increasingly common in the adolescent** years, particularly after puberty. It **primarily affects females** with a female to male ratio of 5:1 prior to puberty and 9:1 during the reproductive years. It is typically diagnosed within the first 6 months of disease onset because of its acute symptomatology. However, the diagnosis can be delayed given the variety of symptoms that do not usually present simultaneously. The diagnostic criteria have been established by the American College of Rheumatology and **four criteria are required** for the diagnosis of SLE. While not needed for diagnosis, **ANA positivity is present in 95% to 99% of children** with SLE. This test, though, has poor specificity as up to 20% of healthy individuals have a positive result. ANA titers do not correlate with disease severity. **Anti–double-stranded** (ds) DNA levels are more specific, and in some individuals, levels do correlate with disease severity. Serum complement levels, C3 and C4, are also important markers of active disease although abnormalities are not specific for SLE.

Constitutional symptoms of malaise, fatigue, anorexia, fever, and weight loss are frequent. The arthritis is nonerosive, usually transient, migratory, and tends to involve the small joints of the hands, wrists, elbows, shoulders, knees, and ankles. **Renal disease is often asymptomatic so if hypertension, elevated creatinine, or findings of nephritis on urinalysis are noted, biopsy is required** for staging the level of disease. **Involvement of other organs may present as cerebritis, pleuritis, pericarditis, hepatitis,** and **hypersplenism.** Hematologic abnormalities include **cytopenias and antiphospholipid antibodies.**

The differential diagnosis for SLE is extensive. Juvenile idiopathic arthritis (JIA) is an important consideration for a child presenting with arthritis because it is the most common rheumatologic disorder in children. Systemic-onset JIA can present with fever, arthralgias, rash, hepatosplenomegaly, pericarditis, and encephalopathy but in contrast to SLE, renal involvement is not seen. Dermatomyositis, another immune-complex mediated vasculitis, is distinguishable from SLE by the presence of proximal muscle weakness, Gottron papules, erythema over the elbows and knees, and the finding of malar rash crossing the nasolabial folds. Reactive and postinfectious arthritis are diagnosed when a sterile inflammatory joint reaction after a recent infection occurs. The term "reactive arthritis" is used if the infection was in the gastrointestinal or genitourinary tract, whereas "postinfectious arthritis" is diagnosed after an upper respiratory tract bacterial pathogen or virus (such as parvovirus).

Treatment of the cutaneous manifestations of SLE includes avoiding sun exposure. **Hydroxychloroquine** is recommended for children with mild SLE. NSAIDs can be useful for management of arthralgia and arthritis. **Glucocorticoids** are used for acute exacerbations and moderate disease; however, their use is limited by potential side effects. Steroid-sparing immunosuppressive agents (cyclophosphamide, rituximab, methotrexate, and mycophenolate mofetil) are used in the treatment of severe disease including evidence of renal or neurologic involvement. SLE is often managed by a pediatric rheumatologist and nephrologist.

COMPREHENSION QUESTIONS

51.1 Which antibody is NOT part of the diagnostic criteria for systemic lupus erythematosus (SLE)?

A. Anti-Sm

B. Rapid plasma reagin (RPR)

C. Rheumatoid factor (RF)

D. Anticardiolipin

E. Lupus anticoagulant

51.2 A 12-year-old boy is suspected of having SLE because of his malar rash, migratory polyarticular arthritis, positive antinuclear antibody (ANA), and positive anti-ds DNA. His complete blood count (CBC) is normal. He is normotensive and a review of systems is positive only for arthritis and the rash. Which of the following tests is indicated in his evaluation?

A. Rapid plasma reagin (RPR)

B. Hepatitis panel

C. Skin biopsy

D. Urinalysis with microscopy

E. Rheumatoid factor (RF)

51.3 A 13-year-old girl is brought to the emergency room for altered mental status. She is not oriented to place or time and perseverates in talking about "demons" that are chasing her. The parents report she has been withdrawn for the past month, sleeping a lot, and exhibiting anorexia and compulsive behavior such as washing her hands multiple times a day. She is afebrile. Her urine drug screen and rapid HIV test are negative. Her CBC shows lymphopenia with absolute lymphocyte count of 400/mm^3. Chest radiography shows bilateral pleural effusions and an enlarged heart. Electrocardiogram shows diffuse ST elevation in all leads consistent with pericarditis. What is the most appropriate next step in management?

A. Rapid strep test

B. Anti-ds DNA

C. Hematology consult

D. Psychiatry consult

E. Broad-spectrum intravenous antibiotics

51.4 A 6-year-old boy is seen by the pediatrician for evaluation of fatigue and a 5-lb weight loss noted over the previous 4 months. He has complained of different sites of arthralgia over the same time interval and the mother has noticed the knee and then the hands appeared swollen on various occasions. After going outdoors, he has been developing pink papules on the sun-exposed areas of his body that he reports "sting." His urinalysis and CBC are normal. What are the most appropriate next diagnostic tests?

A. Antinuclear antibody (ANA), anti-dsDNA

B. Gram stain and culture of synovial fluid

C. Chest radiograph and electroencephalogram (EEG)

D. Rapid strep test and echocardiogram

E. Rheumatoid factor (RF) and hepatitis panel

ANSWERS

51.1 **C.** Rheumatoid factor is not part of the diagnostic criteria for SLE.

51.2 **D.** Identification of nephritis and proteinuria is essential at the time of diagnosis of SLE. Renal disease is a common cause of mortality for patients with SLE.

51.3 **B.** The patient has three criteria of SLE: lymphopenia, serositis (pleuritis and pericarditis), and psychosis. Further specific testing for SLE should be done.

51.4 **A.** The patient has two criteria for SLE: nonerosive arthritis and photosensitivity. If he is ANA and anti-DNA positive, he will have four of the criteria and should be referred to a rheumatologist.

CLINICAL PEARLS

▶ SLE is a multisystem disease with symptoms primarily due to an immune-complex mediated vasculitis which can affect any organ system.

▶ The typical presentation of a child with SLE is after 5 years of age and most cases are during adolescence.

▶ In order to diagnose SLE, four of the American College of Rheumatology criteria are required.

▶ ANA positivity is seen in 95% to 99% of children with SLE but anti-ds DNA is more specific.

REFERENCES

Ardoin SP, Schanberg LE. Systemic lupus erythematosus. In: Kliegman RM, Stanton BF, St. Geme III J, Schor N, Behrman R, eds. *Nelson Textbook of Pediatrics*. 19th ed. Philadelphia, PA: WB Saunders; 2011:841-845.

Cassidy JT. Rheumatic diseases of childhood. In: McMillan JA, Feigin RD, DeAngelis C, Jones MD, eds. *Oski's Pediatrics: Principles and Practice*. 4th ed. Philadelphia, PA: Lippincott Williams & Wilkins; 2006:2543-2546.

Wolff K, Johnson R, Saavedra AP. The Skin in immune, autoimmune, and rheumatic disorders. In: Wolff K, Johnson R, Saavedra AP, eds. *Fitzpatrick's Color Atlas and Synopsis of Clinical Dermatology*. 7th ed. New York, NY: McGraw-Hill; 2013:sec 14. http://accessmedicine.mhmedical.com. ezproxyhost.library.tmc.edu/content.aspx?bookid=682&Sectionid=45130146. Accessed July 14, 2014.

A 14-year-old Hispanic boy presents with a 3-day complaint of "brown urine." He has been your patient since birth and has experienced no major illnesses or injuries, is active in band and cross-country, and denies drug use or sexual activity. Two weeks ago he had 2 days of fever and a sore throat, but he improved spontaneously and has been well since. His review of systems is remarkable only for his slightly puffy eyes, which he attributes to late-night studying for final examinations. On physical examination, he is afebrile, his blood pressure is 135/90 mm Hg, he is active and nontoxic in appearance, and he has some periorbital edema. The urine dipstick has a specific gravity of 1.035 and contains 2+ blood and 2+ protein. You spin the urine, resuspend the sediment, and identify red blood cell casts under the microscope.

▶ What is the most likely cause of this patient's hematuria?
▶ What laboratory tests would support this diagnosis?
▶ What is the prognosis of this condition?

ANSWERS TO CASE 52:

Acute Poststreptococcal Glomerulonephritis

Summary: A healthy adolescent boy with a preceding pharyngitis has periorbital edema and mild hypertension, and has developed tea-colored urine that on microscopy reveals red blood cells and casts.

- **Most likely diagnosis:** Acute poststreptococcal glomerulonephritis (APSGN).

- **Laboratory studies:** C_3 (low in 90% of cases), C_4 (usually normal); antistreptolysin-O (ASO) enzyme antibodies, and antideoxyribonuclease B (anti-DNase B) antibodies provide evidence of recent streptococcal infection.

- **Prognosis:** Excellent; 95% to 98% of affected children recover completely.

ANALYSIS

Objectives

1. Recognize the typical presentation of APSGN.

2. Know the different diagnostic possibilities for a patient with dark urine.

3. Discuss appropriate follow-up care for the patient with APSGN.

Considerations

This patient is otherwise healthy, had a recent pharyngitis, and now has hematuria, proteinuria, edema, and hypertension. Although APSGN is likely, other possibilities must be considered. Strenuous activity can cause rhabdomyolysis and dark urine, but patients with these conditions often will have muscle aches, fatigue, nausea and vomiting, and fever. Immunoglobulin A (Berger) nephropathy is characterized by recurrent painless hematuria, usually preceded by an upper respiratory tract infection. Henoch-Schönlein purpura (HSP) is a relatively common cause of nephritis in pediatrics, but most cases occur in younger children, peaking in incidence between 4 and 5 years of age. Lupus nephritis (systemic lupus erythematosus [SLE]) can present as described and is considered if the hematuria does not resolve or if the C_3 level does not normalize in 6 to 12 weeks.

APPROACH TO:
Acute Poststreptococcal Glomerulonephritis

DEFINITIONS

GLOMERULONEPHRITIS: Glomerular inflammation resulting in the triad of hematuria, proteinuria, and hypertension.

RED CELL CASTS: Injured glomeruli have increased permeability and leak red cells and proteins into the proximal convoluted tubule; the material subsequently clumps in the distal convoluted tubule and in the collecting ducts. When passed, these cell clumps retain the shape of the tubule in the urine. Red cell casts are markers for glomerular injury.

CLINICAL APPROACH

Acute poststreptococcal glomerulonephritis (APSGN) is the most common of the postinfectious nephritides, comprising 80% to 90% of cases. Other bacteria, viruses, parasites, and fungi also have been implicated. Males are more commonly affected; it is most common in children between the ages of 5 and 15 years, and is rare in toddlers and infants. The group A β-hemolytic *Streptococcus* (GABHS) infection can be in the form of either pharyngitis ("strep throat") or a superficial skin lesion (impetigo). Not all GABHS infections result in APSGN; certain GABHS strains are nephritogenic and are more likely to result in APSGN. Rheumatic fever only rarely occurs concomitantly with APSGN. **Antibiotic use during the initial GABHS infection may reduce the subsequent rheumatic fever risk, yet has not been shown to prevent APSGN.** The nephritis risk after infection with a nephritogenic strain of GABHS remains 10% to 15%.

   Generally the interval between GABHS pharyngitis and APSGN is 1 to 2 weeks; the interval between GABHS impetigo and APSGN is 3 to 6 weeks. Symptom onset is abrupt. Although almost all patients have **microscopic hematuria,** only 30% to 50% develop gross hematuria. In addition, 85% present with edema and 60% to 80% develop hypertension.

   The **most important laboratory test** in patients with APSGN is measurement of **serum C_3 and C_4 levels. C_3 is low in 90% of APSGN cases, whereas C_4 usually is normal.** If both levels are low, an alternate diagnosis is considered. Urinalysis typically reveals high specific gravity, low pH, hematuria, proteinuria, and red cell casts. Documentation of a recent streptococcal infection is helpful; **serum markers include the presence of ASO enzyme antibodies and anti-DNase B antibodies.** ASO antibodies are found in 80% of children with recent GABHS pharyngitis but in less than 50% of children with recent GABHS skin infection. ASO titers are positive in 16% to 18% of normal children. **Anti-DNase B antibodies assays are more reliable;** they are present in almost all patients after GABHS pharyngitis and in the majority of patients after GABHS skin infection. Antibodies to other streptococcal antigens (nicotamide adenosine dinucleotide glycohydrolase [NADase], hyaluronidase, and streptokinase) may also be assayed. Renal biopsy is no longer routine.

Treatment is generally supportive. Fluid balance is crucial; diuretics, fluid restriction, or both may be necessary. Sodium and potassium intake may require restriction. **Hypertension** usually is easily controlled with **calcium channel blockers.** Strict bed rest and corticosteroid medications are not helpful. Dialysis is rarely required.

Resolution usually is rapid and complete. The edema resolves in 5 to 10 days, and patients usually are normotensive within 3 weeks. C_3 levels usually normalize in 2 to 3 months; a persistently low C_3 level is uncommon and suggests an alternate diagnosis. Microscopic hematuria may persist for 1 to 2 years.

CASE CORRELATION

- See also Case 51 (SLE) which may present with a plethora of vague signs and symptoms, among which are renal abnormalities that may be confused with poststreptococcal glomerulonephritis.

COMPREHENSION QUESTIONS

52.1 A 13-year-old adolescent presents for follow-up 3 months after a diagnosis of acute poststreptococcal glomerulonephritis. Laboratory testing at this visit reveals microscopic hematuria and a persistently low C_3. Based on these findings, what diagnosis should you consider at this time?

A. Acute poststreptococcal glomerulonephritis

B. IgA vasculitis (Henoch-Schönlein purpura [HSP])

C. IgA nephropathy

D. Nephrolithiasis

E. Membranoproliferative glomerulonephritis

52.2 The parents of a healthy 12-year-old girl bring her to you for a physical examination required for school sports participation. She was recently treated with antibiotics for a throat infection. Vital signs are significant for a blood pressure of 135/85 mm Hg. Urine dipstick testing is positive for blood. Microscopic examination of the urine revealed red cell casts. Family history is negative for renal disease. Which of the following is the most likely diagnosis?

A. Acute poststreptococcal glomerulonephritis

B. IgA nephropathy

C. Benign familial hematuria

D. Goodpasture syndrome

E. Henoch-Schönlein purpura (HSP) nephritis

52.3 A 17-year-old adolescent girl has joint tenderness for 2 months; the pain has affected her summer job as a lifeguard. In the morning, she awakens with bilateral knee pain and swelling, and right hand pain. The pain eases during the day but never completely resolves. Nonsteroidal anti-inflammatory drugs help slightly. She also wants a good "face cream" because "her job has worsened her acne." On physical examination, you notice facial erythema on the cheeks and nasolabial folds. She has several oral ulcers that she calls cold sores and bilateral knee effusions, and her right distal interphalangeal joints on her hand are swollen and tender. Her liver is palpable 3 cm below the costal margin. She has microscopic hematuria and proteinuria. Which of the following laboratory data is consistent with the most likely diagnosis?

A. Low C_3, low C_4

B. Low C_3, normal C_4

C. Normal C_3, normal C_4

D. Normal C_3, low C_4

E. Normal C_3, high C_4

52.4 A 17-year-old boy comes to your clinic for evaluation of 3 days of "dark urine." Of note, he recently competed in a local marathon. He had previous episodes of dark urine, all following strenuous exercise, which resolved without intervention. Physical examination reveals an alert, thin boy in no respiratory distress. Blood pressure and heart rate are normal for age. The remainder of the physical examination is benign with the exception of eczematoid rash in the antecubital fossa bilaterally. Urinalysis reveals the presence of blood and protein with many red blood cells. Which of the following is the most likely diagnosis?

A. Alport syndrome

B. IgA vasculitis

C. Rhabdomyolysis

D. Exercise-induced hematuria

E. IgA nephropathy

ANSWERS

52.1 **E.** This patient was diagnosed with acute poststreptococcal glomerulonephritis (APSGN) likely based on clinical presentation, because biopsy is no longer routine for diagnosis. However, at this visit, his C_3 remains low. In APSGN, it is expected that the C3 levels will normalize in 2 to 3 months. Because this patient continues to have depressed C_3, he was likely misdiagnosed initially. Persistent hypocomplementemia is suggestive of membranoproliferative glomerulonephritis.

Recurrent painless gross hematuria, frequently associated with an upper respiratory tract infection, is typical of IgA nephropathy. These patients often develop chronic renal disease over decades. The classic triad associated with IgA vasculitis (HSP) is purpuric rash, arthritis, and abdominal pain. Nephrolithiasis can produce hematuria, but is almost always painful.

52.2 **A.** This history and presentation is consistent with APSGN. Following an episode of pharyngitis, this patient presents with hypertension, hematuria, and proteinuria, all characteristic of APSGN.

IgA nephropathy is represented by painless recurrent hematuria associated with an upper respiratory infection. Benign familial hematuria, an autosomal dominant condition, causes either persistent or intermittent hematuria without progression to chronic renal failure. Biopsy reveals a thin basement membrane; in some cases the biopsy is normal. Goodpasture syndrome is an autoimmune disease in which antibodies attack the lung and kidneys causing pulmonary hemorrhage and nephritis, respectively. This patient has no pulmonary involvement. The story is not consistent with HSP.

52.3 **A.** Systemic lupus erythematosus affects more women than men, and nephritis is a common presenting feature. Her rash, photosensitivity, oral ulcers, hepatomegaly, arthritis, and nephritis combine to make this a likely diagnosis. A positive antinuclear antibody test and low C_3 and C_4 levels would help to confirm the diagnosis. Low C_3 and normal C_4 are consistent with APSGN. Normal C_3 and normal C_4 represent resolution of APSGN with normal complement values seen about 2 to 3 months after diagnosis.

52.4 **D.** This adolescent presents with dark urine following strenuous exercise. Of the choices listed, this is most likely due to exercise-induced hematuria. This patient's hematuria has resolved in the past without development of chronic disease. This patient has no symptomatology consistent with IgA vasculitis or HSP. In rhabdomyolysis, urine studies are positive for blood, but negative for red blood cells. The myoglobin, from muscle breakdown, causes a false positive on the urine dipstick test. IgA nephropathy is usually following illness and will progress to chronic kidney disease. Alport syndrome is a genetic defect in collagen synthesis that leads to abnormal basement membrane formation; patients will develop hematuria, proteinuria, and renal failure.

CLINICAL PEARLS

▶ Poststreptococcal glomerulonephritis is the most common postinfectious nephritis and has a good prognosis.

▶ Confirming the diagnosis of APSGN requires evidence of invasive streptococcal infection such as an elevated anti-DNase B titer.

REFERENCES

Barron CS. Henoch-Schönlein purpura (anaphylactoid purpura). In: Rudolph CD, Rudolph AM, Lister GE, First LR, Gershon AA, eds. *Rudolph's Pediatrics.* 22nd ed. New York, NY: McGraw-Hill; 2011:810-812.

Eddy AA. Glomerular diseases. In: Rudolph CD, Rudolph AM, Lister GE, First LR, Gershon AA, eds. *Rudolph's Pediatrics.* 22nd ed. New York, NY: McGraw-Hill; 2011:1710-1722.

Eison TM, Ault BH, Jones DP, Chesney RW, Wyatt RJ. Post-streptococcal acute glomerulonephritis in children: clinical features and pathogenesis. *Pediatr Nephrol.* 2011;26:165-180.

Kashtan CE. Denys-Drash syndrome. In: Rudolph CD, Rudolph AM, Lister GE, First LR, Gershon AA, eds. *Rudolph's Pediatrics.* 22nd ed. New York, NY: McGraw-Hill; 2011:1731.

Lum GM. Glomerulonephritis. In: Hay WW, Levin MJ, Sondheimer JM, Deterding RR, eds. *Current Diagnosis & Treatment Pediatrics.* 20th ed. New York, NY: McGraw-Hill; 2011:679-681.

Pan CG, Avner ED. Acute poststreptococcal glomerulonephritis. In: Kliegman RM, Stanton BF, St. Geme JW, Schor NF, Behrman RE, eds. *Nelson Textbook of Pediatrics.* 19th ed. Philadelphia, PA: Elsevier; 2011:1783-1785.

Pan CG, Avner ED. Isolated glomerular diseases with recurrent gross hematuria. In: Kliegman RM, Stanton BF, St. Geme JW, Schor NF, Behrman RE, eds. *Nelson Textbook of Pediatrics.* 19th ed. Philadelphia, PA: Elsevier; 2011:1781-1783.

Silverman ED. Systemic lupus erythematosus. In: Rudolph CD, Rudolph AM, Lister GE, First LR, Gershon AA, eds. *Rudolph's Pediatrics.* 22nd ed. New York, NY: McGraw-Hill; 2011:814-818.

A 15-year-old boy presents to your office with a chief complaint of persistent abdominal pain and nausea. He has no past medical history. His review of systems is remarkable for diarrhea, fatigue, cramping abdominal pain, nausea, fevers, and occasional rectal bleeding. You note in the patient's chart that he had been growing along the 70th percentile on his growth curve, but then at the age of 12 his growth velocity declined and he is now at the 25th percentile. On physical examination, auscultation of the abdomen reveals normoactive bowel sounds and the abdomen is nondistended and nontender to palpation. Perianal examination is significant for a skin tag. The rest of the physical examination is within normal limits. Serum laboratory values are significant for leukocytosis, anemia, and an elevated C-reactive protein (CRP) and erythrocyte sedimentation rate (ESR).

► What is the most likely diagnosis?
► What is the best diagnostic test for this disorder?

ANSWERS TO CASE 53:

Inflammatory Bowel Disease

Summary: A 15 year-old boy presents with persistent abdominal pain, nausea, and weight loss found to have a perianal skin tag on examination and elevated serum inflammatory markers, as well as anemia.

- **Most likely diagnosis:** Inflammatory bowel disease (IBD) (Crohn disease [CD] and ulcerative colitis)

- **Best diagnostic test:** Endoscopy, colonoscopy

ANALYSIS

Objectives

1. Describe signs and symptoms of IBD.

2. Contrast CD with ulcerative colitis.

3. Understand key differences in prognosis and complications.

Considerations

Abdominal pain in children can be a frustrating symptom. Frequently the pain is not associated with any serious condition. However, this patient had fallen off the growth curve; growth failure should always trigger further investigation.

APPROACH TO:

Inflammatory Bowel Disease

DEFINITIONS

CROHN DISEASE: Involves the entire gastrointestinal tract from mouth to anus. Transmural inflammatory process. Tendency for strictures, fistulas, and abscesses. May include skip lesions.

ULCERATIVE COLITIS: Only affects the colon and rectum. Characterized by crypt abscesses.

TOXIC MEGACOLON: Complication characterized by fever, abdominal distention and pain, dilated colon, anemia, and hypoalbuminemia. The condition is life threatening.

CLINICAL APPROACH

Patients with **inflammatory bowel disease** (IBD) may present with complaints of diarrhea, rectal bleeding, cramping, urgency, abdominal pain, early satiety, or nausea.

The majority of children will present with weight loss that may or may not be accompanied by loss of linear growth velocity due to decreased caloric absorption or increased caloric demand of chronic inflammation. Affected patients may also demonstrate a delay in bone development or puberty. Weight loss can be reversed once nutrition is restored. Patients may also have vitamin or mineral deficiencies such as vitamin B_{12}, folate, and iron secondary to malabsorption, anorexia, and chronic inflammation. Other systemic signs may include fever and fatigue. When the colon is affected, children may present with a sense of urgency, tenesmus, and waking from sleep to have a bowel movement.

Description

Crohn disease (CD) involves the entire gastrointestinal tract from mouth to anus. The ileum is involved in 70% of cases. Involvement of the mouth, esophagus, and stomach is much less common. Twenty-five percent of patients have anal involvement. The terminal ileum is affected in 90% of patients. The physical examination should include rectal examination for perianal abscesses, skin tags, fistulas, and fissures. Oral aphthae may be present. Extraintestinal manifestations are less common but may include erythema nodosum, pyoderma gangrenosum, arthritis, digital clubbing, arthralgias, and uveitis.

Ulcerative colitis (UC) involves a continuous section of bowel, unlike CD which can affect different areas (ie, skipped sections) of bowel. UC is a disease only of the rectum and colon. Almost all patients have involvement of the rectum and most children will present with pancolitis. Extraintestinal manifestations are likewise uncommon and may include primary sclerosing cholangitis, arthritis, uveitis, pyoderma gangrenosum, arthritis of large joints, and erythema nodosum.

Incidence

The **incidence of CD** in children/adolescents is 4.56 per 100,000 population. Peak incidence is in the second and third generations of life, then again in the sixth generation of life. Smoking doubles the risk.

The **incidence of UC** in children/adolescents is estimated to be 2.14 cases per 100,000, or about half that of CD. Peak incidence is in the second decade of life. Unlike CD, smoking halves the risk of UC.

Diagnosis

Crohn disease is diagnosed by physical examination, serum and stool laboratory tests, imaging, and colonoscopy. An abdominal radiograph may reveal an abnormal gas pattern or dilation of bowel, or may be normal. Mucosa of patients with CD is characterized by transmural inflammation that often involves the bowel mesentery. Characteristic findings of mucosa during colonoscopy include inflammation with deep fissures, cobblestoning, pseudopolyp formation, skip lesions, and aphthous ulcers. Noncaseating granulomas are present in about 50% of patients on histology. An upper GI with follow through may be performed to evaluate small intestine or a barium enema may be indicated if no evidence of severe colitis is present. CT scans may be performed if no evidence of disease is seen on other studies; thickening of the bowel wall or abscesses are characteristic findings.

An esophagogastroduodenoscopy (EGD) is indicated if upper GI involvement is suspected by the physical examination or the patient's symptoms.

Ulcerative colitis is also diagnosed by physical examination, serum and stool laboratory tests, imaging, and colonoscopy. Barium enema may reveal a "lead pipe" appearance, caused by a loss of haustral markings; or "thumb-printing," indicating inflammation.

Characteristic findings of mucosa during colonoscopy may include protrusions of granulation tissue and regenerating epithelium called *pseudopolyps*. Other findings may include cryptitis and crypt abscesses. UC may result in shortening of the colon or postinflammatory colonic strictures. Fistulas and perianal disease are not seen as in CD. The histology of UC lesions demonstrates both acute and chronic inflammation with mucosal and submucosal infiltration by inflammatory cells, which do not often extend beyond the muscularis layer (unlike CD which involved the full thickness of the bowels). In severe disease in which the mucosal epithelium has been destroyed, inflammation in UC may extend beyond the muscularis mucosae into the submucosa.

Laboratory Values

IBD: Serum laboratory values of patients with IBD may reveal leukocytosis, hypoalbuminemia, anemia, and elevated ESR. Some patients may also have vitamin and mineral deficiencies.

Approximately 10% to 25% of patients with CD are perinuclear neutrophil cytoplasmic antibody (p-ANCA) positive, while 50% to 80% of patients with UC are pANCA positive. Approximately 50% to 70% of patients with CD are positive for anti–*Saccharomyces cerevisiae* antibody (ASCA), whereas only 5% of patients with UC are positive for ASCA.

TREATMENT

Treatment of CD can include immune modifying drugs such as azathioprine, 6-mercaptopurine, or methotrexate. Additional agents used are antibiotics and biologics such as tumor necrosis factor-α inhibitors. Surgery may be required if the symptoms are uncontrolled with medication; however, disease may recur.

Treatment of UC includes aminosalicylate drugs such as sulfasalazine, olsalazine, or balsalazide. Additional agents used are immune modifying drugs such as azathioprine, 6-mercaptopurine, and methotrexate. Antibiotics may also be used. Surgical colectomy is also an option if symptoms are uncontrolled with medication.

MAJOR COMPLICATIONS

Complications of CD may include strictures; fibrosis; fistulas between bowel, bladder, or vagina; strictures; stenosis; and abscesses. If the colon is extensively involved, the risk of colonic cancer is increased, although not to the degree of UC.

The most significant complication of UC is toxic megacolon. This occurs in less than 5% of patients but requires immediate medical and surgical attention. Megacolon is often accompanied by fever, tachycardia, hypokalemia, hypomagnesemia, hypoalbuminemia, and dehydration. Patients may develop colonic perforation or massive hemorrhage.

> **CASE CORRELATION**
>
> - See also Case 10 (Failure to Thrive) which can present with any chronic medical condition. The patient with inflammatory bowel disease may present with rectal bleeding (Case 15) as one of the signs or symptoms. Cystic fibrosis (Case 18) may present with diarrhea and failure to thrive, along with other signs, although classically described as having evidence of pulmonary disease as well. Many of the organisms that cause bacterial enteritis (Case 28) present with diarrhea and mucous in the stool, but also classically with fever.

COMPREHENSION QUESTIONS

53.1 A 14-year-old established patient presents to the office with recurrent painful mouth sores. She notes that for the previous 2 years she has had occasional small sores inside her mouth. She is concerned because her best friend has Crohn disease and has similar ulcers. On examination, you note an afebrile, well-developed adolescent girl with appropriate growth over the previous several years. She has two shallow round, tender ulcers with a grayish base on her left buccal mucosa. The rest of her examination is unremarkable. Her white blood cell count and peripheral smear are normal. The most appropriate next step in her management is:

A. Send blood for perinuclear neutrophil cytoplasmic antibodies (p-ANCA) and anti-Saccharomyces cerevisiae antibodies (ASCA).

B. Refer to gastroenterology for an outpatient colonoscopy.

C. Provide patient and parental reassurance.

D. Culture the ulceration.

E. Initiate oral clindamycin.

53.2 A 17-year-old girl is admitted to the hospital for abdominal pain, fever, bloody diarrhea, and tenesmus. She has no recent travel and no known exposures. Her last illness was 2 weeks ago when she was treated for a folliculitis with clindamycin; she has otherwise been well. Physical examination reveals a tender, nonfocal abdomen. Imaging shows a markedly dilated colon. The likely etiology of this girl's condition is which of the following?

A. Ulcerative colitis (UC)

B. *Clostridium difficile* colitis

C. *Salmonella typhi* colitis

D. Hirschsprung disease

E. Irritable bowel syndrome

53.3 A mother brings her 8-month-old girl to your office with anorexia, abdominal distension, discomfort, weight loss, and intermittent emesis. The mother notes the symptoms began about a month prior as isolated diarrhea. The child has been in day care since 6 weeks of age, but has no known illness contacts there or at home. You note that the child's growth has been poor since the 6-month visit. The mother reports exclusive use of commercially available cow's milk–based formula for the first 6 months of life, adding cereal and other baby food in the previous month. Antitissue transglutaminase IgA antibodies are present. Of the following, which is considered the most appropriate next step?

A. Initiate a lactose-free diet.

B. Initiate a gluten-free diet.

C. Replace the formula with hydrolyzed protein formula.

D. Biopsy of the distal colon.

E. Biopsy of the distal duodenum.

53.4 A 4-month-old formula-fed infant presents with rectal bleeding without emesis or diarrhea. She was the product of a benign term pregnancy and has not been previously ill. Her weight gain has been appropriate since birth, tracking in the 75th percentile on standardized growth curves. The child is afebrile, with normal vital signs, and appears normal on examination. Of the following which is the most likely diagnosis?

A. Necrotizing enterocolitis

B. Ulcerative colitis (UC)

C. Swallowed maternal blood

D. Salmonella gastroenteritis

E. Milk protein allergy

ANSWERS

53.1 **C.** While aphthous stomatitis can be associated with inflammatory bowel disease (more commonly Crohn disease than ulcerative colitis), aphthous ulcers can occur for any number of reasons, including trauma, food sensitivity, and stress. These ulcers are also seen in more uncommon conditions such as immunodeficiency, periodic fever, aphthous stomatitis, pharyngitis, adenitis syndrome (PFAPA), and malignancy-associated acute febrile neutrophilic dermatosis (Sweet syndrome). Her normal growth points away from inflammatory bowel disease, so invasive procedures and extensive laboratory testing are not required. A culture would likely reveal normal oral flora. With no other symptoms and a normal white count, reassurance and observation are appropriate management.

53.2 **B.** Toxic megacolon, or toxic colitis, is a potentially lethal condition. Signs and symptoms may include fever, tachycardia, leukocytosis, anemia, hypotension, colonic dilation on radiography, dehydration, electrolyte abnormality, and altered mental status. While toxic colitis is historically thought to be associated with UC, it can occur with any colitis, including pseudomembranous colitis. Her recent use of clindamycin makes pseudomembranous (ie, *Clostridium difficile*) colitis more likely. Hirschsprung likely would not go unnoticed this long. Irritable bowel syndrome is a relatively benign condition and would not have these radiographic findings. *Salmonella typhi* can cause toxic colitis, but without a travel or exposure history, this is less likely.

53.3 **E.** This child probably has celiac disease, an immune-mediated inflammation of the small intestine in response to dietary gluten. The symptoms in this patient began when additional items were added to the diet around 6 months of age. Commercial formulas are typically gluten free, so symptoms will typically appear between 6 and 24 months of age once parents introduce gluten-containing foods. Grains known to cause symptoms include wheat, barley, and rye. Oats may be involved as well. While presentation in childhood is "classic," many children and adults will first present at an older age, some with constipation, with bulky and foul-smelling stools. Antibody screening has become quite reliable, but diagnosis requires a duodenal biopsy, and must be done while the child is on a gluten-containing diet. Initiating a gluten-free diet before biopsy may make diagnosis difficult.

53.4 **F.** The most common causes of rectal bleeding in the infant period are a milk protein allergy and an anal fissure. The patient in the case presentation has no physical examination finding, so milk protein allergy is more likely. Necrotizing enterocolitis (NEC) is typically seen in premature infants. NEC can rarely occur in term infants with an associated infection. However, with a normal physical examination and no emesis, this diagnosis is unlikely. Retained maternal blood in the baby's gastrointestinal (GI) tract is seen in the immediate postpartum period. Patients with UC do not gain weight well, and salmonella infection typically results in other symptoms such as fever and emesis.

CLINICAL PEARLS

▶ Abdominal pain with weight loss or poor weight gain requires further investigation.

▶ Ulcerative colitis (UC) affects a continuous area of the colon; Crohn disease (CD) can affect multiple discontinuous areas along the entire GI tract.

▶ Both conditions convey an increased risk of colon cancer, although UC is associated with a higher risk than CD.

REFERENCES

Grossman AB, Baldassano RN. Inflammatory bowel disease. In: Kliegman RM, Stanton BF, St. Geme JW, Schor NF, Behrman RE, eds. *Nelson Textbook of Pediatrics*. 19th ed. Philadelphia, PA: Elsevier; 2011:1294-1304.

Rufo PA, Denson LA, Sylvester FA, et al. Health supervision in the management of children and adolescents with IBD: NASPGHAN recommendations. *J Pediatr Gastroenterol Nutr*. 2012;55:93-108.

Stephens MC, Kugathasan S, Sato TT. Inflammatory bowel disease. In Rudolph CD, Rudolph AM, Lister GE, First LR, Gershon AA, eds. *Rudolph's Pediatrics*. 22nd ed. New York, NY: McGraw-Hill; 2011:1460-1467.

A 15-year-old girl is seen by the pediatrician complaining of abdominal pain and vomiting. The abdominal pain is periumbilical, started 12 hours prior, is 9 out of 10 on the pain scale, and is constant, dull, and achy in nature. The pain is aggravated by walking and changing positions. The acetaminophen her mother gave her did not reduce the pain, but is diminished only by lying supine. She is not hungry and has had one episode of nonbilious emesis 2 hours after the onset of the pain and one small, loose bowel movement. She denies dysuria, urinary frequency, and her last menses a week ago was normal; she denies having any sexual contact. On examination, she appears uncomfortable, has a heart rate of 110 beats/min, and a temperature of 100°F (37°C). The lung fields are clear to auscultation bilaterally. Her abdominal examination reveals hypoactive bowel sounds, right rectus abdominis muscle rigidity, and tenderness to palpation, particularly in the periumbilical region. Her pelvic examination shows neither vaginal discharge nor cervical motion tenderness, but she has some abdominal tenderness with gentle bimanual palpation. She has pain at the right lower quadrant when she flexes the right thigh and extends the hip to place her leg into the stirrup for the bimanual examination.

▶ What is the most likely diagnosis?
▶ What is the next step in the management of this patient?

ANSWERS TO CASE 54:
Appendicitis

Summary: A 15-year-old girl with periumbilical pain of 12-hour duration, followed by anorexia and emesis. She has no dysuria or sexual activity, and the pain appears unrelated to her menses. Her physical examination shows a quiet, rigid, tender abdomen, and positive psoas sign.

- **Most likely diagnosis:** Appendicitis.

- **Next step in management:** A surgeon should be consulted once the diagnosis of appendicitis is suspected. Abdominal ultrasound has high sensitivity for diagnosis of appendicitis in experienced pediatric centers, but abdominal computed tomography (CT) is more often used. Ancillary tests include a **complete blood count (CBC) that may show leukocytosis**, a metabolic panel (to identify diabetes, hypercalcemia, abnormal creatinine, transaminitis), pancreatic enzymes, and **a urinalysis** to eliminate other causes of the pain. Despite this adolescent's denial of sexual activity, a urine pregnancy test should always be obtained in postmenarchal females.

ANALYSIS

Objectives

1. Recognize the presenting clinical signs for appendicitis.

2. Know the differential diagnosis for appendicitis.

3. Know the appropriate management for appendicitis.

Considerations

The definitive diagnosis of appendicitis is made once the pathologist finds inflammation histologically on the appendix specimen obtained by surgical removal. For this patient, the initial periumbilical **abdominal pain followed by anorexia and vomiting** suggests appendicitis. **The pain of appendicitis classically begins periumbilically and then migrates to the right lower quadrant with maximal discomfort at McBurney point.** However, the pain can occur laterally if the appendix is retrocecal or it can become diffuse if perforation occurs.

If a patient presents early in the disease process, is lacking the characteristic physical examination findings, has inconclusive imaging findings, and thus has a questionable diagnosis, the child may be observed and undergo serial abdominal examinations for a few hours. However, once appendicitis seems likely, surgical management should occur in a timely fashion; perforation rates exceed 65% if diagnosis is delayed beyond 36 to 48 hours from symptom onset. The most common complications of appendicitis are wound infection and intra-abdominal abscess or phlegmon formation, all of which occur more frequently with appendiceal perforation. Other serious complications are sepsis, shock, ileus, peritonitis, and adhesions causing small bowel obstruction.

APPROACH TO:

Appendicitis

DEFINITIONS

MCBURNEY POINT: The junction of the lateral and middle third of the line joining the right anterior superior iliac spine and the umbilicus (Figure 54–1); typically this area is of greatest discomfort in acute appendicitis.

PSOAS SIGN: Irritation of the psoas muscle caused by active right thigh flexion or passive right hip extension in patients with appendicitis.

OBTURATOR SIGN: Irritation of the obturator muscle caused by passive internal rotation of the right thigh in patients with appendicitis.

ROVSING SIGN: Palpation of the *left* lower quadrant causes pain at the *right* lower quadrant in patients with appendicitis.

CLINICAL APPROACH

Appendicitis is a common reason for emergent surgery in children. A person's lifetime risk of appendicitis has been estimated at 6% to 20%, with the **peak incidence in adolescence** and a slight predilection for males. Appendicitis can develop via several mechanisms but a frequent cause is when the appendiceal lumen becomes obstructed, leading to vascular congestion followed by ischemia, gangrene, and ultimately perforation with spillage of contaminated material into the peritoneum. Obstruction can be caused intrinsically by inspissated fecal material (a fecalith) or by external compression from enlarged lymph nodes associated with bacterial or viral infections.

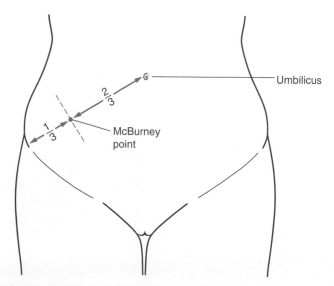

Figure 54–1. McBurney point.

A broad differential diagnosis exists for acute abdominal pain in children (Table 54–1). A thorough history of the illness with close attention to symptoms in other organ systems can help identify these causes; for example, subacute weight loss, sore throat, dysphagia, cough, jaundice, rash, vaginal discharge, and arthralgias do not typically occur with appendicitis. However, diarrhea can be present with appendicitis due to bowel inflammation or because enteric infection may have led to the initial appendiceal inflammation. A comprehensive physical examination can identify pharyngitis, tonsillitis, icterus, a scarlatiniform or purpuric rash, Murphy sign, costovertebral angle tenderness, cervical motion

Table 54–1 • PARTIAL DIFFERENTIAL DIAGNOSIS OF ACUTE ABDOMINAL PAIN IN CHILDREN BEYOND INFANCY	
Condition	Signs and Symptoms
Appendicitis	Right lower quadrant pain, abdominal guarding, and rebound tenderness
Bacterial enterocolitis	Diarrhea (may be bloody), fever, vomiting
Cholecystitis	Right upper quadrant pain, often radiating to subscapular region of the back
Constipation	Infrequent, hard stools, and recurrent abdominal pain; sometimes enuresis
Diabetic ketoacidosis	History of polydipsia, polyuria, and weight loss
Ectopic pregnancy	Lower abdominal pain, vaginal bleeding, and an abnormal menstrual history
Gastroenteritis	Fever, vomiting, and hyperactive bowel sounds
Hemolytic-uremic syndrome	Irritability, pallor, bloody diarrhea, anemia, thrombocytopenia, decreased urine output, hypertension
Henoch-Schönlein purpura	Purpuric lesions, especially of lower extremities and joint pain, blood in stool (guaiac positive)
Hepatitis	Right upper quadrant pain and jaundice
Inflammatory bowel disease	Weight loss, diarrhea, and malaise
Mittelschmerz	Sudden onset of right or left lower quadrant pain with ovulation, may have copious mucoid vaginal discharge
Nephrolithiasis	Hematuria, colicky abdominal pain
Ovarian cyst	Acute pain with rupture or torsion; possible hypotension and fainting accompany hemorrhage in the peritoneum
Pancreatitis	Severe, boring mid-epigastric abdominal pain that might radiate to the back or worsen with eating, persistent vomiting, elevated amylase and lipase
Pelvic inflammatory disease	Cervical motion tenderness; white blood cells in the vaginal secretions
Pneumonia	Fever, cough, and crackles on auscultation of the chest
Sickle cell crisis	Anemia and extremity pain
Streptococcal pharyngitis	Fever, sore throat, and headache
Urinary tract infection	Dysuria, fever, vomiting, flank pain, pyuria, urine nitrites

tenderness, or testicular torsion. Many cases of appendicitis do not present with characteristic features so tools such as the pediatric appendicitis scale (PAS) have been developed, but they have not shown an advantage over clinical experience in reducing perforation.

Appendicitis usually **begins with nonspecific symptoms** of malaise and anorexia and then abdominal pain following in a few hours. **Localization to the right lower quadrant may take 12 to 24 hours** to appear, and pain will then be made worse with movement. Observation of the child getting on and off the examination table can be revealing; children with appendicitis avoid sudden movements. They may walk in a manner to decrease movement of the right side of the abdomen, such as a shuffle, refuse to hop off the table, or brace the abdomen against coughing. The abdomen is inspected, auscultated for bowel sounds, followed by gentle palpation for the area of maximal tenderness and rigidity. The examination should be done with the area of tenderness being palpated last. **Gentle finger percussion is the best method to assess for peritoneal irritation ("rebound tenderness").** The utility of a rectal examination for children with suspected appendicitis is debatable so it is not routinely performed; it can, however, be helpful for localizing the pain source in a female adolescent.

Although not a specific finding, **leukocytosis with a predominance of polymorphonuclear cells (a "left shift")** on a CBC supports an inflammatory process. However, the CBC may be normal in the first 48 hours of the illness. Thereafter, it would be expected to be greater than $10,000/mm^3$ and in cases of perforation, it may be greater than $20,000/mm^3$. **Urinalysis is important to evaluate for glucose and large ketones or pyuria with nitrites and bacteria** because these findings suggest diabetic ketoacidosis or urinary tract infection respectively. Mild hematuria or pyuria can occur with acute appendicitis because of irritation of the bladder or ureteral wall. Chest radiographs eliminate pneumonia as an alternate diagnosis. Plain abdominal radiographs can be obtained but are infrequently helpful. Psoas shadow obliteration, right lower quadrant intestinal dilation, scoliosis toward the affected region, and an appendicolith (seen in 10% of cases) support appendicitis. **In a facility experienced in using ultrasonography in children, ultrasound is the preferred imaging modality for a child suspected of having appendicitis.** It is more sensitive than plain films for appendicitis and is particularly useful in female adolescents, in whom the differential diagnosis often includes ovarian cyst rupture or hemorrhage, follicle rupture, torsion, or PID. Its main limitation is that the appendix cannot always be visualized, which can occur if the appendix has already perforated, the patient is obese, or if there is a lot of bowel distention. Therefore, **abdominal CT has become the diagnostic test of choice in most centers** because it is readily available and is particularly helpful for patients who are **neurologically impaired, immunosuppressed, or obese**, or for patients in whom **perforation** is suspected. If pelvic views are included, it can evaluate for ovarian pathology as the cause of the abdominal pain. Its disadvantages are the amount of radiation exposure generated, increased cost, and it may give limited information without the use of contrast.

Electrolyte abnormalities and volume depletion should be corrected preoperatively as surgery within 48 hours from diagnosis does not influence perforation rate but reduces the risk of surgical complications. Analgesia should be given because it has been shown that it does not interfere with identifying the correct diagnosis.

Definitive treatment is surgical removal of the appendix (appendectomy), accomplished ideally in less than 24 hours from the time of diagnosis. For perforated appendicitis, initial management consists of intravenous antibiotics and fluid replacement. Percutaneous catheters can be used to drain any abscess and then appendectomy is performed at a later time.

CASE CORRELATION

- Myriad conditions may be confused with the abdominal pain of appendicitis. Sickle cell disease (Case 13) may present as an abdominal pain crisis or with gall bladder disease. Pneumonia (Case 14) of the lower lobes is classically described as possibly causing abdominal pain similar to appendicitis. In the smaller child with significant lead poisoning (Case 25), abdominal pain along with achy joints, change in behavior, and encephalopathy can be seen. Bacterial enteritis (Case 28), especially when caused by *Campylobacter* or *Yersinia* sp., and the inflammatory bowel disease (Case 53) may cause abdominal pain confused with appendicitis. While malrotation (Case 34) typically occurs in smaller children, the presentation with abdominal pain may be similar; as part of the surgical procedure to correct a malrotation, an appendectomy typically is performed. Diabetic ketoacidosis (Case 42) presents in a variety of ways, among which is abdominal pain; measurement of a serum sugar typically is performed as part of the evaluation of a patient with possible appendicitis. The patient with severe sore throat, abdominal pain, and fever may have streptococcal pharyngitis; the later complication of this condition is poststreptococcal glomerulonephritis (Case 52).

COMPREHENSION QUESTIONS

54.1 A 7-year-old girl has 3 days of right-sided abdominal pain and 1 day of fever to 102°F (38.9°C). Her mother says that she has also had poor appetite and two loose stools the day prior. On examination, her temperature is 101.7°F (38.7°C), heart rate is 130 beats/min, and respiratory rate is 30 breaths/min. She appears ill and lies motionless on the stretcher. Because of the pain, she is unable to sit up for lung auscultation or percussion of the costovertebral angles. She winced as the stretcher is bumped during palpation of the left abdomen. The abdomen is distended and diffusely tense with hypoactive bowel sounds. Percussion over all areas of the abdomen elicits tenderness in the right lower quadrant (RLQ). Which of the following would NOT be indicated at this time?

    A. Abdominal computed tomography (CT)

    B. Abdominal radiograph

    C. Pediatric surgery consult

    D. Intravenous morphine

    E. Normal saline bolus

54.2 A 14-year-old girl presents with a 2-day history of abdominal pain, anorexia, and vomiting and a 1-day history of fever. For which of the following conditions would exclude appendicitis from the differential diagnosis?

A. She has not passed a stool over the 2 days of illness.

B. She has had diarrhea.

C. Her urine pregnancy test is negative.

D. Her complete blood count (CBC) shows a white blood cell (WBC) count of 8,000/mm^3.

E. She has scleral icterus and tender posterior cervical lymph nodes.

54.3 A previously healthy 8-year-old boy presents to the pediatric clinic with 24 hours of worsening abdominal pain, anorexia, and vomiting. The pain is located in the umbilical region. A CBC reveals a white blood count of 17,000 cells/mm^3 with 70% polymorphonuclear cells. A urine dipstick on a clean-catch specimen shows 1+ leukocytes, trace blood, and trace ketones, but no nitrites and no bacteria. Which of the following is the most appropriate management at this point?

A. Obtain a complete chemistry panel and continue to observe him in the office.

B. Send the patient immediately to the pediatric hospital for an abdominal ultrasound.

C. Give him a prescription for trimethoprim-sulfamethoxazole; schedule a follow-up visit in 2 days to reevaluate the urine.

D. Admit him to the hospital for intravenous antibiotics to treat presumed pyelonephritis.

E. Schedule a computed tomography scan of the abdomen for the next morning.

54.4 A 4-year-old girl has 1 day of fever of 102.4°F (39.1°C), anorexia, two episodes of vomiting, and abdominal pain. Which of the following would NOT be part of your examination?

A. Inspection of the oropharynx

B. Auscultation of the abdomen

C. Percussion of the abdomen

D. Digital rectal examination

E. Assessment of gait and self-transferring

ANSWERS

54.1 **B.** This child's presentation is concerning for appendicitis, and she may have already perforated. Abdominal CT is the best imaging tool for confirming the diagnosis, showing any complication, and helping guide management. A suspected diagnosis of appendicitis warrants a surgery consult. Her current management should consist of analgesia and volume repletion. Abdominal radiographs can be included in the evaluation of abdominal pain but is not the appropriate imaging tool when appendicitis is strongly suspected.

54.2 **E.** It is not uncommon for appendicitis to cause stool changes, either obstipation or ileus from the inflammation. Diarrhea can occur by the same mechanism or may be part of the initial illness that created the appendicitis. A negative pregnancy test only excludes ruptured ectopic pregnancy as her diagnosis. The WBC count may be normal in the first 48 hours of acute appendicitis. Scleral icterus and tender posterior cervical lymph nodes are not features of appendicitis.

54.3 **B.** This boy's symptoms and signs can be caused by appendicitis so prompt imaging to further confirm the diagnosis is indicated. His urinalysis is not consistent with a urinary tract infection, especially because he has peripheral leukocytosis; the urine abnormalities are most likely the result of bladder wall or ureter irritation caused by an inflamed appendix. Waiting to perform diagnostic imaging another 24 hours would increase the risk of perforation to 65% or more.

54.4 **D.** Children with abdominal pain require a comprehensive examination but rectal examination is rarely indicated. Inspection of the oropharynx will show pharyngitis or tonsillitis and her age may prevent her from disclosing that she has pain in her throat. Auscultation and percussion of the abdomen should always be done when pain is reported. If you encounter the child supine on the examination table, it is important to watch the child go through changes in position, such as sitting up for the lung examination, transferring off the table, and then her gait.

CLINICAL PEARLS

▶ Acute appendicitis typically causes periumbilical abdominal pain that eventually migrates to the right lower quadrant. Emesis usually follows, rather than precedes, the onset of pain.

▶ Surgical management of appendicitis occurs as soon as the diagnosis is suspected in order to minimize the risk of perforation.

▶ Appendicitis often is not confirmed until surgery. A history and physical examination, urinalysis, CBC, and abdominal ultrasound or computed tomography scan are the most useful tools for eliminating other preoperative considerations.

REFERENCES

Aiken JJ, Oldham KT. Acute appendicitis. In: Kliegman RM, Stanton BF, St. Geme III J, Schor N, Behrman R, eds. *Nelson Textbook of Pediatrics*. 19th ed. Philadelphia, PA: WB Saunders; 2011:1349-1355.

Egan JC, Aiken JJ. Acute appendicitis, typhlitis, and chronic appendicitis. In: Rudolph CD, Rudolph AM, Lister GE, First LR, Gershon AA, eds. *Rudolph's Pediatrics*. 22nd ed. New York, NY: McGraw-Hill; 2011:1473-1474.

A 19-year-old student presents to the university health center with several days of fever, sore throat, malaise, and a new rash that developed today. She first started feeling ill 10 days ago with general malaise, headache, and nausea. Four days ago she developed a temperature of 103°F (39.4°C) that has persisted. She has worsening sore throat and difficulty swallowing solid foods; she is drinking well. She denies emesis, diarrhea, or sick contacts. She takes an oral contraceptive daily and took two doses of ampicillin yesterday (left over from a prior illness). On examination, she is well developed with a diffuse morbilliform rash. She appears tired but in no distress. Her temperature is 102.2°F (39°C). She has mild supraorbital edema, bilaterally enlarged tonsils that are coated with a shaggy gray exudate, a few petechiae on the palate and uvula, bilateral posterior cervical lymphadenopathy, and a spleen that is palpable 3 cm below the costal margin. Laboratory data include a white blood cell (WBC) count of 17,000 cells/mm³ with 50% lymphocytes, 15% atypical lymphocytes, and platelet count of 100,000/mm³.

▶ What is the most likely diagnosis?
▶ What is the best study to quickly confirm this diagnosis?
▶ What is the best management for this condition?
▶ What is the expected course of this condition?

ANSWERS TO CASE 55:

Acute Epstein-Barr Viral Infection (Infectious Mononucleosis)

Summary: A female college student has 10 days of malaise, headache, and nausea. She now has a fever, sore throat, and morbilliform rash after taking ampicillin. Her examination reveals a fever, rash, tonsillar hypertrophy with exudate, posterior cervical lymphadenopathy, and splenomegaly. She has an elevated WBC count with a lymphocytic predominance and a mild thrombocytopenia.

- **Most likely diagnosis:** Epstein-Barr virus (EBV) infection (infectious mononucleosis).

- **Best study:** Assay for heterophil antibodies (Monospot).

- **Best management:** Symptomatic care, avoidance of contact sports while the spleen is enlarged (usually 1-3 months).

- **Expected course:** Acute illness lasts 2 to 4 weeks, with gradual recovery; splenic rupture is a rare but potentially fatal complication. Rarely, some patients have persistent fatigue.

ANALYSIS

Objectives

1. Describe the presenting signs and symptoms of acute EBV infection.

2. Contrast EBV infection symptoms in young children with those in adolescents and adults.

3. List potential complications of acute EBV infection.

Considerations

This case is typical for adolescents with primary EBV infection, although supraorbital edema occurs in only 10% to 20% of patients. Differential diagnosis includes group A β-hemolytic streptococcal pharyngitis, but streptococcal infection typically does not have a prodrome similar to this case or cause splenomegaly. Acute cytomegalovirus (CMV) infection is another possibility; similarities include splenomegaly, fever, and atypical lymphocytosis, but exudative sore throat and posterior cervical lymphadenopathy occur less frequently. Although the patient denied recent ill contacts, EBV infection has a 30- to 50-day incubation; further questioning revealed that her boyfriend had similar symptoms 6 weeks ago. Rash is seen less commonly in adolescents with EBV, but many patients develop a morbilliform rash in response to ampicillin, amoxicillin, or penicillin.

APPROACH TO:
Epstein-Barr Infection

DEFINITIONS

EPSTEIN-BARR VIRUS (EBV): A double-stranded DNA herpes virus. EBV infects human oropharyngeal and salivary tissues and B lymphocytes. It can cause persistent viral shedding, is associated with oral hairy leukoplakia in HIV-infected adults and lymphoid interstitial pneumonitis in HIV-infected children, and causes several malignancies.

INFECTIOUS MONONUCLEOSIS (IM): The typical EBV presentation in older children and adolescents. Fever, posterior cervical adenopathy, and sore throat are seen in more than 80% of cases.

CLINICAL APPROACH

EBV is ubiquitous in humans. The majority of primary EBV infections throughout the world are subclinical and imperceptible. In developing nations, infection occurs in almost all children by 6 years of age. In the industrialized world, about half of adolescents have serologic evidence of previous EBV infection; 10% to 15% of previously uninfected college students seroconvert each year. Approximately 90% to 95% of adults are EBV seropositive. The virus is excreted in saliva; infection results from mucosal contact with an infected individual or from contact with a contaminated fomite. Shedding of EBV in the saliva after an acute infection can continue for more than 6 months, and occurs intermittently thereafter for life.

   After an infection occurs, EBV replicates in the oropharyngeal epithelium and later in the B lymphocytes. Acute infectious mononucleosis (IM) often begins with a prodromal period that may last for 1 to 2 weeks with vague symptoms such as malaise, headache, and low-grade fever before development of the more definite signs of tonsillitis and/or pharyngitis, cervical lymph node enlargement and tenderness, and moderate to high fever. Affected patients usually have peripheral blood lymphocytosis, composed in large measure of atypical lymphocytes. **Physical findings during an acute infection may include generalized lymphadenopathy, splenomegaly, and tonsillar enlargement with exudate.** Less common findings include a rash and hepatomegaly.

   Primary EBV infection presents as typical IM in older children and adults, but this presentation is less common in young children and infants. In small children, many infections are asymptomatic. In others, fever may be the only presenting sign. Additional acute findings in small children include otitis media, abdominal pain, and diarrhea. Hepatomegaly and rash are seen more often in small children than in older individuals.

   The presence of heterophile antibodies (**Monospot**) **is a useful diagnostic test in children older than 5 years;** the results are unreliable in younger children. Reactive heterophile antibodies in a patient with a compatible syndrome are diagnostic of EBV infection. Early in the illness the heterophile antibodies may be falsely negative (25% in the first week; 5% to 10% in the second week, 5% in the third week). **More definitive testing includes assays of EBV viral capsid antigen, early antigen, and Epstein-Barr nuclear antigen.** In general, **IgM and IgG EBV-VCA** have **high sensitivity and specificity for the diagnosis** of acute IM and are usually present proximate to the onset of illness. IgG VCA antibodies persist for life and are a marker of EBV past infection. IgG antibodies to **early antigen (EA)** are present at the onset of clinical illness. **IgG antibodies to EBV nuclear antigen (EBNA)** form only as the virus establishes latency, beginning to appear 6 to 12 weeks after the onset of illness and persisting throughout life; their presence early in the illness successfully excludes acute EBV infection.

Other laboratory findings include a **lymphocytic leukocytosis,** with approximately **20% to 40% atypical lymphocytes.** Mild **thrombocytopenia** is common, only rarely precipitating bleeding or purpura. More than half of patients with EBV infection develop **mildly elevated liver function tests,** but jaundice is uncommon.

Infection complications are rare but can be life threatening. Neurologic sequelae include Bell palsy, seizures, aseptic meningitis or encephalitis, Guillain-Barré syndrome, optic neuritis, and transverse myelitis. Parotitis, orchitis, or pancreatitis may develop. Airway compromise may result from tonsillar hypertrophy; treatment may include steroids. **Splenomegaly** is seen in approximately half of those with IM; **rupture is rare, but the blood loss is life threatening.**

Typical IM requires only rest. Strict bed rest is not useful except for patients with debilitating fatigue. **Children with splenomegaly should avoid contact sports** to prevent splenic rupture until the enlargement resolves. Acyclovir, which is effective in slowing viral replication, does not affect disease severity or outcome.

Epstein-Barr virus initially was identified from Burkitt lymphoma tumor cells and was the first virus associated with human malignancy. Other associated malignancies include Hodgkin disease, nasopharyngeal carcinoma, and lymphoproliferative disorders. Epstein-Barr virus can stimulate hemophagocytic lymphohistiocytosis. HIV-infected patients may develop oral hairy leukoplakia, smooth muscle tumors, and lymphoid interstitial pneumonitis with EBV infection.

CASE CORRELATION

- See also Case 19 (Leukemia) which also presents with abnormal white blood cells on blood smear, fever, and lymphadenopathy. Typically in Epstein-Barr virus infection, however, the blood abnormalities are limited to one cell line (atypical lymphocytes), whereas in leukemia the abnormalities exist across all three hematologic cell lines. One feature common to Epstein-Barr virus infection and retropharyngeal abscess (Case 46) include the profoundly sore throat.

COMPREHENSION QUESTIONS

55.1 A 17-year-old adolescent boy has left shoulder and left upper quadrant abdominal tenderness and vomiting. He reports having "mono" last month but says he is completely recovered. He was playing flag football with friends when the pain started an hour ago. On examination, his heart rate is 150 beat/min and his blood pressure is 80/50 mm Hg. He is pale, weak, and seems disoriented. He has diffuse rebound abdominal tenderness. Emergent management includes which of the following?

   A. Laparoscopic appendectomy

   B. Fluid resuscitation and blood transfusion

   C. Intravenous antibiotics

   D. Hospital admission for observation

   E. Synchronized cardioversion for supraventricular tachycardia

55.2 You are in a small town practicing pediatrics and have been asked to see a 2-year-old boy in consultation. His general practice doctor admitted him to the hospital 2 days ago because of 3 days of fever. He has generalized lymphadenopathy but is otherwise well. Results of Monospot, HIV testing, and cytomegalovirus (CMV) antigen tests are negative; his liver function test values are mildly elevated. His physician diagnosed the boy's 7-year-old sibling with "mono" the month prior. You should suggest which of the following?

   A. Start intravenous immunoglobulin and obtain an echocardiogram; the patient likely has Kawasaki disease.

   B. Send an Epstein-Barr virus (EBV) culture for confirmation of the physician's suspicions.

   C. Acyclovir treatment because he has an exposure history positive for EBV.

   D. Obtain EBV-VCA IgG and IgM, EBV-EA, and EBV-NA tests.

   E. Liver imaging with ultrasonography or computed tomography.

55.3 The mother of a 15-year-old adolescent girl recently diagnosed with infectious mononucleosis calls for more information. She reports that her daughter, although tired, seems comfortable and is recovering nicely. She remembers that her 20-year-old son had "mono" when he was 10 years old, and he received an oral medicine. She requests the same medication for her daughter. Which of the following is the most appropriate course of action?

   A. Explain that medications are not routinely used in EBV infection.

   B. Call the pharmacy and order oral prednisone 50 mg daily for 5 days (1 mg/kg/d).

   C. Call the pharmacy and order oral acyclovir 250 mg four times per day (20 mg/kg/d).

   D. Have her come to the clinic for a single dose of 50-mg intravenous methylprednisolone (1 mg/kg).

   E. Call the pharmacy and order oral amoxicillin 250 mg three times per day for 7 days.

55.4 A teenage boy arrives for a checkup. His friend recently was diagnosed with mononucleosis. He is worried he will contract it. Which of the following is true regarding transmission of EBV?

A. It is common among casual friends.

B. It occurs only in immunodeficient individuals.

C. It requires close contact with saliva (ie, kissing or drinking from the same cup).

D. It is passed only through sexual contact with an infected individual.

E. It does not occur after the infected person recovers from the initial infection.

ANSWERS

55.1 **B.** The patient described is in hypovolemic shock and likely has splenic rupture with intraperitoneal bleeding. He will die shortly if not aggressively resuscitated with fluids and blood. Evaluation by a surgeon for potential removal of the ruptured spleen should follow quickly. Note that recent surgical literature suggests that many patients with splenic injury may be observed; removal of the spleen is not always required.

55.2 **D.** The Monospot heterophil antibody test, useful in older children, is not so reliable in younger children. Antibodies against specific EBV antigens are more helpful in this age group. No imaging study is diagnostic for EBV, and acyclovir is not indicated for EBV exposure. EBV culture is not readily available except in reference laboratories; the antibody studies described typically are adequate to make the diagnosis. While Kawasaki disease must be considered in patients with persistent fever, the exposure history makes EBV more likely.

55.3 **A.** Supportive care alone usually is required for a patient with acute EBV infection. Steroids have been used historically; current literature suggests their use only in impending airway compromise due to tonsillar hypertrophy or other life-threatening complications. Acyclovir suppresses viral shedding acutely but has no long-term benefit and is not routinely recommended. Amoxicillin and ampicillin are ineffective antiviral medications and induce a rash in some EBV-infected patients.

55.4 **C.** EBV is excreted in saliva and is transmitted through mucosal contact with an infected individual (as in kissing) or through a contaminated object. Virus is shed for a prolonged period after symptoms resolve and is intermittently reactivated and shed for years asymptomatically.

CLINICAL PEARLS

▶ Most adults show evidence of past Epstein-Barr virus (EBV) infection; it is a common infection worldwide.

▶ Children in industrialized nations usually are infected with EBV infection later in life than are children in developing countries.

▶ Diagnosis of EBV infection in young children is best achieved by specific antibody assays.

▶ Infectious mononucleosis is self-limited and usually does not require treatment. Occasional complications of EBV infection may require steroid administration.

REFERENCES

Hunt WG, Brady MT. Epstein-Barr virus mononucleosis. In: Rudolph CD, Rudolph AM, Lister GE, First LR, Gershon AA, eds. *Rudolph's Pediatrics*. 22nd ed. New York, NY: McGraw-Hill; 2011: 1154-1158.

Hurt C, Tammaro D. Diagnostic evaluation of mononucleosis-like illnesses. *Am J Med*. 2007;120(10): 911.e1.

Jenson HB. Epstein-Barr virus. In: Kliegman RM, Stanton BF, St. Geme JW, Schor NF, Behrman RE, eds. *Nelson Textbook of Pediatrics*. 19th ed. Philadelphia, PA: Elsevier; 2011:1110 1115.

Levine MJ, Weinburg A. Infectious mononucleosis (Epstein-Barr virus). In: Hay WW, Levin MJ, Sondheimer JM, Deterding RR, eds. *Current Diagnosis & Treatment Pediatrics*. 20th ed. New York, NY: McGraw-Hill; 2011:1131-1133.

Luzuriaga K, Sullivan JL. Infectious mononucleosis. *N Engl J Med*. 2010;362(21):1993.

A previously healthy 17-year-old boy presents to the emergency department complaining of dark reddish brown urine and severe thigh and calf pain after running a marathon earlier in the day. Physical examination reveals temperature of 101°F (38.3°C), heart rate of 110 beats/min, and blood pressure of 124/72 mm Hg. He has tenderness to palpation and 4/5 strength in his bilateral lower extremities. Laboratory studies include a urine dipstick with 3+ blood and 1+ protein. Urine microscopy shows few red blood cells (RBCs).

▶ What is the most likely diagnosis?
▶ What laboratory tests would you order to support the diagnosis?
▶ What would be the initial step in treatment?

ANSWERS TO CASE 56:

Rhabdomyolysis

Summary: A 17-year-old boy has dark urine, myalgias, fever, and tachycardia after marked physical exertion.

- **Most likely diagnosis:** Rhabdomyolysis.

- **Laboratory studies:** Serum creatine kinase (CK) elevated to at least five times the upper limit of normal (confirms the diagnosis), urine microscopy with few RBCs ("blood" on dipstick is due to myoglobin, not hemoglobin), and urine myoglobin elevated (urine findings not required for diagnosis).

- **Initial treatment:** Aggressive IV fluid resuscitation, correction of electrolyte abnormalities.

ANALYSIS

Objectives

1. Recognize the typical presentation of rhabdomyolysis.

2. List traumatic, "nontraumatic exertional," and "nontraumatic nonexertional" causes of rhabdomyolysis.

3. Discuss basic management principles of rhabdomyolysis.

Considerations

This patient experienced pigmenturia, myalgias, fever, and tachycardia after physical exertion, and his diagnosis is confirmed by a markedly elevated CK. Many causes of rhabdomyolysis exist, including trauma (crush injury, immobilization, muscle compression, compartment syndrome, high voltage electrical injury), exertion (physical effort, seizures, psychotic agitation, metabolic myopathies, thermal extremes), and nontraumatic, nonexertional causes (drugs, toxins, infections, electrolyte abnormalities, endocrine disorders, inflammatory myopathies). It is imperative to remove the offending agent, if one can be identified, to prevent further muscle necrosis. In addition to removing triggering events, management includes intravenous fluid administration, correction of electrolyte abnormalities, and prompt recognition of compartment syndrome, when present.

APPROACH TO:
Rhabdomyolysis

DEFINITIONS

RHABDOMYOLYSIS: Muscle cell necrosis and death with release of intracellular material into circulation causing elevated CK levels, typically accompanied by myalgias and myoglobinuria.

CLINICAL APPROACH

Signs and Symptoms of Rhabdomyolysis

Rhabdomyolysis most classically presents with myalgias, weakness, and dark urine. However, patients with more severe cases may also report fever, tachycardia, malaise, abdominal pain, nausea, and vomiting. If the underlying etiology of rhabdomyolysis involves drugs, toxins, electrolyte abnormalities, or trauma, altered mental status may also be present. On physical examination, muscle tenderness and weakness may be present and occasionally muscle swelling is seen.

Because of muscle cell necrosis and the associated release of breakdown products (such as myoglobin) into circulation, **additional clinical manifestations of rhabdomyolysis include electrolyte abnormalities (most commonly hyperkalemia, hyperphosphatemia, hypocalcemia, hyperuricemia), renal failure, hepatic injury, and cardiac dysrhythmias secondary to hyperkalemia. Late complications include acute kidney injury (AKI), compartment syndrome, and disseminated intravascular coagulation (DIC).** The incidence of AKI in patients with rhabdomyolysis is about 15% to 50%, and is less frequent in patients with relatively lower CK levels at the time of presentation. Renal damage is secondary ischemia (due to hypovolemia from third spacing), as well as tubular injury related to pigment casts and free iron. Compartment syndrome may develop after fluid resuscitation as the muscle becomes more edematous. In rare cases, DIC develops after release of prothrombotic elements from the injured muscle.

Evaluation

When rhabdomyolysis is suspected, initial workup should include creatine kinase, urine dipstick with microscopy, CBC with differential and platelets, electrolytes, BUN, creatinine, calcium, phosphate, albumin, and uric acid. Clinical presentation may dictate further studies, such as drug and toxin screens. **While a markedly elevated CK confirms the diagnosis, a normal level should prompt consideration of other diagnoses.** Urinalysis should be used to identify myoglobinuria; however, myoglobin is rapidly cleared and, therefore, may be absent in the urine in 25% to 50% of patients with rhabdomyolysis. Patients with rhabdomyolysis should be monitored for electrolyte abnormalities, renal and hepatic function, cardiac dysrhythmias, and DIC. In addition to the laboratory studies listed previously, an electrocardiogram (ECG) should be obtained to rule out cardiac rhythm abnormalities. **Muscle biopsy, electromyography (EMG), and magnetic resonance imaging (MRI) are not required for diagnosis.**

TREATMENT

Management of rhabdomyolysis focuses on correction of fluid and electrolyte abnormalities with aggressive rehydration to help prevent AKI and severe metabolic disturbances. Any inciting factors should be removed, and patients should be monitored closely for compartment syndrome. In most cases, the patient can be discharged from the hospital with instructions for continued oral rehydration when the CK has dropped to less than 5000 IU/L.

CASE CORRELATION

- See also Case 52 (Post-streptococcal Glomerulonephritis) which has positive urine for blood due to heme from the red blood cells in contrast to the positive urine for blood due to myoglobin in rhabdomyolysis. While the most commonly seen etiology for rhabdomyolysis is physical exertion or infection, substance abuse (Case 49) in adolescents or adults also is a well-described cause.

COMPREHENSION QUESTIONS

56.1 The adolescent in the initial vignette is found to have a creatine kinase (CK) of 124,000 IU/L and is admitted to the pediatric floor for aggressive IV fluid administration. Which of the following laboratory tests should be ordered for further evaluation?

A. Basic metabolic panel, including electrolytes, blood urea nitrogen (BUN), creatinine (Cr)

B. Calcium and phosphorous

C. Complete blood count (CBC) with differential and platelets

D. Uric acid

E. All of the above

56.2 The patient's laboratory test results return and are significant for potassium level of 6.9. Which of the following is the most appropriate next step in management?

A. Observe and recheck potassium level in 8 hours.

B. Echocardiogram.

C. Electrocardiogram (ECG).

D. Increase the IV fluid rate.

E. Decrease the IV fluid rate.

56.3 You continue to check a BMP and CK level every 8 hours. The potassium level and CK have been trending down with your current therapy, and the remainder of the electrolytes is within normal limits. You have been monitoring kidney function and urine output has been normal, but you are concerned with preventing acute kidney injury (AKI). What is the most important intervention for preventing renal failure in this patient?

A. Discontinue the IV fluids to prevent volume overload.

B. Continue aggressive fluid resuscitation.

C. Perform renal ultrasound to rule out structural abnormalities.

D. Begin renal dialysis if the BUN and creatinine begin to rise.

E. Administer systemic steroids.

56.4 After several hours of fluid administration, the patient begins to complain of severe right calf pain. On examination, the calf appears edematous, the skin over the affected area appears tight, and the posterior tibial and dorsal pedal pulses are not palpable. What is the next step in management?

A. Magnetic resource imaging (MRI) of the right lower extremity

B. Doppler ultrasound of right lower extremity

C. Administration of anticoagulation therapy

D. Immediate surgical consultation for fasciotomy

E. Close observation

ANSWERS

56.1 **E.** Once the diagnosis of rhabdomyolysis is made, additional studies should be sent to assess for further abnormalities and complications. BMP, calcium, and phosphate should be checked for electrolyte abnormalities and renal function, CBC for infection, and uric acid for baseline level (it is expected to be elevated).

56.2 **C.** Hyperkalemia puts the patient at risk for cardiac dysrhythmias, so an ECG is the first step in evaluation. An echocardiogram would not be warranted at this stage in the workup. Aggressive IV fluid administration should continue, but alteration of the rate based on the potassium is not required. Observation would be inappropriate in this context.

56.3 **B.** Aggressive IV fluid administration prevents acute kidney injury by correcting volume depletion, leading to better renal perfusion and less ischemic injury. In addition, it may help wash out heme pigment casts from the renal tubules; increased urine output will aid in potassium excretion. Discontinuing IV fluids would put the patient at more risk for AKI. Renal ultrasound, dialysis, and steroids would not be indicated at this time.

56.4 **D.** Compartment syndrome is a known complication of rhabdomyolysis, and it is considered a surgical emergency. The patient should be evaluated by a surgeon as soon as possible, because increased ischemia to the area will lead to more muscle and tissue necrosis. MRI and ultrasound would support your clinical diagnosis but would delay surgical intervention. Anticoagulation is not indicated for the treatment of compartment syndrome.

CLINICAL PEARLS

▶ Rhabdomyolysis and its complications are caused by release of muscle breakdown products being released into circulation after muscle cell necrosis.

▶ Typical presentation includes myalgias and dark-colored urine, and the diagnosis is confirmed with markedly elevated CK level.

▶ Important findings and complications include electrolyte abnormalities, AKI, and compartment syndrome.

▶ The most important treatment is aggressive IV fluid administration.

REFERENCES

Bosch X, Poch E, Grau JM. Rhabdomyolysis and acute kidney injury. *N Engl J Med*. 2009;361:62.

Counselman FL, Lo BM. Rhabdomyolysis. In: Tintinalli JE, Stapczynski J, Ma O, Cline DM, Cydulka RK, Meckler GD, T. eds. *Tintinalli's Emergency Medicine: A Comprehensive Study Guide*. 7th ed. New York, NY: McGraw-Hill; 2011:chap 92.

Giannoglou GD, Chatzizisis YS, Misirli G. The syndrome of rhabdomyolysis: Pathophysiology and diagnosis. *Eur J Intern Med*. 2007;18:90.

Hellmann DB, Imboden JB, Jr. Rheumatologic & immunologic disorders. In: Papadakis MA, McPhee SJ, Rabow MW, eds. *CURRENT Medical Diagnosis & Treatment 2014*. New York, NY: McGraw-Hill; 2014:chap 20.

Huerta-Alardín AL, Varon J, Marik PE. Bench-to-bedside review: Rhabdomyolysis—an overview for clinicians. *Crit Care*. 2005;9:158.

Khan FY. Rhabdomyolysis: a review of the literature. *Neth J Med*. 2009;67:272.

Knochel JP. Rhabdomyolysis. In: Lerma EV, Berns JS, Nissenson AR, eds. *CURRENT Diagnosis & Treatment: Nephrology & Hypertension*. New York, NY: McGraw-Hill; 2009: chap 11.

Mandt MJ, Grubenhoff JA. Emergencies & injuries. In: Hay WW, Jr, Levin MJ, Deterding RR, Abzug MJ, Sondheimer JM, eds. *CURRENT Diagnosis & Treatment: Pediatrics*. 21st ed. New York, NY: McGraw-Hill; 2012: chap 12.

McMillan JA, Feigin RD, DeAngelis C, Jones DM. *Oski's Pediatrics*. 4th ed. Philadelphia, PA: Lippincott Williams & Wilkins; 2006:69, 2549.

Schwartz MW, Bell LM, Bingham PM, et al. *5-Minute Pediatric Consult*. 4th ed. Philadelphia, PA: Lippincott Williams & Wilkins; 2008:720-721.

Warren JD, Blumbergs PC, Thompson PD. Rhabdomyolysis: a review. *Muscle Nerve*. 2002;25:332.

A 16-year-old adolescent girl presents to your clinic complaining of very heavy menstrual bleeding for the last 6 months. She notes that her cycles are regular, occurring every 29 days, but they last for 10 days and she goes through 10 to 12 pads per day. Her last period ended a week ago, and she now complains of dizziness when she stands up. She denies concurrent vaginal discharge or abdominal pain. Her past medical and family histories are negative for bleeding problems. Her menarche was at 12 years of age, and she started having regular menstrual cycles at 14 years of age. She denies all forms of sexual activity. Her examination is significant for mild resting tachycardia and orthostatic hypotension. Her nail beds and conjunctiva are pale. A urine pregnancy test is negative, and her hemoglobin is 8 g/dL.

▶ What is the most likely diagnosis?
▶ How would you manage this patient?

ANSWERS TO CASE 57:

Abnormal Uterine Bleeding

Summary: An adolescent girl complains of heavy but regular menstrual bleeding that has resulted in anemia and orthostatic hypotension.

- **Most likely diagnosis:** Abnormal uterine bleeding (AUB)

- **Management:** Iron supplement and monophasic low-dose oral contraceptive pills (OCPs) for 3 to 6 months with a follow-up hemoglobin in 6 weeks

ANALYSIS

Objectives

1. List the diagnostic possibilities for AUB.

2. Describe the appropriate evaluation of AUB.

3. Differentiate between the different managements of AUB based on symptoms and type of bleeding.

Considerations

Menstrual bleeding that leads to anemia and orthostatic hypotension is not typical, and requires further investigation. Excessive bleeding may be caused by pregnancy; although she denies sexual activity, a urine pregnancy test should be part of the evaluation. Sexually transmitted diseases, bleeding disorders, malignancy, and trauma should also be considered.

APPROACH TO:

Abnormal Uterine Bleeding

DEFINITIONS

The terminology for this disorder has changed over the last several years. In place of the historical terms such as menorrhagia and metrorrhagia, international consensus has been reached on four general categories of menstrual disturbances:

REGULARITY: Irregular menstrual bleeding (variation of cycle length of more than 20 days over the course of a year); also includes amenorrhea.

FREQUENCY: Infrequent menstrual bleeding/oligomenorrhea (one or two episodes in a 3-month period) or frequent menstrual bleeding (more than four episodes in a 3-month period).

HEAVINESS OF FLOW: Excessive menstrual blood loss that interferes with the woman's quality of life.

DURATION OF FLOW: Prolonged bleeding (exceeding 8 days on a regular basis) or shortened bleeding (no more than 2 days).

CLINICAL APPROACH

Abnormal uterine bleeding (AUB) is defined as abnormal menstrual flow, not caused by pelvic pathology, medications, systemic disease, or pregnancy that occurs either excessively in a prolonged or regular cycle, or irregularly and not related to the normal menstrual flow. The four descriptive characteristics, outlined earlier, include regularity, frequency, heaviness of flow, and duration of flow. In adolescents, AUB is usually due to immaturity of the hypothalamic-pituitary-ovarian axis, specifically lack of the midcycle luteinizing hormone (LH) surge, which results in anovulation. Abnormal uterine bleeding is a diagnosis of exclusion; other diagnoses must be considered first. Of young women presenting with abnormal vaginal bleeding in the United States requiring hospitalization, 46% of cases were due to anovulation, 33% were due to hematologic causes, 11% due to infection, and 11% due to chemotherapy. Organic causes, such as ectopic pregnancy or threatened abortion are found in about 9% of cases. Other potential causes include infections (cervicitis, human papillomavirus [HPV], trichomonas), trauma, hormonal contraceptives and other medications, hypothyroidism, foreign body, coagulopathy, or malignancy. The remainder of women will have no demonstrable cause for their bleeding and are diagnosed with abnormal (formerly dysfunctional) uterine bleeding. The key to differentiating these causes is the presence of pain, which is usually absent in anovulatory bleeding and present in organic or infections causes.

The typical presentation is that of a teen with regular menstrual cycles that then develops prolonged or heavy menstrual bleeding, or irregular bleeding. The bleeding is usually painless. Important aspects of the history include prior episodes of bleeding, the length of the woman's cycle, the number of days of bleeding, and the severity of the bleeding (can be established by asking about the number of pads or tampons used per day). Family history should include others with bleeding problems, such as excessive hemorrhage after surgery and women requiring hysterectomy after child birth.

After verifying that the patient is not pregnant, the next most important laboratory evaluation is the hemoglobin and hematocrit. The degree of anemia helps categorize the severity of bleeding and helps guide management (Figure 57–1). Women with hemoglobin greater than 12 g/dL are considered to have mild bleeding, and may be managed with iron supplements and careful follow-up alone. A hemoglobin of 9 to 12 g/dL is considered a result of moderately severe bleeding; treatment includes iron and monophasic OCP. Women with hemoglobin less than 7 g/dL or less than 10 g/dL with significant orthostatic blood pressure changes are considered to have severe bleeding, and may need hospitalization and blood transfusion. Intravenous estrogen (Premarin) and high-dose oral contraceptives are used until the bleeding stops; further bleeding despite these measures may require dilation and curettage. Although these high doses of estrogen raise theoretical concerns about thrombotic events, none have been reported with the short-term use required in this condition.

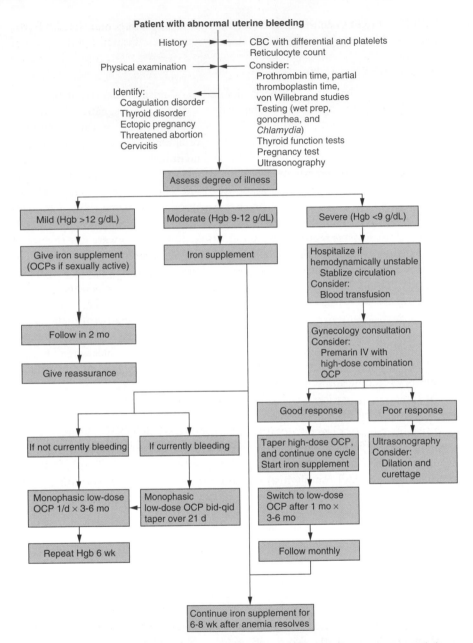

Figure 57–1. Evaluation of dysfunctional uterine bleeding. (CBC, complete blood count; Hgb, hemoglobin; OCP, oral contraceptive pills.) (*Reproduced, with permission, from Hay WW, Levin MJ, Sondheimer JM, Deterding RR, eds. Current Diagnosis and Treatment in Pediatrics, 19th ed. New York: McGraw-Hill, 2009:128. Figure 3-8.*)

Patients with AUB continue oral contraceptives for 3 to 6 months. After the menstrual cycle is regular and irregular bleeding has ceased, careful withdrawal of the OCP may be attempted if desired with close follow-up. Iron supplementation should be continued for 2 months after the anemia is resolved.

COMPREHENSION QUESTIONS

57.1 A 15-year-old adolescent girl presents to the local hospital emergency center complaining of several days of left-sided abdominal pain, mild vaginal bleeding, and dizziness. Upon further questioning you learn that she has had near-syncopal episodes the last few times she has tried to stand up. She denies fever, sexual activity, previous episodes of midcycle vaginal bleeding, and abdominal or genitourinary trauma. On examination, she is pale and tachycardic. She has abdominal pain with rebound and guarding in the upper and lower left quadrants that radiates to the back. Her hemoglobin is 5 g/dL, her white count is 12,000/mm^3, and her platelet count is 210,000/mm^3. Her serum β-HCG is 1800 mIU/mL. Which of the following is the most likely diagnosis?

A. Metrorrhagia with subsequent anemia

B. Pelvic inflammatory disease

C. Salicylate overdose

D. Ruptured ectopic pregnancy

E. Uterine malignancy

57.2 A 13-year-old adolescent girl comes to the office for a preparticipation sports physical before the start of the basketball season. She has no complaints, but wants to discuss the human papillomavirus (HPV) vaccine some of her friends have received. Which of the following is an accurate statement about HPV and the vaccine?

A. The HPV vaccine is indicated only once a woman becomes sexually active.

B. HPV types 6 and 11 are high-cancer risk serotypes and are included in the vaccine.

C. HPV vaccine helps prevent cervical cancer but not genital warts.

D. HPV types 16 and 18 are associated with the majority of cervical cancers.

E. Syncope after injection has been reported and is a unique adverse reaction to HPV vaccine.

57.3   A 16 year old presents to your clinic with a complaint of persistent vaginal bleeding. She had been seen 3 months ago when you noted a mild anemia of 13 g/dL, diagnosed her with abnormal uterine bleeding, and started her on iron supplements. Today she is listless and pale. Her hemoglobin in your clinic is 6 g/dL, her platelet count is normal, and her urine pregnancy test remains negative. You admit her to your local hospital and order a transfusion of packed red blood cells. In addition to stabilizing her circulatory system, which of the following is the most appropriate next step in the acute management of her condition?

   A.   Monophasic low-dose oral contraceptive (OCP)

   B.   Intravenous conjugated estrogens (Premarin) and high-dose combination OCP

   C.   Hysterectomy

   D.   Discharge after transfusion with iron supplementation

   E.   Triphasic low-dose OCP

57.4   A 19-year-old adolescent girl presents with a temperature of 101.2°F (38.4°C), lower abdominal pain, bloody vaginal discharge, and dyspareunia. She has no nausea or vomiting, and is tolerating fluids well. She has cervical motion tenderness on examination. Her urine pregnancy test is negative, and an ultrasound of her right lower quadrant is negative for appendicitis. Which of the following is the appropriate outpatient management for her likely condition?

   A.   Levofloxacin, 500 mg orally once a day for 14 days as monotherapy

   B.   Ofloxacin, 400 mg orally twice a day for 14 days as monotherapy

   C.   Ceftriaxone, 250 mg IM in a single dose as monotherapy

   D.   Levofloxacin, 500 mg orally once a day, and doxycycline, 100 mg orally twice a day, both for 14 days

   E.   Ceftriaxone, 250 mg IM as a single dose and doxycycline, 100 mg orally twice a day for 14 days

ANSWERS

57.1   **D.** The classic triad of abdominal pain, vaginal bleeding, and amenorrhea only occurs in about 50% of cases of ectopic pregnancy. Because ectopic pregnancy is the leading cause of pregnancy-related death in the first trimester, a physician must consider the diagnosis for any woman of childbearing age with abdominal pain. Risk factors for an ectopic pregnancy include pelvic inflammatory disease (PID), intrauterine device (IUD), previous ectopic pregnancy, previous tubal surgery, increasing age, use of fertility drugs, and smoking. Because this patient is hemodynamically unstable, admission and surgery are indicated; however, hemodynamically stable patients with an unruptured ectopic pregnancy and good follow-up may be managed expectantly or treated with methotrexate.

57.2 **D.** Quadrivalent HPV vaccine (Gardasil) was licensed in 2006, and is indicated for the prevention of HPV types 6, 11, 16, and 18. Types 6 and 11 cause about 90% of all genital warts, but carry a low risk of malignancy. Types 16 and 18 cause about two-thirds of all cervical cancer cases. Immunization before sexual debut is ideal, but even women who are sexually active may benefit from the vaccine; because there is no commercially available screening test to determine the serotypes to which a woman has been exposed, the vaccine may still provide some protection. Boys, too, receive this vaccination beginning at the age of 11 years in the effort to prevent warts and spread of the virus. The vaccine is a three-dose series. Common side effects include headache and pain at the injection site. Anaphylaxis to yeast is a contraindication. Syncope has been reported in the adolescent population with all vaccines; current recommendations suggest observing adolescents for 15 minutes after immunization.

57.3 **B.** Based on her anemia, this adolescent's abnormal uterine bleeding is classified as severe and warrants hospitalization. Stabilization of her circulatory system is the first priority, and then steps must be taken to stop the bleeding. Intravenous conjugated estrogens (Premarin) in conjunction with a high-dose OCP is the next step. If this treatment is successful in decreasing the bleeding, she can be continued on high-dose OCP for a month and then moved to a low-dose OCP. If she continued to have bleeding after IV Premarin and a high-dose OCP, dilation and curettage may be necessary.

57.4 **E.** More than one million women develop pelvic inflammatory disease (PID) in the United States each year, and more than a quarter of these require hospitalization. PID is most common in the teen population, with decreasing incidence with increasing age. Because presenting signs and symptoms are variable, diagnosis can be difficult. The Centers for Disease Control and Prevention (CDC) recommends that empiric treatment should be started if a young woman at risk for PID presents with lower abdominal or pelvic pain, no other cause for the pain can be identified, and the woman has: (1) cervical motion tenderness, (2) uterine tenderness, or (3) adnexal tenderness. Treatment is aimed at both gonorrhea and chlamydia. Recent surveillance by the CDC has shown fluoroquinolone-resistant gonorrhea is widespread in the United States, so fluoroquinolones are no longer recommended in the treatment of PID.

CLINICAL PEARLS

▶ Pregnancy and sexually transmitted diseases (STDs) must be considered in any adolescent with abnormal vaginal bleeding.

▶ Abnormal uterine bleeding can be excessive flow with normal intervals (menorrhagia) or flow with irregular intervals (metrorrhagia).

▶ Cessation of bleeding can usually be achieved through the use of oral contraceptives; occasionally, intravenous estrogen is required.

REFERENCES

Buzzini SR, Gold MA. Menstrual disorders. In: McMillan JA, Feigin RD, DeAngelis CD, Jones MD, eds. *Oski's Pediatrics: Principles and Practice*. 4th ed. Philadelphia, PA: Lippincott Williams & Wilkins; 2006:561-566.

Cromer B. Abnormal uterine bleeding. In: Kliegman RM, Stanton BF, St. Geme JW, Schor NF, Behrman RE, eds. *Nelson Textbook of Pediatrics*. 19th ed. Philadelphia, PA: Elsevier; 2011:688-690.

Cunningham FG, Leveno KJ, Bloom SL, et al. Ectopic pregnancy. *Williams Obstetrics*. 23rd ed. New York, NY: McGraw-Hill; 2010. http://www.accessmedicine.com/content.aspx?aID=6020319. Accessed April 24, 2012.

Daley MF, O'Leary ST, Simoes EA, Nyquist A-C. Immunization. In: Hay WW, Levin MJ, Sondheimer JM, Deterding RR, eds. *Current Diagnosis & Treatment Pediatrics*. 20th ed. New York, NY: McGraw-Hill; 2011:267-268.

Edman JC, Shafer M. Dysfunctional uterine bleeding. In: Rudolph CD, Rudolph AM, Lister GE, First LR, Gershon AA, eds. *Rudolph's Pediatrics*. 22nd ed. New York, NY: McGraw-Hill; 2011:298-299.

Fraser IS, Critchley HO, Broder M, Munro MG. The FIGO recommendations on terminologies and definitions for normal and abnormal uterine bleeding. *Semin Reprod Med*. 2011;29:383-390.

Sass AE, Kaplan DW. Dysfunctional uterine bleeding. In: Hay WW, Levin MJ, Sondheimer JM, Deterding RR, eds. *Current Diagnosis & Treatment Pediatrics*. 20th ed. New York, NY: McGraw-Hill; 2011:132, 134-135.

Workowski KA, Berman S. Centers for Disease Control and Prevention. Sexually transmitted diseases treatment guidelines, 2010. *MMWR Recomm Rep*. 2010;59(No. RR-12):63-67.

A 13-year-old girl complains about "zits" on her face and shoulders. She has tried over-the-counter benzoyl peroxide for 2 months to no avail, and has stopped eating chocolate and French fries on her mother's advice. She has been invited to an upcoming school dance and wants to look her best. She complains about blackheads, but also lesions that are deep and painful.

▶ What is the diagnosis?
▶ What is the best treatment for her condition?

ANSWERS TO CASE 58:

Acne Vulgaris

Summary: An adolescent girl presents with acne on her face and shoulders.

- **Most likely diagnosis:** Combination acne with mixed comedonal and inflammatory lesions.

- **Best therapy:** First-line therapy includes antibacterial soap, keratolytic agent (benzoyl peroxide), comedolytic agent (tretinoin), and/or topical antibiotic (erythromycin). Oral antibiotics (tetracycline) are a secondary option. Isotretinoin (oral tretinoin) is reserved for severe, resistant nodulocystic acne.

ANALYSIS

Objectives

1. Understand the various types of acne vulgaris.

2. Know the treatments for various types of acne.

3. Discuss the potential side effects of isotretinoin.

Considerations

Acne vulgaris has the potential to be as damaging to the psyche as it can be to the skin. Managing acne successfully involves promoting patient understanding of the basics behind its development, creating thoughtful treatment regimens tailored to each patient, and periodically reassessing acne control in an effort to prevent possible emotional and physical scarring.

APPROACH TO:

Acne Vulgaris

DEFINITIONS

COMEDONE: Open comedones (blackheads) are composed of compacted melanocytes; closed comedones (whiteheads) contain purulent debris.

CYST: Dilated and often tender intradermal follicle.

PAPULE: Small, erythematous, and inflamed "bump" under the skin due to sebum, fatty acids, and bacteria reacting within a follicle.

NODULE: Papule greater than 5 mm penetrating deep into the dermis.

PUSTULE: Elevated focus of inflammation and purulent exudate around a comedone, occurring in the superficial dermis.

CLINICAL APPROACH

Roughly 70% to 85% of adolescents have some form of acne. **Pubertal hormonal surges lead to an increase in sebum production by sebaceous glands.** Proliferation of the bacterium *Propionibacterium acnes* leads to distention of follicular walls, causing obstruction of sebum flow. Follicles reach a maximum capacity and rupture, releasing their inflammatory contents. Neutrophils and liposomal enzymes are released, causing further inflammation. Scarring and pitting often may result.

Acne lesions are categorized as inflammatory or noninflammatory. Noninflammatory lesions consist of open and closed comedones. Inflammatory lesions are characterized by the presence of papules, pustules, nodules, or cysts. Physical examination of the patient with acne should include a thorough observation and description of lesion type(s) and distribution across the body (face, chest, back).

Of note, other skin disorders can mimic acne. Examples include tinea barbae pustules composed of dermatophytes under the beard of a rancher working with livestock and requiring an antifungal (griseofulvin); erythematous and papulopustular rosacea with undetermined etiology on the nose and cheeks of a teenager usually responding to a topical antibacterial (metronidazole); and allergic dermatitis with inflammatory papules on the chin of a toddler often controlled with an emollient or an occasional low-strength topical steroid (hydrocortisone).

Acne treatment goals are elimination of lesions and diminishment of scarring (Table 58–1). Improvement may not be noticed for at least a month after therapy is initiated, with flare-ups possible during treatment. Patients should be discouraged from manipulating skin lesions because doing so will increase inflammation and promote scarring. The affected skin should be gently washed using antibacterial soap and rinsed well to prevent soap buildup on the skin surface. Scrubbing agents and harsh soaps should not be used, because they may stimulate more oil production and promote acne. Oil-based cosmetics, sunscreens, and moisturizers also may worsen acne. Evidence-based guidelines for acne treatment, based on severity and lesion type, were issued by the American Acne and Rosacea Society and endorsed by the American Academy of Pediatrics in 2013.

First-line management should begin with topical benzoyl peroxide or a comedolytic agent such as a retinoid (Retin-A). The combination of benzoyl peroxide in the morning and a comedolytic agent at night may be effective when either alone has failed. Benzoyl peroxide must be washed off prior to application of tretinoin or the retinoid will be rendered ineffective. Benzoyl peroxide is bactericidal and

Table 58–1 • TREATMENT OF VARIOUS TYPES OF ACNE	
Acne Type	**Treatment[a]**
Pure comedonal acne	Topical tretinoin or adapalene at night
Mild papular acne	Benzoyl peroxide in the morning and at night
Papulopustular and cystic (inflammatory) acne	Benzoyl peroxide and/or topical antibiotics in the morning, and topical tretinoin or adapalene at night
Severe pustulocystic acne	Benzoyl peroxide and oral antibiotic
Severe cystic acne	Oral retinoid (isotretinoin)

[a]Wash all types with antibacterial soap in the morning and at night.

keratolytic, causing follicular desquamation. It is available in over-the-counter preparations with variable uniformity, stability, and efficacy. Although these over-the-counter preparations eliminate bacteria at the skin surface, they do not have a carrier vehicle that allows deep follicular penetration. Therefore, 2.5% to 10% prescription preparations are preferable, with gels being more efficacious although more irritating at times; starting at the lowest concentration is recommended. A benzoyl peroxide wash is beneficial when lesions are widely distributed or when adherence to a treatment plan is problematic. Washes are applied in the shower and then rinsed off after approximately 30 seconds. Benzoyl peroxide can bleach fabric, so careful and thorough rinsing and drying is recommended.

Topical tretinoin, a vitamin A derivative, inhibits the formation of microcomedones and increases cell turnover. Therapy should begin conservatively at 0.025%, with 3 to 4 weeks allowed for accommodation. Patients should use a mild soap (Dove, Cetaphil) and allow the skin to dry 20 to 30 minutes prior to applying nightly tretinoin. Mild redness and peeling can occur, and patients should avoid sun exposure and use sunscreens. Adapalene 0.1% (Differin) is a retinoid formulation that causes less irritation and photosensitivity, has more activity, and can be used concomitantly with benzoyl peroxide preparations. A combination product combining adapalene and benzoyl peroxide (Epiduo Gel 0.1%/2.5%) is available. Tazarotene 0.1% (Tazorac) is a retinoid that is active against psoriasis. This agent is teratogenic and causes irritation, so it should be used with caution. Some believe that azelaic acid applied twice daily for 4 to 6 months may provide acne relief, especially for those sensitive to other agents, and theoretically can reduce scarring.

Topical, rather than systemic, antibiotics are preferred because of their fewer side effects. Topical antibiotics (erythromycin, clindamycin) often are applied to affected areas twice daily or in combination with benzoyl peroxide or tretinoin. Long-term topical or oral antibiotic monotherapy is not recommended due to the potential development of bacterial resistance. Combination benzoyl peroxide and topical antibiotic preparations can be particularly beneficial, and do not typically promote resistance. Oral antibiotics (doxycycline, erythromycin, tetracycline) are used when moderate to severe inflammatory and pustular acne does not respond to topical treatment. Tetracycline is the most frequently used oral antibiotic because it is inexpensive and has few side effects. To minimize the potential for antibiotic resistance, oral antibiotics ideally should be discontinued after a few months. Antibiotics, irrespective of the formulation, should be discontinued once inflammatory lesions are under good control.

Isotretinoin (Accutane) is the **treatment of choice for severe, resistant nodulocystic acne.** A 5-month course often clears a severe case of acne. It is highly teratogenic and has many side effects, including **mood dysregulation, cheilitis, conjunctivitis, hyperlipidemia, blood dyscrasias, elevated liver enzymes, and photosensitivity.** Lipid levels, liver enzymes, and complete blood counts should be monitored monthly during the course. Females should have a negative pregnancy test immediately before isotretinoin is initiated and should maintain effective contraception before, during, and after therapy. Prescribers and patients must be registered in the iPLEDGE pregnancy prevention and risk management program.

Oral contraceptives (Ortho Tri-Cyclen) are approved for treatment of acne, and intralesional steroid therapy is sometimes used in unresponsive cases.

CASE CORRELATION

- See also Case 45 (Precocious Puberty) which may be heralded by unexpected and early acne development. The facial rash of system lupus erythematosus (Case 51) is occasionally confused with acne, although the "butterfly, malar" distribution of systemic lupus erythematosus (SLE) is classically described whereas acne tends to be found beyond those boundaries.

COMPREHENSION QUESTIONS

58.1 A teenager with severe cystic acne started using isotretinoin a month ago. Initially her acne worsened, but is now starting to improve. However, she reports "not feeling normal." She does not want to go to school, cries frequently, and feels hopeless, but declares no suicidal thoughts. She also feels "achy" all over. Which of the following is the best course of action?

 A. Continue isotretinoin and see her in follow-up in a week.

 B. Prescribe an antidepressant.

 C. Discontinue isotretinoin and refer her to a psychiatrist.

 D. Decrease her isotretinoin dose to determine if the side effects resolve.

 E. Counsel her that these symptoms will resolve over time.

58.2 A teenage boy complains of a several-week history of facial "zits" that are painful and itchy. There are no other breakouts. He has inflammatory papules and pustules in the beard and moustache area and has mild cervical lymphadenopathy. He occasionally works weekends on a farm. Which of the following therapies is appropriate?

 A. Topical retinoid

 B. Oral steroid

 C. Oral antifungal

 D. Topical antibacterial

 E. Oral antiviral

58.3 A 7-day-old infant is brought to clinic because of "pimples" on his cheeks and forehead. He is breast-feeding well, and the parents have no other concerns. The skin around the pimples and elsewhere is unremarkable, as is the rest of his examination. Which of the following is appropriate advice or therapy?

 A. Recommend a different soap.

 B. Prescribe topical triamcinolone.

 C. Prescribe topical erythromycin.

 D. Recommend no treatment.

 E. Recommend more frequent bathing.

58.4 A 17-year-old girl is prescribed oral tetracycline, topical tretinoin, and topical benzoyl peroxide for her combination acne. She is sexually active and takes an oral contraceptive. You should counsel her to do which of the following?

A. Take the tetracycline with food or milk.

B. Use a second form of birth control in addition to her oral contraceptive.

C. Get some sun to help dry up her acne.

D. Avoid chocolate and fried foods.

E. Avoid water-based sunscreen.

ANSWERS

58.1 **C.** Depression is a rare side effect of isotretinoin, but it can be severe and suicides have been reported. Myalgias and arthralgias have also occurred. It would be best to stop the drug and have the patient evaluated for depression.

58.2 **C.** Tinea barbae is caused by various dermatophytes and closely resembles tinea capitis. It can be acquired through animal exposure and is more common in farmers. Topical antifungal preparations are ineffective; oral antifungals are required.

58.3 **D.** Approximately 20% of normal neonates develop at least a few comedones within the first month of life. The cause of neonatal acne is unknown, but has been attributed to placental transfer of maternal androgens, hyperactive adrenal glands, and a hypersensitive neonatal end-organ response to androgenic hormones. Such patients may be predisposed to adolescent acne. In most cases, a prescription or change in skin care is not warranted.

58.4 **B.** Oral antibiotics may decrease the effectiveness of oral contraceptive pills. Tretinoin can lead to photosensitivity; patients should avoid sun exposure or use sunscreen. Diet has not been found to have an effect on acne. Tetracycline should be taken on an empty stomach; milk products bind tetracycline.

CLINICAL PEARLS

▶ Acne is a disorder of the sebaceous follicle in which excess sebum, keratinous debris, and bacteria accumulate, producing microcomedones that may become inflamed.

▶ Treatment of acne depends on its severity and distribution, and may involve a regimen of oral or topical agents, alone or in combination.

REFERENCES

Baldwin HE, Friedlander SF, Eichenfield LF, Mancini AJ, Yan AC. The effects of culture, skin color, and other nonclinical issues on acne treatment. *Semin Cutan Med Surg.* 2011;30:S12-S15.

Dill SW, Cunningham BB. Acne and other disorders of the pilosebaceous unit. In: Rudolph CD, Rudolph AM, Lister G, First LR, Gerson AA, eds. *Rudolph's Pediatrics.* 22nd ed. New York, NY: McGraw-Hill; 2011:1287-1288.

Friedlander SF, Baldwin HE, Mancini AJ, Yan AC, Eichenfield LF. The acne continuum: an aged-based approach to therapy. *Semin Cutan Med Surg.* 2011;30:S6-S11.

Habif TP. *Clinical Dermatology.* 5th ed. St. Louis, MO: Mosby-Year Book; 2010.

Mancini AJ, Baldwin HE, Eichenfield LF, Friedlander SF, Yan AC. Acne life cycle: the spectrum of pediatric disease. *Semin Cutan Med Surg.* 2011;30:S2-S5.

Morelli JG. Acne. In: Kliegman RM, Stanton BF, St. Geme JW, Schor NF, Behrman RE, eds. *Nelson Textbook of Pediatrics.* 19th ed. Philadelphia, PA: Elsevier Saunders; 2011:2322-2328.

Tunnessen WW, Krowchuk DP. Acne. In: McMillan JA, Feigin RD, DeAngelis CD, Jones MD, eds. *Oski's Pediatrics: Principles and Practice.* 4th ed. Philadelphia, PA: Lippincott Williams & Wilkins; 2006:875-877.

Yan AC, Baldwin HE, Eichenfield LF, Friedlander SF, Mancini AJ. Approach to pediatric acne treatment: an update. *Semin Cutan Med Surg.* 2011;30:S16-S21.

The mother of a healthy 8-year-old boy is concerned about his school performance. At the last parent–teacher conference, his teacher noted that he is easily distracted and routinely fails to complete both homework assignments and classroom papers. His mother states that at home he also has difficulty in completing tasks and he fidgets constantly. Although the child is very talkative, he does not answer questions clearly. His physical examination is significant only for fidgeting.

▶ What is the most likely diagnosis?
▶ What is the next step in management?

ANSWERS TO CASE 59:
Attention Deficit Hyperactivity Disorder

Summary: An 8-year-old easily distractible, hyperkinetic boy who cannot complete school work or stay on task at home.

- **Most likely diagnosis:** Attention deficit hyperactivity disorder (ADHD).

- **Next step in management:** An ADHD evaluation, which includes information regarding his behavior obtained from both the caregiver and the classroom teacher.

ANALYSIS

Objectives

1. Know the clinical criteria for ADHD.

2. Understand the basic evaluation of the child with symptoms of ADHD.

3. Know the various treatment options available for this condition.

Considerations

This boy exhibits ADHD behaviors, including easy distractibility, inability to focus and complete tasks, and excessive fidgeting. The next step is a complete ADHD evaluation as described. If data suggest ADHD, he should undergo developmental and psychological evaluations for coexisting psychiatric conditions or learning disability. Target outcomes can then be identified and a behavioral therapy, classroom modification, and possibly medication treatment plan designed.

APPROACH TO:
Attention Deficit Hyperactivity Disorder

DEFINITION

ATTENTION DEFICIT HYPERACTIVITY DISORDER (ADHD): A condition with a persistent pattern of inattention and/or hyperactivity-impulsivity that interferes with functioning or development.

CLINICAL APPROACH

The *Diagnostic and Statistical Manual of Mental Disorders, Fifth Edition (DSM-V)* describes **criteria** of **inattentiveness** and **hyperactivity/impulsivity** necessary to make an **ADHD diagnosis.** Attention deficit hyperactivity disorder is estimated to affect 5% to 10% of school-aged children with a significant male predominance; 25% of ADHD patients have an affected primary relative. The pathophysiology of ADHD remains to be elucidated, but decreased dopamine activity of certain brain regions in the prefrontal cortex and basal ganglia may be responsible.

Inattention criteria of ADHD include careless mistakes, having difficulty paying attention, not listening, not completing assigned tasks, avoiding sustained mental effort, frequently losing things, easy distractibility, and forgetfulness.

Hyperactivity criteria of ADHD include frequent fidgeting, being out of one's seat frequently, running or climbing excessively, having difficulty playing quietly, and often talking excessively.

Impulsivity criteria of ADHD include blurting out answers, having difficulty waiting for his or her turn, and interrupting or intruding frequently.

Attention deficit hyperactivity disorder is subdivided into three types:

- ADHD/predominantly inattention (**at least six of nine** inattention behaviors for children up to age 16, but only five of nine for children aged 17 and older)

- ADHD/predominantly hyperactive-impulsive (**at least six of nine** hyperactive/impulsive behaviors for children up to age 16, but only five of nine for children aged 17 and older)

- ADHD/combined (**at least six of nine** of both the inattention and hyperactive/impulsive behaviors for children up to age 16, but only five of nine for children aged 17 and older). In addition, the following conditions must be met:

  ○ Several inattentive or hyperactive-impulsive symptoms were present **before age 12**.

  ○ Several symptoms are present for **at least 6 months.**

  ○ Several symptoms are present in **two or more settings** (eg, at home, school, or work; with friends or relatives; in other activities).

  ○ Clear evidence exists that the symptoms **interfere with social, school, or work functioning.**

  ○ The symptoms are not better explained by another mental disorder (eg, psychotic disorder, mood disorder, anxiety disorder, dissociative disorder, or a personality disorder).

Caregivers and classroom teacher(s) provide the critical information by completing checklists, such as the Conners rating, the AHDH index, the Swanson, Nolan, and Pelham (SNAP) checklist, or the ADD-H comprehensive teacher rating scale (ACTeRS). Alternatively, information can be surmised through narratives or descriptive interviews.

Psychological and developmental testing is part of the evaluation of an ADHD child; coexisting psychological and learning disorders occur frequently. Common coexisting conditions include oppositional-defiant disorder (35.2%), conduct disorder (25.7%), anxiety disorder (25.8%), and depressive disorder (18.2%). Approximately 12% to 60% of ADHD children have concurrent learning disorders and may benefit from special education services.

Management includes the implementation of a long-term treatment program in collaboration with caregivers and teachers. The care plan includes setting specific goals such as increasing independence, decreasing disruptive behavior, improving academic performance, organization, and task completion, and improving relationships with family members, teachers, and peers.

Behavioral modification can be used alone or in conjunction with pharmacologic therapy. Positive reinforcement (providing rewards or privileges) and negative consequences (time-out or withdrawal of privileges) emphasize appropriate behavior. Small class size, structured work, stimulating schoolwork, and appropriate seating arrangements can help **decrease disruptive classroom behaviors. Medications are often used to assist in treatment. Stimulant medications are considered first-line pharmacologic therapy to decrease ADHD behaviors.** Commonly used stimulant medications include **methylphenidate and dextroamphetamine. Atomoxetine (Strattera) is a nonstimulant, selective norepinephrine reuptake inhibitor** approved for use in adults and children. Tricyclic antidepressants, clonidine and bupropion, often prescribed under the direction of a psychiatrist or neurologist, are also used.

Long-term sequelae of ADHD include poor peer relationships, poor fine motor control, and increased risk of accidents. Adolescents may develop substance abuse problems as a comorbid condition, but this comorbidity does not seem to be related to treatment of ADHD with stimulants. Approximately 50% of children function well in adulthood; others demonstrate continued inattention and impulsivity symptoms.

CASE CORRELATIONS

- See also Case 41 (Klinefelter) which is an example of intellectual deficiency (with hyperactivity as a component) caused by a chromosome abnormality. The patient with obstructive sleep apnea (Case 43) also may present with a history of attention deficit disorder (ADD). And the adolescent with substance abuse disorder (Case 49) may have signs and symptoms of ADD. Thus, in all patients who are considered for the diagnosis of attention deficit disorder other diagnostic possibilities must be considered.

COMPREHENSION QUESTIONS

59.1 An 8-year-old boy presents because his mother is concerned that he has attention deficient hyperactivity disorder (ADHD). At home he is always restless, never seems to pay attention, and is always losing things. In the clinic, the child is cooperative and has a normal examination. Which of the following is the best next step in management?

A. Give the child a 2-week trial of stimulant medication.

B. Obtain further information from the parents and teachers.

C. Reassure the child's mother that this behavior is age appropriate.

D. Send the child for psychological assessment.

E. Send the child for psychiatric evaluation.

59.2 A 7-year-old boy appears distracted. His mother notes that he daydreams "all of the time," and when he is daydreaming he does not respond to her. She describes the episodes as short (lasting several seconds) and occurring many times per day. When he is not daydreaming, he is attentive and can complete tasks. His behavior in class is not disruptive. Which of the following is the best next step in management?

   A. Obtain further information from his parents and teachers with the Conners rating scale.

   B. Begin a program of behavioral modification.

   C. Reassure the child's mother that this behavior is age appropriate.

   D. Send the child for an electroencephalogram.

   E. Send the child for psychological assessment.

59.3 An 8-year-old boy has completed the initial ADHD evaluation, which demonstrates that he meets seven of the nine criteria for inattention and that he also has many impulsive behaviors. Which of the following is the most appropriate next step in management?

   A. Give the child a 2-week trial of stimulant medication.

   B. Arrange for special education placement.

   C. Send the child for a complete psychoeducational assessment.

   D. Send the child for an electroencephalogram.

   E. Reassure the child's mother that this behavior is age appropriate.

59.4 A 16-year-old adolescent girl is brought for evaluation after teachers have complained that for the past 8 months her academic performance has declined. They say she has difficulty paying attention and is easily distractible. She is noted to not listen in class or complete assigned tasks. She tries to avoid sustained mental effort, is frequently losing things, and is very forgetful. Parents note seeing similar changes at home over the same period of time. They are also concerned that she does not smile as often and stays in her room not interested in activities that used to make her happy. Her appetite has decreased and she has had trouble sleeping. Which of the following diagnoses best describe this girl?

   A. ADHD/predominantly hyperactive-impulsive

   B. ADHD/predominantly inattention

   C. ADHD/combined

   D. Dissociative disorder

   E. Depression

ANSWERS

59.1 **B.** A physical examination (with emphasis on the neurologic component) is completed to identify any soft signs of neurologic conditions. If none are found, he should undergo an ADHD evaluation with ADHD-specific behavior information obtained from caregivers and teachers. A diagnosis is considered if he has ADHD-specific behaviors in two or more settings. His ability to maintain focus during a brief visit to your clinic does not preclude the diagnosis of ADHD.

59.2 **D.** This child does not fit the classic ADHD pattern. Episodes of "daydreaming," which last several seconds, may be petit mal or absence seizures; an electroencephalogram is needed.

59.3 **C.** Prior to developing a management plan, the child is assessed for coexisting psychiatric and learning disorders (psychoeducational testing). Management can include stimulant medication, behavioral modification, and therapy appropriate for coexisting conditions.

59.4 **E.** While she does fulfill six of the nine inattention criteria, her symptoms can also be better explained by her likely mood disorder (which is an exclusion criteria). Also, while her symptoms have occurred for over 6 months, it is suggested that these are recent changes that were not occurring prior to age 12. In general, common coexisting psychiatric conditions for ADHD include oppositional-defiant disorder (35.2%), conduct disorder (25.7%), anxiety disorder (25.8%), and depressive disorder (18.2%).

CLINICAL PEARLS

▶ Attention deficit hyperactivity disorder (ADHD) is considered in children who have specific behaviors in two or more settings, such as at home and school or work.

▶ Children with ADHD frequently have coexisting psychiatric or learning disorders, including oppositional-defiant disorder, conduct disorder, anxiety disorder, and depression.

▶ Commonly used pharmacologic agents for the treatment of ADHD are methylphenidate and dextroamphetamine.

REFERENCES

American Academy of Pediatrics. Clinical practice guideline: diagnosis and evaluation of the child with attention-deficit/hyperactivity disorder. *Pediatrics.* 2000;105:1158-1170.

American Academy of Pediatrics. Clinical practice guideline: treatment of the school-aged child with attention-deficit/hyperactivity disorder. *Pediatrics.* 2001;108:1033-1044.

American Psychiatric Association. *Diagnostic and Statistical Manual of Mental Disorders.* 5th ed. Arlington, VA. American Psychiatric Association; 2013.

Cunningham NR, Jensen P. Attention deficit hyperactivity disorder. In: Kliegman RM, Stanton BF, St. Geme JW, Schor NF, Behrman RE, eds. *Nelson Textbook of Pediatrics.* 19th ed. Philadelphia, PA: WB Saunders; 2011:108-112.

Cutting LE, Mostofsky SH, Denckla MB. School difficulties. In: McMillan JA, Feigin RD, DeAngelis CD, Jones MD, eds. *Oski's Pediatrics: Principles and Practice.* 4th ed. Philadelphia, PA: Lippincott Williams & Wilkins; 2006:674-680.

Stein MT, Reiff MI. Hyperactivity and inattention. In: Rudolph CD, Rudolph AM, Lister GE, First LR, Gershon AA, eds. *Rudolph's Pediatrics.* 22nd ed. New York, NY: McGraw-Hill; 2011:321-327.

A 14-year-old boy is seen in the pediatrician's office at the request of his high school athletic trainer to be cleared to return to play football. He is the star quarterback and the state championship game is in 6 days. During last night's game, he was tackled from the side, sustaining a blow from the other player against his left shoulder. When he fell, he struck the right side of his head against the ground but did not lose consciousness. He remembers hitting his head and events of the game before and after the tackle. Subsequently he has had a dull, throbbing headache (described in intensity as 5 out of 10), located globally. He denies associated visual disturbance, photophobia, phonophobia, nausea, vomiting, and dizziness. He described no exacerbating factor for the headache and it is relieved with ibuprofen. He reports he felt "a little woozy" after the initial hit but feels tired only this morning. His mother says he slept an extra hour today but was not difficult to awaken; he has shown no change in his behavior. He has had no previous head injury. Examination of his head, neck, cranial nerves, strength, range of motion of all joints, sensation, gait, balance, coordination, and deep tendon reflexes is normal. He is oriented to month, date, day of week, year and time, able to recall five words immediately, but when asked to recall them 5 minutes later he can only remember three of the words.

▶ What is the most likely diagnosis?
▶ What is the next step in management?

ANSWERS TO CASE 60:

Concussion

Summary: An adolescent boy complains of headache after a head injury during his football game. The only other symptom is fatigue with a corresponding increase in his sleep. His examination is normal except for demonstrating difficulty with memory recall.

- **Most likely diagnosis:** Concussion.

- **Next step in management:** Physical and cognitive rest until he is asymptomatic for 24 hours without the use of any medications. He may then begin a graduated return-to-play protocol in which he must remain asymptomatic before advancing to each subsequent phase.

ANALYSIS

Objectives

1. Recognize symptoms of concussion.

2. Describe the management of concussion.

3. List factors associated with a concussion that warrant further evaluation with imaging.

Considerations

This boy has a sport-related concussion, an injury which accounts for almost 10% of all athletic injuries during high school. Most occur during football. Concussion is a functional injury so imaging is not routinely done nor required for diagnosis. Instead, signs and symptoms indicating a concussion will involve one or more of the following areas: somatic, cognitive, emotional, or sleep (Table 60–1). Some of the symptoms will be immediate, such as his dizziness and the mental "fogginess," a somatic and a cognitive symptom, respectively, which may worsen, subside, or fully resolve only to be followed by new findings. He now has symptoms from each of the categories: headache (somatic), anterograde amnesia (cognitive), fatigue (emotional), and increased sleep.

APPROACH TO:

Concussion

DEFINITIONS

CONCUSSION: A complex process involving a decline in neurologic or cognitive function that is induced by traumatic mechanical force to the person's head, neck, or body.

Table 60–1 • SYMPTOMS OF CONCUSSION			
Somatic/Physical	**Cognitive**	**Emotional/Affective**	**Sleep**
Dizzy/dysequilibrium	Amnesia	Anxious	Decreased sleep
Headache	Confused/disoriented	Fatigued	Increased sleep
Nausea/vomiting	Drowsy	Irritable	Trouble falling asleep
Phonophobia	Loss of consciousness	Labile	
Photophobia	Mental "fog"	Sad	
Visual disturbance	Poor concentration Slowed motor/verbal responses Slurred speech Staring		

Modified from Centers for Disease Control and Prevention. Heads Up To Clinicians: Addressing Concussion in Sports among Kids and Teens. http://www.cdc.gov/headsup/providers/training/index.html. Accessed July 29, 2015.

COGNITIVE REST: Limiting mental exertion during tasks such as homework, testing, video games, and even TV viewing in order to prevent worsening of concussive symptoms.

GRADUATED RETURN-TO-PLAY PROTOCOL: A **stepwise approach** for athletes to demonstrate symptom-free intervals before increasing the level of physical and cognitive exertion. The athlete must remain **symptom free for 24 hours at each level without any medication before advancing.**

SECOND IMPACT SYNDROME: If an individual is still recovering from a concussion and receives a second concussion, **increased cerebral vascular congestion and edema may occur which can lead to death.**

CLINICAL APPROACH

Concussions are common in the pediatric and adolescent population. These injuries can be more significant than in professional athletes because the developing brain is more vulnerable and the cervical and shoulder musculature is less developed. The immediate assessment of the child or adolescent with head injury begins at the time of the trauma. **Loss of consciousness (LOC) is infrequent,** occurring in only 10% of sport-related concussions. Sideline evaluation tools are available for older children, and assess for the signs and symptoms that define a concussion. The athlete should be removed from play and **is not to return to any level of activity on the same day a concussion is sustained.** If LOC is for more than 30 seconds, cervical pain, vomiting, or a loss in range of motion or sensation in any extremity is identified, the athlete must be taken to the emergency room to be evaluated. Otherwise the child's caregiver should be informed of the event, the definition of a concussion, and instructed to observe the child for 24 to 48 hours. Emergent care is to be obtained if increasing headache, vomiting, confusion, or unusual behavior develops.

While **most concussions resolve within a 7- to 10-day period**, some signs or symptoms may linger much longer. Younger athletes demonstrate longer recovery time compared to older athletes. Cognitive exertion or physical activity can cause worsening of symptoms, so the best management after a concussion is **physical and cognitive rest**. A concussion is more of a **functional brain injury** than a structural injury so **neuroimaging is usually normal**. Imaging with computed tomography (CT) or magnetic resonance imaging (MRI) should be used only when a serious structural pathology is suspected such as with focal findings on the neurologic examination, prolonged or severe headache, persistent amnesia, seizure, Glasgow coma scale (GCS) less than 15, persistent emesis, or signs of skull fracture.

For optimal patient safety, **graduated return-to-play protocols** have been developed and provide guidelines for a stepwise approach to advance activity while monitoring for symptoms. The protocol is not initiated until the athlete has been **asymptomatic for 24 hours without the use of any medications**, including acetaminophen, ibuprofen, or aspirin. Within these protocols, a 24-hour symptom-free period is also required before advancing to the next level. It takes a **minimum of 5 days to complete the protocol** and no limit exists on how long the athlete may remain at a certain level. Signs and symptoms of concussions have been documented to worsen with activity so if recurrence is noted, the protocol is discontinued until the athlete is asymptomatic for a 24-hour period. Then the protocol can be resumed at the level the athlete was at before symptom onset.

Failure to properly manage concussions can lead to serious long-term consequences ranging from second impact syndrome to chronic traumatic encephalopathy. All reported cases of second impact syndrome have been in athletes younger than 20 years. Returning to play too early and/or repeat concussions can be detrimental; it is important to educate the child or adolescent and parent about the dangers of returning to activity before the concussion has resolved. Athletes who have symptoms lasting over 3 months or who sustain three concussions in a single season should be disqualified from return to the sport.

CASE CORRELATION

- Concussion generally is describing a condition of traumatically induced altered mental status. Thus, the child with failure to thrive (Case 10) due to child abuse (Case 38) may have symptoms of head injury. Secondary headache (Case 48) is a common complaint among those who have sustained a concussion-producing injury. Acute onset of neurologic symptoms in the patient with sickle cell disease (Case 13) may be confused with concussion, especially if the stroke causes a fall with resultant head injury. The adolescent with substance abuse disorder (Case 49) often participates in high-risk activities, thus has a higher rate of accidents and concussion.

COMPREHENSION QUESTIONS

60.1 A 13-year-old girl is seen in the pediatrician's office with her mother follow-ing a head injury 3 days prior. She initially had a headache when the injury occurred but it resolved and her energy level has returned to normal. She has now gone back to school but gets a headache about 20 minutes after she starts her first class of the morning. She does not get the headache if she takes acetaminophen before leaving for school. The headache recurs in the afternoon as she tries to do her homework. Her physical examination is normal. Her mother is concerned because school standardized testing is beginning in 48 hours and her daughter seems to be falling behind in her studies. Which of the following is the next best step in management?

A. Reassure the mother that her daughter will be fine and there is no reason to be concerned about the testing.

B. Recommend continued treatment with acetaminophen or ibuprofen for symptom relief, and obtain a more thorough history regarding the head-ache to determine if she has migraines.

C. Explain to the mother that the persistent headache is still secondary to the concussion and provide documentation to the school for the girl to have reduced assignments and defer the testing until she recovers.

D. Perform a vision test and restrict the amount of time she can use the computer.

E. Ask the girl if she is in danger of failing and ask the mother if her daugh-ter might be trying to avoid taking the tests for fear of a poor performance.

60.2 Which of the following symptoms after a concussion would warrant further evaluation with neuroimaging?

A. Decreased appetite

B. Nausea but no vomiting

C. Fatigue

D. Unable to remember the locker combination

E. Difficulty falling asleep

60.3 A high school soccer player suffered his first head injury during a game 4 days prior to being seen in the pediatrician's office. He denies loss of consciousness, nausea, vomiting, or amnesia. He had a headache initially but it resolved with a single dose of ibuprofen. He has been strictly following your orders of physical and cognitive rest and has been asymptomatic for 2 days. He is wondering when he can return to play. Which of the following is the next best step in management?

A. Allow him to start the graduated return to play protocol with his athletic trainer since he has been asymptomatic.

B. Obtain a head computed tomography (CT) and if normal, allow him to return to play.

C. Allow him to return to practice immediately because his symptoms are resolved.

D. Tell him he will not be allowed to return to play this season.

E. Allow him to participate in practice only if he promises not to strike the ball with his head.

60.4 Which of the following statements for counselling an athlete who has sustained a concussion is NOT correct?

A. Second impact syndrome is a rare but potentially lethal complication of sustaining another concussion in close proximity to a prior concussion that is not fully recovered.

B. The earliest an athlete should anticipate returning to play is within 5 days, and this timeframe would presume the symptoms of the concussion had already resolved for 24 hours.

C. Even if no loss of consciousness is sustained at the initial injury, a concussion requires the athlete to be removed from play that day.

D. Initial management of a concussion includes rest from physical activity, not just the competitive training, and also rest from academic work.

E. A shorter recovery time is expected in a younger child because their concussions are milder because they cannot really hit as hard as older athletes.

ANSWERS

60.1 **C.** The patient is still exhibiting symptoms of her concussion which is not unexpected since most take 7 to 10 days to resolve. Cognitive and physical rest is the mainstay of therapy for concussion management. Standardized testing should be discouraged during the recovery phase because it is not cognitive rest and some studies have documented lower scores result.

60.2 **D.** Persistent amnesia would warrant further evaluation with imaging. Nausea, fatigue, and difficulty falling asleep are symptoms of concussion that can last several months but do not require imaging.

60.3 **B.** An asymptomatic period without the use of any medications for over 24 hours suggests a graduated return to play protocol may be initiated. Imaging is not useful for determining the phase of recovery from concussion. Graduated return to play is best because symptoms of concussion often worsen or can recur with exertion. Because this injury is his first concussion, it is unlikely he would be out for the season.

60.4 **E.** Younger athletes generally require longer recovery time and they are at higher risk for more severe injuries due to a developing brain and less developed cervical and shoulder musculature.

CLINICAL PEARLS

▶ A concussion is a functional brain injury defined by the presence of a symptom in any of the following categories: somatic, cognitive, emotional, or sleep.

▶ Concussions in the pediatric and adolescent population should be managed conservatively with physical and cognitive rest.

▶ Graduated return-to-play protocols should be utilized for every athlete; these protocols require the athlete to be asymptomatic for a 24-hour period without the use of medications before advancing to each subsequent level.

REFERENCES

Halstead ME, Walter KD. Council on Sports Medicine and Fitness. Clinical report—sport-related concussion in children and adolescents. *Pediatrics.* 2010;126(3):597-615.

Landry GL. Head and neck injuries. In: Kliegman RM, Stanton BF, St. Geme III J, Schor N, Behrman R, eds. *Nelson Textbook of Pediatrics.* 19th ed. Philadelphia, PA: Elsevier, 2011:2418-2419.

US Department of Health and Human Services; Centers for Disease Control and Prevention. *Heads Up To Clinicians: Addressing Concussion in Sports among Kids and Teens.* www.cdc.gov/headsup/providers/training/index.html. Accessed July 29, 2015.

Review Questions

R-1. An 18-month-old girl is seen by the pediatric nurse practitioner for an episode of cyanosis and a concern for poor eating. The family reports that they are extremely worried that for the previous several months she "refuses to eat enough." Rather, they report that she will eat a few bites of chicken nuggets, a French fry or two, and then insists on getting down from the table and going to play with her toys. Earlier in the day when she was forced to sit at the table to eat she proceeded to scream loudly, turn blue, and then fall off her chair. About 10 seconds later she was back to her baseline. She was born vaginally at term after an uncomplicated pregnancy to a 28-year-old gravida 1 woman; birth weight was 3900 g (8.6 lb). She was exclusively breast-fed until about 4 months of age when solids were introduced, and she was switched from breast to whole milk at 1 year of age. She has had no previous hospitalizations and takes no medications. Her mother reports that she is able to climb, throw a ball, and walk up and down stairs with assistance. She uses some two-word phrases. On physical examination, she is a healthy, active, normal-appearing child. Temperature is 37.5°C (98.9°F), heart rate 90 beats/min, respiratory rate 16 breaths/min, and blood pressure 100/70 mm Hg. Weight is 12 kg (26.5 lb; 75th percentile), height 80 cm (31.5 in; 50th percentile), and head circumference 47 cm (18.5 in; 50th percentile). Mucous membranes are pink, moist, and without lesions. The chest is clear. The heart has a normal S1 and S2 without murmur. The abdomen is soft and nontender. No hepatosplenomegaly or adenopathy is noted. Extremities and neurologic examination are normal. Which of the following is the most appropriate next step?

A. Begin daily multivitamins to include iron and vitamin D.

B. Advise the family to force the child to eat all food before allowing play time.

C. Reassure the family of the child's normalcy and provide disciplinary guidance.

D. Begin oral high-calorie toddler nutritional supplementation.

E. Obtain a pulse oxygen saturation, electrocardiogram (ECG), and echocardiogram.

R-2. A 15-month-old boy is seen by the pediatrician for a well-child checkup. The family has no complaints other than his being a picky eater choosing to drink about 48 oz of whole milk daily instead of eating other foods. He was a term infant born to a 22-year-old woman whose pregnancy was complicated by gestational hypertension. He has had neither previous serious illness nor hospitalization and takes no medications. On physical examination, his vital signs are normal. He is at the 75th percentile for weight, 50th percentile for height, and 55th percentile for head circumference. Mucous membranes are pale, moist, and without lesions. The chest is clear. The heart has a normal S1 and S2 without murmur. The abdomen is soft and nontender. No hepatosplenomegaly or adenopathy is noted. Extremities are without lesions. Neurologic and developmental examinations are normal. Laboratory data show:

Hemoglobin 9.7 g/dL

Hematocrit 29.2%

Mean corpuscular volume (MCV) 51 fL

Many microcytes noted on smear

White blood count 8000/mm³

Segmented neutrophils 40%

Band forms 1%

Lymphocytes 59%

Platelet count 195,000/mm³

Serum lead level 4 µg/dL

Which of the following is the most likely diagnosis?

A. Sickle cell disease

B. Folate deficiency

C. Lead toxicity

D. Iron deficiency

E. Leukemia

R-3. An 8-year-old girl is seen in the emergency department for diabetic ketoacidosis (DKA). Her initial electrolytes were:

Sodium 128 mEq/L

Potassium 5.9 mEq/L

Chloride 90 mEq/L

Bicarbonate 13 mEq/L

Glucose 830 mg/dL

Six hours after initiation of treatment with insulin and fluid boluses her electrolytes are:

Sodium 132 mEq/L

Potassium 5.8 mEq/L

Chloride 92 mEq/L

Bicarbonate 12 mEq/L

Glucose 310 mg/dL

She complained of a headache about 1 hour prior and now is difficult to arouse. She is currently receiving 0.1 units/kg/h of regular insulin as well as normal saline. Which of the following is the most appropriate next step?

A. Continue current therapy.

B. Infuse intravenously 1 g/kg of mannitol over 20 minutes.

C. Stop intravenous insulin therapy and begin subcutaneous insulin administration.

D. Continue intravenous insulin therapy and administer bicarbonate.

E. Stop intravenous insulin therapy and administer bicarbonate.

R-4. A 5-year-old boy is seen in the emergency department for new-onset right arm weakness. His mother reports that he had previously been in good health when he awoke 3 hours previously with the symptoms. She reports he has had no nausea, vomiting, fever, or other symptoms. His past medical history is positive for sickle cell disease with one previous hospitalization for pain crisis involving his left knee. Medications include daily penicillin and folate. On physical examination, the temperature is 37.5°C (98.9°F), heart rate 90 beats/min, respiratory rate 18 breaths/min, and blood pressure 100/70 mm Hg. Weight, height, and head circumference are at the 50th percentile for age. Mucous membranes are pale, moist, and without lesions. The chest is clear. The heart has a normal S1 and S2 with II/VI SEM at left lower sternal border. The abdomen is soft and nontender. No hepatosplenomegaly or adenopathy is noted. The right arm has considerable weakness but no focal pain. Other extremities and the rest of the neurologic examination are normal. Cerebellar and cerebral functions are normal. Which of the following is the most appropriate next step in his management?

A. Order a stat transcranial Doppler (TCD) study.

B. Obtain an ultrasound of the spleen.

C. Order a hemoglobin electrophoresis.

D. Prepare for an emergency partial exchange transfusion.

E. Begin broad-spectrum antibiotics after obtaining a lumbar puncture for cultures.

R-5. An 8-month-old girl is seen by the emergency department physician for bloody stools. The father reports that she was in her normal state of good health until about 4 hours previously when he noted a large amount of dark red blood in her diaper. He denies recent fever, vomiting, abdominal pain, trauma, and change in activity or diet. She completed a course of amoxicillin for otitis media 3 weeks prior. She was born vaginally at term; she has had no previous serious illnesses or hospitalizations. She is breast-fed with supplemental baby foods and takes daily vitamin D drops. On physical examination, the temperature is 37°C (98.6°F), heart rate 124 beats/min, respiratory rate 16 breaths/min, and blood pressure 99/68 mm Hg. Her height, weight, and head circumference are at the 75th percentile for age. The head is normocephalic without lesions. Mucous membranes are pale, moist, and without lesions. The chest is clear. The heart has a normal S1 and S2 and a 2/6 systolic ejection flow murmur at the left lower sternal border. Capillary refill is 4 to 5 seconds. The abdomen is soft and nontender. No hepatosplenomegaly is noted. The rectum and vagina are without trauma, but there is dark red blood around the anus. Which of the following is the most likely diagnosis?

A. Malrotation of the intestines

B. Shigellosis

C. Intussusception

D. Meckel diverticulum

E. Peptic ulcer disease

R-6. A term African American infant is seen at 36 hours of life by the neonatologist for routine care. The infant was born at term by Cesarean due to failure to progress to a 33-year-old woman whose pregnancy was complicated by scant prenatal care and poorly controlled gestational diabetes. Apgar scores were 5 and 8 at 1 and 5 minutes, respectively. Birth weight was 4200 g (10 lb, 12 oz). The hospital course has been notable for an initial glucose in the normal newborn nursery of 34 mg/dL which improved to 52 mg/dL after breast-feeding. The infant has been breast-feeding well every 2½ to 3 hours and has voided but has not yet stooled. The initial examination at approximately 18 hours of life was normal. On current physical examination, the temperature is 37°C (98.6°F), heart rate 144 beats/min, respiratory rate 30 breaths/min, and blood pressure 99/68 mm Hg. She is asleep but easily arousable. Height, weight, and head circumference are at the 95th percentile. Skin is slightly icteric. The head is normocephalic without lesions. Mucous membranes are moist, pink, and without lesions. The chest is clear. The heart has a normal S1 and S2 without murmur. The abdomen is soft, full in appearance, and nontender. No hepatosplenomegaly is noted. The rectum and vagina are patent. Which of the following is the current diagnosis of most concern?

A. Polycythemia

B. Hypocalcemia

C. Small left colon syndrome

D. Cystic fibrosis

E. Caudal regression syndrome

R-7. A previously healthy 2-year-old child is seen by the pediatrician for a 1-week history of cough. The family reports that he had been in good health until the sudden onset of coughing about 1 week prior for which he was diagnosed with and treated for pneumonia at a local urgent care center. He has no current fever, vomiting, diarrhea, or change in behavior. He was born vaginally at term to a 22-year-old woman whose pregnancy was complicated by prolonged rupture of membranes. He takes no medications, has had no serious illnesses, and has had no prior hospital-izations. Growth and development have been normal as compared to the mothers' other child. On physical examination, the temperature is 37°C (98.6°F), heart rate 100 beats/min, respiratory rate 16 breaths/min, and blood pressure 100/70 mm Hg. His height, weight, and head circumfer-ence are at the 75th percentile age. Nose is patent without discharge. The heart has normal S1 and S2 with normal pulses. The chest has good air movement on the left. On the right decreased air movement during inspiration and no air movement upon expiration is found. No wheezes, rhonchi, or rales are heard. The abdomen is soft, nontender, and with normal bowel sounds. No hepatosplenomegaly is noted. Extremities are without clubbing. Which of the following is the most likely mechanism of disease?

A. Mutation of a protein transmembrane conductance regulator gene

B. Aspiration of a foreign body into the airway

C. Infection of the alveoli with bacteria

D. Hyperresponsiveness of the bronchial tree

E. Remodeling of the airways due to chronic obstruction

R-8. An 18-hour-old infant is seen by the pediatrician for "jaundice." The child was delivered vaginally at 39 weeks of gestation to a 28-year-old G1 woman whose pregnancy was complicated by an *Escherichia coli* urinary tract infec-tion during the second trimester. He has been eating about 20 to 30 cc of standard infant formula every 2 to 3 hours without difficulty. He has stooled twice and voided three times. The mother reports no familial ill-ness; the father of the baby has not been involved during the pregnancy. On physical examination, the temperature is 37°C (98.6°F), heart rate 145 beats/min, and respiratory rate 33 breaths/min. His weight, length, and head circumference are at the 45th percentile. Skin is icteric without bruising. The head is normocephalic with minimal molding. Mucous mem-branes are moist and without lesions. The chest is clear. The heart has a normal S1 and S2 without murmur. The abdomen is soft and nontender. The liver is felt about 1 cm below the right costal margin; the spleen is palpable 4 cm below the left costal margin. Extremities and neurologic examinations are normal. Laboratory data reveal:

Maternal blood type O-positive, antibody screen negative

Baby blood type O-positive, Coombs negative

Serum bilirubin

Total 14.8 mg/dL

Direct 0.2 mg/dL

Hemoglobin 12 g/dL

Hematocrit 36%

Platelet count 278,000/mm^3

White blood count 23,000/mm³

    Segmented neutrophils 49%

    Band forms 0%

    Lymphocytes 51%

Peripheral blood smear

    Anisocytosis as well as red cells that appear to be small in size with lack of central pallor

Reticulocyte count 14.5%

Which of the following is the most likely mechanism of disease?

A. Rh or ABO hemolytic disease

B. Physiologic jaundice

C. Sepsis

D. Hereditary spherocytosis

E. Biliary atresia

R-9. A 6-month-old boy is brought via ambulance to the emergency department intubated and with cardiopulmonary resuscitation (CPR) in progress. After 30 minutes of resuscitation, the infant temporarily regains normal sinus rhythm. The parents report that he had been healthy and that they put him to bed as usual for the night at about 8 PM. He did not awaken for his normal nightly feeding. When they next saw him in the morning, he was not breathing. Physical examination in the emergency department shows only evidence of resuscitation including abrasions on his chest, an endotracheal tube from the mouth, and an intraosseous line in the left leg. An emergency computed tomography (CT) scan of the head shows a right-sided subdural hematoma. Shortly after arrival to the PICU, he becomes unstable, becomes bradycardic, and despite an additional 40 minutes of CPR is pronounced dead. Which of the following is the most likely diagnosis?

A. Hemophilia

B. Ruptured arteriovenous malformation

C. Sudden infant death syndrome (SIDS)

D. Idiopathic thrombocytopenia

E. Abuse

R-10. A 12-hour-old infant in the well-baby nursery is seen by the pediatric nurse practitioner. The staff has just completed the mandatory newborn hearing test when the child develops cyanosis. The infant was born by Cesarean section after a failed induction at 41 weeks of gestation to a 24-year-old gravida 2 woman whose pregnancy was uncomplicated. Apgar scores were 8 and 9 at 1 and 5 minutes, respectively. The infant has been breastfeeding well, and has voided and stooled. On physical examination, the temperature is 36.7°C (98.0°F), heart rate 155 beats/min, respiratory rate 55 breaths/min, and BP 89/63 mm Hg. Weight, length, and head circumference are at the 45th percentile for gestational age. The head is normocephalic. Fontanelles are flat. The chest has good air movement without distress. The heart has normal S1 and S2. No murmur is heard. Distal pulses are normal. Capillary refill is less than 3 seconds. The abdomen is soft and nontender. No hepatosplenomegaly is noted. Oxygen saturation is 65% on room air and 63% on 10 L/min oxygen face mask. Which of the following is the most appropriate next step in management?

A. Obtain blood cultures and initiate antibiotic therapy.

B. Infuse indomethacin intravenously.

C. Begin an adenosine infusion.

D. Start a prostaglandin E_1 infusion.

E. Give 10-CC/kg normal saline fluid bolus and a dose of digoxin.

R-11.   A 2-month-old infant is seen by the pediatrician for a well-child checkup. The family has no concerns. He has been breast-feeding well, voiding and stooling regularly, and developing normally as compared to their other children. He was a vaginal delivery after a term, uncomplicated pregnancy. Initial hospital stay was for 24 hours. He has experienced no previous illness or hospitalizations, and takes vitamin D drops only. On physical examination, the temperature is 36.7°C (98.0°F), heart rate 135 beats/min, respiratory rate 30 breaths/min, and BP 90/65 mm Hg. Weight, length, and head circumference are at the 55th percentile for age. The head is normocephalic. Fontanelles are flat. The chest has good air movement without distress. The heart has normal S1 and a fixed split S2. The right ventricle impulse is increased. A 3/6 SEM is noted over the left upper sternal border. Distal pulses are normal. Capillary refill is less than 3 seconds. The abdomen is soft and nontender. No hepatosplenomegaly is noted. Oxygen saturation is 95% to 99% on room air. Which of the following is the most likely mechanism of disease?

A. Congenital switch of the pulmonary and aortic vessels

B. Ongoing patency of the ductus arteriosus

C. Congenital absence of the pulmonary valve with an intact ventricular septum

D. Hypoplastic development of the left ventricle

E. Failed closure of the ostium secundum atrial septum

R-12.   A 2-year-old girl is seen in an urgent care center for difficulty breathing and a sore throat. Her father states that over the previous 48 hours she complained of a sore throat, developed a fever to touch, and had some rhinorrhea. He states that the sore throat seems to have progressed over the previous 4 hours such that she now refuses to take liquids or to swallow. He states that she has developed difficulty breathing in the last 1 hour. The child has had no previous serious illnesses, takes no medications, and has had normal development compared to her siblings. She is current with her immunizations. On physical examination, she is lying on the examination table, wary of strangers but easily consoled. Vital signs show temperature of 39.3°C (102.8°F), heart rate 150 beats/min, respiratory rate 24 breaths/min, blood pressure 102/71 mm Hg, and oxygen saturation of 95% on room air. The head is normocephalic. Movement of the head from side to side is limited. Ear canals are clear; the tympanic membranes are translucent. Mucous membranes are moist; saliva is noted dripping from the mouth. The tongue and tonsils are of normal size. The posterior pharynx is full and red. The uvula is midline. The nares have clear discharge bilaterally. The heart has normal S1 and S2; no murmur is heard. The chest and abdominal examinations are normal. Neurologic and musculoskeletal examinations are normal. Infection of which of the following structures is the most likely etiology of these findings?

A. Retropharyngeal space

B. Peritonsillar spaces

C. Epiglottis

D. Remnant of a thyroglossal duct

E. Meninges

R-13. An 18-month-old child is brought by helicopter to the emergency department after having been found by passersby in a locked car in a convenience store parking lot. The helicopter crew report that when the fire department entered the vehicle, the child was obtunded, was covered in emesis, and his clothing was soaked from sweat. On physical examination, the temperature is 41°C (105.9°F), heart rate 150 beats/min, respiratory rate 40 breaths/min, and BP 80/55 mm Hg. The head is normocephalic. Fontanelles are closed. The chest has good air movement without distress. The heart has normal S1 and S2. No murmur is heard. Distal pulses are normal. Capillary refill is less than 5 seconds. The abdomen is soft and nontender. No hepatosplenomegaly is noted. Glasgow coma scale is 6 (somewhat responsive to pain). Which of the following laboratory findings is most likely to be present and to be life threatening?

A. Serum creatinine kinase level of 35,000 U/L

B. Serum phosphate level of 2 mg/dL

C. Serum potassium level of 8.2 mg/dL

D. Serum calcium level of 6.4 mg/dL

E. Positive urine dip for blood

R-14. A 15-year-old boy is seen by the pediatrician for a 3-day history of groin pain. He reports that for the previous 2 weeks he has had a limp, but in the prior 3 days he has also developed pain in the right groin which he describes as dull and difficult to pinpoint. He is a tackle for his high school football team; practice makes the pain worse. Ibuprofen every 6 hours has had minimal impact on the pain. He denies fever, vomiting, headache, or weight loss. He denies tobacco, alcohol, and other drugs. He is sexually active with one partner and reports frequent condom use. Past medical history is positive for a broken arm at age 7 years when he fell from a tree. On physical examination, the temperature is 37.5°C (98.9°F), heart rate 90 beats/min, respiratory rate 16 breaths/min, and blood pressure 132/88 mm Hg. Height is 178 cm (5' 10"), weight 100 kg (220 lb), and body mass index (BMI) 31.6. The mucous membranes are pink, moist, and without lesions. Extraocular eye movement and fundoscopic examinations are normal. The chest is clear. The heart has a normal S1 and S2 without murmur. The abdomen is soft and nontender. No hepatosplenomegaly or adenopathy is noted. The left hip has reduced internal rotation, abduction, and flexion; the preferred position is passive external rotation. Gait has Trendelenburg and antalgic pattern. Sensation and deep tendon reflexes are normal. Genitourinary examination shows normal Tanner 4 development, no urethral discharge, and testes without pain or masses. Anteroposterior and frog-leg radiographs of the hips show:

Widening of the physis and posteriorly displaced femoral epiphysis overlying the femoral head.

Which of the following is the most likely mechanism for his condition?

A.   Disruption of blood flow to the femoral head

B.   Hematologic dissemination of a sexually acquired infection

C.   Bone marrow infiltration of leukemic cells

D.   Disruption through the growth plate of the femoral neck from the femoral head

E.   Deposition of immune complexes in the joint space

R-15.   An obtunded 10-year-old boy is air lifted from an outside emergency department to the intensive care unit of a local children's hospital. The patient had been in good health until that morning when his mother reported that he awoke feeling poorly, had a fever, and had a rash on his arms and legs. While driving him to the outside emergency room, the mother noticed spreading of the rash. The mother denies travel, exposure to illnesses, previous serious illness, or intake of medications. On physical examination, he is minimally responsive to painful stimuli. Temperature is 39.7°C (103.5°F), heart rate 155 beats/min, respiratory rate 30 breaths/min, and blood pressure of 78/40 mm Hg. The head is normocephalic without trauma. The oral and ocular mucosae are moist and pale. Throat is without lesions or redness. The chest is clear. The heart has normal S1 and S2 without murmur. Capillary refill is 8 seconds. The abdomen is nondistended and bowel sounds are absent. No hepatosplenomegaly or masses are found. Normal male genitalia and descended testes are noted. Skin has numerous purple nonblanching patches scattered over her body, especially on the arms and legs. Laboratory data show:

Hemoglobin 9 g/dL

Hematocrit 27%

Platelet count 15,000/mm³

> White blood count 1000/mm³
>> Segmented neutrophils 60%
>>
>> Band forms 30%
>>
>> Lymphocytes 10%

Which of the following is the most likely mechanism of disease?

A. Infection by a rickettsial agent

B. Infection by a bacterial agent

C. Infection by a viral agent

D. Platelet destruction by circulating antiglycoprotein IIb/IIIa antibodies

E. Vasculitis of medium-sized arteries

REVIEW QUESTIONS 16 TO 19

For each clinical scenario of respiratory distress in a neonate below, select the most likely diagnosis. Each lettered option may be used once, more than once, or not at all.

A. Transient tachypnea of the newborn

B. Group B streptococcus (GBS) infection

C. Herpes simplex virus infection

D. Polycythemia

E. Opioid narcosis

F. Primary surfactant deficiency (Infant Respiratory Distress Syndrome)

G. Listeria pneumonia

H. Congenital diaphragmatic hernia

I. H-type tracheoesophageal fistula (TE) fistula

R-16. An infant is seen by the neonatal transport team in the delivery room immediately after birth for respiratory distress. The child was born by Cesarean section at 34 weeks of gestation to a 29-year-old gravida 3 woman who has severe hypertension. The mother reports no illness or problems with the pregnancy but she has had no prenatal care. On physical examination in the delivery room the infant is cyanotic and has severe subcostal and supraclavicular retractions. The chest has reduced breath sounds on the left and good air movement on the right. Heart sounds are best heard on the right side revealing a distant but normal S1 and S2. The abdomen is scaphoid. He is intubated and moved to the neonatal intensive care unit for further evaluation.

R-17. A 2-hour-old infant in the normal newborn nursery develops tachypnea, grunting, and retractions. The child was born vaginally at 31 weeks of gestation to a 32-year-old woman whose pregnancy was complicated by poorly controlled diabetes and gestational hypertension. On physical examination, the temperature is 37°C (98.6°F), heart rate 150 beats/min, respiratory rate 60 breaths/min, and blood pressure of 90/60 mm Hg. The head is normocephalic without trauma. The fontanelles are flat. The oral and ocular mucosae are moist and pink. Nasal flaring is noted. The chest examination shows reduced air excursion, subcostal and intercostal retractions, and expiratory grunting. The heart has normal S1 and S2 without murmur. Capillary refill is 3 seconds. The abdomen is nondistended and bowel sounds are active. No hepatosplenomegaly or masses are found. Laboratory data show:

> Hemoglobin 15 g/dL
>
> Hematocrit 45%
>
> Platelet count 155,000/mm^3
>
> White blood count 18,500/mm^3
>
>> Segmented neutrophils 65%
>>
>> Band forms 3%
>>
>> Lymphocytes 32%

Chest radiograph shows bilateral, diffuse, ground-glass appearance with air bronchograms and poor lung expansion.

R-18. A 14-day-old infant is seen in the emergency department for fever, lethargy, and irritability. The family reports he was a term vaginal delivery after an uncomplicated pregnancy. He was discharged on the second day of life, was breast-feeding well, and had shown no signs of illness until 8 hours prior when he became warm to the touch and had reduced intake. He has no known sick exposures. On physical examination, he is irritable and difficult to console. Temperature is 38.6°C (101.5°F), heart rate 155 beats/min, respiratory rate 30 breaths/min, and blood pressure of 60/40 mm Hg. The head is normocephalic without trauma. The fontanelles are bulging. The oral and ocular mucosae are moist. The chest is clear. The heart has normal S1 and S2 without murmur. Capillary refill is 5 seconds. The abdomen is nondistended and bowel sounds are reduced. No hepatosplenomegaly or masses are found. Normal male genitalia and descended testes are noted. Skin is pale and mottled. Laboratory data show:

> Hemoglobin 10 g/dL
>
> Hematocrit 31%
>
> Platelet count 55,000/mm^3
>
> White blood count 1500/mm^3
>
>> Segmented neutrophils 65%
>>
>> Band forms 35%
>>
>> Lymphocytes 10%
>
> Cerebral spinal fluid
>
>> Glucose 10 mg/dL
>>
>> Protein 100 mg/dL
>>
>> White blood count 1000/mm^3 with 90% segmented neutrophils
>>
>> Red blood count 10/mm^3

R-19. A 4-day-old infant is transferred to the normal newborn nursery from the neonatal intensive care unit after having undergone a sepsis evaluation for maternal fever. The 36-week gestation infant was born vaginally to a 22-year-old woman whose pregnancy was complicated by scant prenatal care, a 2-week history of leaking amniotic fluids, and a 4-day history of maternal fever to 39.7°C (103.5°F). The mother's physical examination was normal. The infant underwent a sepsis evaluation immediately after birth, was started on antibiotics, and was sent to the normal nursery after all cultures proved to be negative. During his stay in the NICU the infant's vital signs were normal, and he was eating, voiding, and stooling well. About 8 hours after arrival to the normal newborn nursery he began to have some lethargy, reduced intake, and a temperature to 38.6°C (101.5°F). Repeat sepsis evaluation demonstrated:

> Hemoglobin 15 g/dL
>
> Hematocrit 45.3%
>
> Platelet count 125,000/mm³
>
> White blood count 3300/mm³
>> Segmented neutrophils 70%
>>
>> Band forms 0%
>>
>> Lymphocytes 30%
>
> Cerebral spinal fluid (nontraumatic)
>> Glucose 85 mg/dL
>>
>> Protein 65 mg/dL
>>
>> White blood count 60/mm³
>>
>> Red blood count 1950/mm³

REVIEW QUESTIONS R-20 TO R-23

For each clinical scenario of an apparent hematologic condition in a young child, select the most likely diagnosis. Each lettered option may be used once, more than once, or not at all.

   A. Immune thrombocytopenic purpura

   B. Leukemia

   C. Megaloblastic anemia

   D. Child abuse

   E. Sickle cell disease

   F. Wiskott-Aldrich syndrome

   G. Neuroblastoma

   H. Cystic fibrosis

R-20.   A 6-month-old white male infant is seen by the pediatrician for well-child evaluation. The infant is noted to be at the 5th percentile for weight, the 25th percentile for length, and the 50th percentile for head circumference. He was born vaginally at 39 weeks of gestation to a 28-year-old woman whose pregnancy was uncomplicated. Discharge was at 48 hours of age once he had his first stool. He has been exclusively breast-fed since birth and has been given vitamin D and iron drops. On physical examination, he is small for his age and is pale.

R-21.   A 4-month-old Asian male infant is seen by the pediatrician for fever and otitis media. The child was born by Cesarean section at 40 weeks of gestation, was discharged at 3 days of age, and had an uneventful newborn course other than prolonged bleeding from the circumcision site. He has been breast-fed since birth. Medications include daily vitamin D drops and topical steroids. He has had four episodes of otitis media and one hospitalization for a superficial staphylococcal skin infection.

R-22.   A 9-month-old African American female infant is seen by the emergency department physician for the sudden onset of pallor. Her father reports that she was in her normal state of good health until about 2 hours ago when she became pale, lethargic, and her abdomen began to swell. On physical examination, she is pale, tachycardic, and has profound splenomegaly.

R-23.   A 1-year-old American Indian boy is seen in the emergency room for bruising. The child had been in good health until the previous day when he began to develop a limp and fever. On physical examination, he is pale, has bruising on his arms and legs, periorbital ecchymosis, and an abdominal mass.

REVIEW QUESTIONS R-24 TO R-27

For each clinical scenario of a child being seen for well-child evaluation and with poor school performance, select the most likely diagnosis. Each lettered option may be used once, more than once, or not at all.

   A.   Obstructive sleep apnea
   B.   Klinefelter syndrome
   C.   Migraine headache
   D.   Conversion disorder
   E.   Brain tumor
   F.   Drug abuse
   G.   Tension headache
   H.   Noonan syndrome

R-24.   A 14-year-old boy is seen with school complaints that his grades have fallen in the past 6 months and that he often is seen to fall asleep in class.

On physical examination, the temperature is 37.5°C (98.9°F), heart rate 90 beats/min, respiratory rate 16 breaths/min, and blood pressure 132/88 mm Hg. Height is 178 cm (5' 10"), weight 100 kg (220 lb), and BMI 31.6. The mucous membranes are pink, moist, and without lesions. Extraocular eye movement and fundoscopic examinations are normal. The chest is clear. The heart has a normal S1 and S2 without murmur. The abdomen is soft and nontender. No hepatosplenomegaly or adenopathy is noted. Extremities are without lesions; joints are normal. Genitourinary examination shows normal Tanner 4 development, no urethral discharge, and testes without pain or masses.

R-25. A 14-year-old boy is clumsy and has poor penmanship. He had delayed speech and has been diagnosed with minor learning difficulties. On physical examination, the temperature is 37.5°C (98.9°F), heart rate 90 beats/min, respiratory rate 16 breaths/min, and blood pressure 110/70 mm Hg. Height is 182 cm (5' 11"), weight 64 kg (140 lb), and BMI 19.5. The mucous membranes are pink, moist, and without lesions. Extraocular eye movement and fundoscopic examinations are normal. The chest is clear. Gynecomastia is noted. The heart has a mid-to-late systolic click and a mid-to-late systolic murmur at the cardiac apex. The abdomen is soft and nontender. No hepatosplenomegaly or adenopathy is noted. Extremities are without lesions; joints are normal. Genitourinary examination shows Tanner 2 development with sparse hair as well as small and firm testis.

R-26. A 14-year-old girl has headaches and a drop in school performance since her recent move into the area. Her mother reports that at her previous school she was a good student and participated in a variety of extracurricular activities. At the new school she is disinterested in academics and does not join in extracurricular activities. Her mother reports that toward the end of almost every weekend she complains of a headache and stomach ache. She reports no nausea, vomiting, diarrhea, fever, or weight loss. On physical examination, her temperature and vital signs are normal. Height and weight are at the 50th percentile for age. The mucous membranes are pink, moist, and without lesions. Extraocular eye movement and fundoscopic examinations are normal. The chest is clear. The heart has normal S1 and S2; no murmur is heard. The abdomen is soft and nontender. No hepatosplenomegaly or adenopathy is noted. Extremities are normal without lesions; joints are normal. Genitourinary examination shows Tanner 4 development. Neurologic examination is normal.

R-27. A 14-year-old girl has worsening of headaches and new-onset nausea and vomiting. The family reports that over the previous 5 days her occasional headaches have worsened, and that over the previous 5 days she developed nausea and vomiting due to a "stomach bug" going around the school. She has had no fever, diarrhea, or weight loss. They report that her school performance has deteriorated over the previous 6 weeks. On physical examination, her temperature and vital signs are normal. Height and weight are at the 50th percentile for age. The mucous membranes are pink, moist, and without lesions. She has loss of sensation over the left side of her face. Extraocular eye movement is normal and upbeating nystagmus is noted. Fundoscopic examination is not tolerated. The chest is clear. The heart has normal S1 and S2; no murmur is heard. The abdomen is soft and nontender. No hepatosplenomegaly or adenopathy is noted. Extremities are normal without lesions; joints are normal. Genitourinary examination shows Tanner 4 development. Neurologic examination shows truncal ataxia and an unsteady gait.

REVIEW QUESTIONS R-28 TO R-31

For each clinical scenario of an adolescent with altered mental status, select the most likely diagnosis. Each lettered option may be used once, more than once, or not at all.

A. Concussion
B. Poststreptococcal glomerulonephritis
C. Isotretinoin-associated intracranial hypertension
D. Lupus encephalitis
E. Subdural hematoma
F. Brain tumor
G. Bacterial meningitis

R-28. A 12-year-old boy is seen by the pediatrician for malaise, generalized weakness, headache, and anorexia. On physical examination, the blood pressure is 180/110 mm Hg. He has generalized edema, especially of the lower extremities and distant heart sounds on cardiac auscultation.

R-29. A 16-year-old girl is seen in the emergency room for new-onset delirium. Her mother reports that for the last several weeks she has had fever, arthralgia, and weight loss. She has had to discontinue her afterschool job as a lifeguard due to unrelenting sunburns.

R-30. A 15-year-old boy is seen by the pediatrician for a well-adolescent visit. He complains that he has severe headache and double vision since starting a new medication prescribed by his dermatologist 2 months prior. Over the past several weeks he has become withdrawn and no longer enjoys playing football.

R-31. A 14-year-old girl is seen in the emergency department for fever. She was in her normal state of health until 8 hours prior when she developed fever, headache, nausea, and vomiting. Her mother reports that she began to hallucinate on the way to the hospital. On physical examination, she has tachycardia, hypotension, and a nonblanching purpuric rash on her extremities.

ANSWERS TO REVIEW QUESTIONS

R-1.   Correct Answer: C (see Cases 10 and 23)

This child's growth and development are perfectly normal. The cyanotic episode was caused by a breath-holding spell and not a cardiac abnormality such as tetralogy of Fallot. Observation, parental reassurance, and disciplinary guidance are the most appropriate approaches. While poor appetite and picky eating are exceedingly common complaints from parents of toddlers, the number of normally developing children offered adequate nutrition who then develop failure to thrive or vitamin deficiencies is exceedingly small. When a toddler's diet is evaluated over a week or so, all necessary nutrients are eventually ingested. Appropriate advice for the adequately growing child might include offering healthy food options at each meal, avoiding supplementation with high-calorie foods (such as chocolate milk or ice cream), wasting money on unnecessary vitamins, and developing an unrealistic expectation of "eating all the food." Rather mealtime should include setting a routine, being patient if the child is a slow eater, and ending mealtime when the child begins to play with his or her food. Forcing the child to sit at the table until all food is eaten results in a power struggle that will result in no winners and all unhappy participants.

R-2.   Correct Answer: D (see Cases 11, 13, 19, and 24)

The history is suggestive of a normal child who is a picky eater and has a high intake of whole milk, an especially poor source of iron. The physical examination shows a normally growing and developing child with pallor. The laboratory data identify a microcytic anemia, an MCV less than 80, slight thrombocytosis, and normal white blood cell lines. Thus, iron-deficiency anemia is the most likely diagnosis. Therapy for this child is oral iron supplementation for several months. Failure of this child with microcytic anemia to respond to oral iron therapy would prompt an evaluation for other causes of microcytic anemia such as lead poisoning (unlikely because the lead level is low), sideroblastic anemia, thalassemia, hemoglobin E or C syndrome, or chronic disease (unlikely in a normally growing and developing child). Folate deficiency from poor nutrition alone is unusual and results in a megaloblastic anemia in contrast to the microcytic anemia presented in this case. Leukemia may present with pallor, but also may have bruising or gum bleeding as a presenting symptom. The laboratory data likely would show abnormalities on the red, white, and platelet cell lines. The child with sickle cell disease may have a history of painful crisis, pallor, and splenomegaly (especially in the younger child with splenic sequestration) on physical examination, and anemia with sickled cells on the blood smear. Hemoglobin electrophoresis done at birth (or repeated if results not known) would be diagnostic of the condition.

R-3.   Correct Answer: B (see Cases 42 and 48)

Cerebral edema is a rare but potentially fatal complication that arises in the treatment of DKA. Early signs and symptoms of cerebral edema include change in level of consciousness, headache, lethargy, decorticate or decerebrate posturing, cranial nerve palsy, hypertension, and bradycardia. Magnetic resonance imaging (MRI) can confirm the diagnosis, but early treatment with mannitol or hypertonic saline should be initiated if symptoms are present. The cause is felt to be partially due to idiogenic osmoles, which have developed in the brain to keep brain cells from shrinking while the DKA episode was developing. Overly aggressive hypotonic fluid resuscitation with rapid drop in serum osmolality (rapid drop in glucose) has been postulated to be a contributing factor.

The "hyponatremia" noted in the case is as expected: serum Na concentration falls by about 1.6 mEq/L for every 100 mg/dL (5.55 mmol/L) increase in the plasma glucose level above normal.

R-4.   Correct Answer: D (see Cases 13, 30, and 48)

Patients with sickle cell disease (SCD) have a variety of known complications, among which is ischemic stroke. Stroke typically presents with hemiparesis, but may also present with seizures. Appropriate therapy to prevent stroke extension is partial exchange transfusion to reduce the percentage of circulating sickled cells to less than 30%. Subsequent therapy for this child would include an ongoing chronic transfusion program because the incidence of subsequent stroke approaches 90%. Patients at risk for developing a stroke can be identified by screening all SCD patients prior to symptoms with transcranial Doppler studies. A repeat hemoglobin electrophoresis will confirm what is already known and unnecessarily delays definitive treatment. Splenic sequestration occurs in the first 5 years of a SCD patient's life when symptoms of life-threatening anemia present due to rapid enlargement of their spleen owing to trapped sickled cells. SCD patients have auto-infarction of their spleen and an increased incidence of infection caused by encapsulated organisms, especially *Streptococcus pneumoniae*. Such an infection is heralded by signs and symptoms of sepsis such as fever, stiff neck, headache, petechiae, and hypotension.

R-5.   Correct Answer: D (see Cases 15, 28, and 34)

A child who presents with a large amount of painless bleeding from the rectum raises the suspicion of Meckel diverticulum. The appropriate test is the technetium-99m pertechnetate scintiscan.

A Meckel diverticulum, heterotopic gastric mucosa in the intestine that secretes gastric acid and causes damage to adjacent tissue, typically presents in children as painless dark red/maroon or bright red hematochezia. A less common presentation in children (although more common in adults) is obstruction with the Meckel tissue serving as a lead point for intussusception. In most cases, the examination is normal unless blood loss results in signs and symptoms of anemia. In the case presented, the bleed is substantial and is resulting in tachycardia and mild hypotension; therapy would involve fluid resuscitation. The diagnosis can be made with a Meckel scan (technetium-99m pertechnetate scintiscan) to identify the aberrant gastric tissue.

Shigellosis is a bacterial enteritis whose symptoms include fever, crampy abdominal pain, fever, and bloody diarrhea. Intussusception classically causes vomiting (initially nonbilious but later bilious as obstruction worsens), abdominal pain, rectal bleeding, lethargy, and abdominal mass. Peptic ulcer disease is uncommon in an 8 month old, and typically presents as chronic abdominal pain, hematemesis, and melena.

R-6.   Correct Answer: C (see Cases 2 and 18)

The infant born to a poorly controlled diabetic mother is at risk for a variety of conditions including small left colon syndrome (with delayed stooling as in this case), macrosomia (as in this case), early hypoglycemia (as noted in the case), hypocalcemia, polycythemia (and resultant hyperbilirubinemia), a higher incidence of surfactant deficiency at later gestational ages that results in respiratory distress, cardiomyopathy (especially left ventricular outflow obstruction), and caudal regression syndrome (complete or poorly developed lower extremities). Cystic fibrosis (CF) also causes delayed stooling (meconium ileus), but the incidence of CF is significantly lower in African American children. Should small left colon syndrome not be found in this child born to the poorly controlled diabetic mother, an evaluation for cystic fibrosis would be another consideration to then pursue.

R-7.   Correct Answer: B (see Cases 14, 18, and 20)

Recurrent unilateral pneumonias in an otherwise healthy child should suggest the potential for anatomic blockage of an airway. In the patient in this question, the acuteness of the disease onset and the findings on clinical examination suggest a foreign body in the airway. Inspiratory and expiratory films early in the disease course can be helpful. Routine inspiratory films are likely to appear normal or near normal. Expiratory films will identify unilateral air trapping behind the foreign body. It is uncommon for the foreign body to be visible on the plain radiograph; a high index of suspicion is necessary to make the diagnosis. Recurrent unilateral pneumonia is unlikely to be cystic fibrosis (caused by a mutation of a protein transmembrane conductance regulator gene) which rather presents classically with delayed stooling at birth, recurrent pneumonias, nasal polyps, failure to thrive, and large, bulky, malodorous stools. Infection of the alveoli with bacteria (pneumonia) typically results in fever, cough, rales, and radiographic findings of infiltrates. Asthma is caused in part by hyperresponsiveness of the bronchial tree that ultimately causes remodeling of the airways due to chronic obstruction; signs and symptoms are of episodes of bilateral wheezing that are responsive to bronchodilator or steroid therapy.

R-8.   Correct Answer: D (see Cases 3, 4, and 6)

The case represents an infant jaundiced in the first 24 hours of life, a condition considered pathologic until proven otherwise. The physical examination shows minimal molding but splenomegaly along with visible jaundice. The laboratory data show a significant indirect hyperbilirubinemia, a complete blood count (CBC) with anemia and abnormally shaped cells (spherocytes), a lack of ABO or Rh incompatibility, and an elevated reticulocyte. All suggest ongoing hemolysis with sequestration of the cells in the spleen. A family history of spherocytosis would be an additional clue, but the osmotic fragility test will confirm the diagnosis. A more common cause of pathologic hyperbilirubinemia is ABO or Rh incompatibility which is highly unlikely in this case where the mother and baby have the same blood type and no abnormal antibodies are noted on the maternal antibody screen. With infection, hemolytic and hepatotoxic factors are reflected in the increased levels of both direct and indirect bilirubin along with findings of an ill-appearing infant who has temperature instability, lethargy, and poor feeding. Biliary atresia and neonatal hepatitis can be accompanied by elevated levels of transaminases, but characteristically present as chronic cholestatic jaundice with mixed hyperbilirubinemia after the first week of life. Physiologic jaundice is a diagnosis of exclusion. It becomes apparent on the second or third day of life, peaks to levels no higher than about 12 mg/dL on the fourth or fifth day, and resolves by the end of the first week of life. The rate of rise is less than 5 mg/dL per 24 hours and levels of conjugated bilirubin do not exceed about 1 mg/dL.

R-9.   Correct Answer: E (see Cases 21, 29, 37, and 38)

The CT scan showing a subdural hematoma or plain radiographs showing a fracture (or a radiograph showing multiple fractures in various stages of healing) indicates trauma. This information should be reported to the medical examiner and appropriate social agencies, including the police, so that an investigation can be started and other children in the home or under the care of the same providers can be protected. Although an autopsy (and death-scene investigation) should be done in every such case, there is a tendency for medical examiners to diagnose SIDS without an autopsy, particularly if the parents object to one, unless further information is provided by the ER staff, as in this case. Among the tests that should be done on this child would be clotting studies to eliminate from the differential the rare case of hemophilia as a contributing factor. The autopsy should identify a ruptured arteriovenous malformation, another rare but possible condition that would lead to an intracranial hemorrhage, which would be expected to result in a lesion that is intraparenchymal rather than subdural. Idiopathic thrombocytopenia rarely presents as an acute intracranial hemorrhage. Idiopathic thrombocytopenic purpura (ITP) classically presents in the 2 to 4 year old as petechial rash with a history of a viral illness in the days or weeks before; it does not occur in 6-month-old children.

R-10.   Correct Answer: D (see Cases 2, 22, and 23)

This child likely has a ductal-dependent cyanotic congenital heart lesion. In such conditions, a patent ductus arteriosus is the only route through which oxygenated blood ultimately may be sent to the systemic circulation. When the ductus begins to close, profound cyanosis will develop. The first step in managing a newborn with cyanosis is to give oxygen; when a cyanotic infant does not improve with administration of oxygen (or actually worsens) a structural heart defect that is dependent on a patent ductus may be the etiology for the condition. Because maintaining patency of this critical structure is a priority, transfer to a neonatal intensive care unit and initiation of prostaglandin E_1 (PGE_1) is imperative. Sepsis is always a consideration when a newborn becomes ill, but the rapidity of the onset of cyanosis as the only finding makes this choice less likely. Indomethacin is a medication that closes a patent ductus arteriosus; it is sometimes utilized in the premature infant who is developing evidence of heart failure due to failure of normal closure of this structure. Adenosine is used for supraventricular tachycardia. Digoxin would be appropriate for a child with heart failure.

R-11.   Correct Answer: E (see Cases 2, 22, and 23)

The child with an atrial septal defect (ASD) has blood flow from the left atrium to the right atrium. This increased blood volume then crosses into the right ventricle, across the pulmonary valve, and to the lungs. The extra flow of blood across a normal pulmonary valve results in delayed closure of the pulmonary value (fixed split S2) and the "pulmonary stenosis" murmur described. The lesion is not cyanotic. The murmur of an ASD is NOT due to the turbulence created at the atrial level (the pressure gradient is not high enough) but due to extra flow across the pulmonary valve. If the flow is great enough, a diastolic murmur across the tricuspid valve may also be heard. In contrast, a loud, continuous, machine-like murmur over the left upper sternal border that may obscure the second heart sound and with associated widened pulse pressures are characteristic findings of a persistently patent ductus arteriosus. Transposition of the great vessels, hypoplastic left heart, and pulmonary artery atresia are examples of "ductal dependent lesions," all typically present early in life when the ductus begins to close and deep cyanosis develops.

R-12.   Correct Answer: A (see Cases 27 and 46)

The history of sore throat, fever, difficulty breathing, and refusal to take liquids suggests an upper airway infection. The clinical findings of refusal to move the head from side to side and fullness of the midline posterior pharynx suggests retropharyngeal abscess. Other classical findings of retropharyngeal abscess include a muffled ("hot potato") voice and unilateral lymphadenopathy. Palpation of the abscess might reveal a fluctuant mass, but palpation is not recommended because it also may result in rupture with aspiration of purulent fluid. Lateral neck radiographic findings include widening of the soft tissues with anterior displacement of the airway, sometimes with gas noted in the soft tissue. Surgical drainage may be required.

A peritonsillar abscess presents with similar findings as retropharyngeal abscess but the pharyngeal swelling is asymmetric, lateral, and superior to the affected tonsil. Epiglottitis was a common cause of fever and stridor prior to the introduction of the *Haemophilus influenza* type B vaccine. This disease is classically described as high fever, acute onset of drooling, stridor, muffled voice, and a characteristic "tripod position of sitting," whereby the child refuses to lie down, rather preferring to sit with tongue protruding and their head projected forward. A thyroglossal duct cyst usually presents as an asymptomatic midline mass located at or below the hyoid bone; infection of this mass results in localized and superficial tenderness and overlying redness of the area. Meningitis classically presents with fever, headache, toxicity, and stiff neck as well as a positive Kernig and Brudzinski sign.

R-13.   Correct Answer: C (see Cases 49, 52, and 56)

The child in the question has hyperthermia and rhabdomyolysis (as evidenced by the elevated serum creatinine kinase level and the urine positive for "blood" which is actually myoglobin). Neither of these laboratory findings is immediately life threatening. However, life-threatening electrolyte disturbances can occur, the most common of which is hyperkalemia due to the damaged muscle and to renal failure. Other laboratory findings that may be seen but that are less likely to be fatal include hyperphosphatemia, hypocalcemia, hyperuricemia, and hypoalbuminemia. Accumulation of potassium due to the damaged muscle and the altered renal function is a common and expected consequence of rhabdomyolysis regardless of the underlying etiology for the muscle breakdown.

R-14.   Correct Answer: D (see Cases 19 and 47)

The obese adolescent boy is at especially high risk for developing slipped capital femoral epiphysis (SCFE), a displacement through the growth plate of the femoral neck from the femoral head. The history often is of several weeks of limp and pain, with the pain classically described as being referred to the knee. The examination will demonstrate a preferred position of passive external rotation of the affected hip (more commonly on the left) and reduced internal rotation, abduction, and flexion of the affected side. Trendelenburg gait (dropping of the pelvis of the unaffected side upon heelstrike of the affected side) with a shortened weight-bearing phase on the affected side (antalgic gait) is seen. The evaluation begins with anteroposterior and frog-leg radiographs of the hips. Findings for SCFE include widening of the physis and posteriorly displaced femoral epiphysis overlying the femoral head. Surgical internal fixation of the affected hip is the usual treatment. Bilateral disease is possible. Patients who present before about 10 years of age or after about 16 years of age have a higher incidence of endocrinologic disorders such as hypothyroidism and may require an endocrinology evaluation.

Avascular necrosis of the femoral head (disruption of blood flow to femoral head) typically presents with pain in the groin, knee, or buttocks that is worsened with weight bearing. Classic radiographic findings include sclerosis and radiolucency of the affected femoral head, reduction in size of the femoral head, and flattening/fragmentation of the affected femoral head. Septic joint (hematologic dissemination of a sexually acquired infection) classically presents with painful joint and also with fever, myalgia, and other systemic signs. A urethral discharge may be noted. Malignancy (bone marrow infiltration of leukemic cells) typically presents with additional findings such as fatigue, weight loss, fever, easy bruising, bleeding, and hepatosplenomegaly. The classic description of rheumatologic conditions (deposition of immune complexes in the joint space) include fatigue, morning stiffness, and daytime arthralgia.

R-15. Correct Answer: B (see Cases 27, 37, 39, and 55)

The case description is of fulminant meningococcemia, a rapidly progressive bacterial infection caused by *Neisseria meningitidis*. Classic findings include fever, altered mental status, early shock, and rapid progression of purpura. Despite early intervention with antibiotics and cardiovascular support, mortality is high. Survivors may have loss of digits or limbs due to gangrene. Prevention is with the administration of a meningococcal vaccine, typically initiated at 11 years of age for normal hosts. Rickettsial infection, with Rocky Mountain spotted fever being a prototypical example, requires a history of travel to an endemic area, exposure to the bite of a tick, and the classic clinical findings of fever, headache, myalgia, and a maculopapular rash of the wrists and ankles that then spreads to the trunk and proximal extremities with late involvement of the palms and soles. Many viral agents, such as varicella, rubella, and Epstein-Barr virus, cause rashes of various kinds but most do not commonly present with overwhelming sepsis and purpura as described in the case. Immune thrombocytopenic purpura is caused by antibody-mediated platelet destruction, classically by antiglycoprotein IIb/IIIa antibodies. It typically occurs in the 2- to 4-year-old child as petechiae of the lower extremities and in areas of trauma or less commonly as bleeding from the gums. Vasculitis of medium-sized arteries is a finding of Kawasaki disease which also has a polymorphous rash as part of its diagnostic requirements. It typically occurs in children younger than about 5 years with other clinical features including fever longer than 5 days, changes in the extremities (swelling of the palms and soles followed by desquamation of the finger and toe tips), oropharyngeal changes (crusting and fissuring of lips), bulbar conjunctivitis, and lymphadenopathy.

Correct Answers: (see Cases 1, 2, 4, 6, 7, 8, 14, and 27)

R-16:   H

R-17:   F

R-18:   B

R-19:   C

Transient tachypnea of the newborn classically is described as an increased respiratory rate in a term infant after a Cesarean delivery. The infant typically does not require oxygen, the lungs may sound "wet" on examination, and radiographs of the chest will show streakiness, fluid in the fissure, and a "star burst" pattern consistent with retained fluid. Early-onset Group B streptococcus (GBS) infection typically occurs as overwhelming sepsis in the first 48 hours of life (but before 7 days of age) with rapid onset of poor feeding, temperature instability, tachypnea, and cardiovascular collapse. A history of a mother being GBS positive may be obtained. Late-onset GBS occurs after 7 days of age, often as meningitis, with irritability, fever, poor feeding, and physical examination findings of bulging fontanelle and sepsis. Herpes simplex virus infection is particularly serious in an infant born to a mother whose primary infection occurs just prior to delivery. In such instance, the infant is exposed to a high viral load, no passed IgG immunity from the mother, and is therefore dependent on their innate IgM immunity for protection. Infection may develop a few days after delivery with subtle signs of temperature instability, poor feeding, and evidence of sepsis. Viremia may result in encephalitis, as in the case above, sometimes with increased red blood cell (RBC) count in the spinal fluid. Opioid narcosis typically presents as apnea in the infant whose mother has received narcotics as part of her delivery process. An infant with polycythemia typically is ruddy in appearance and may develop early respiratory distress and hypoglycemia. Exaggerated hyperbilirubinemia may also be noted. Surfactant deficiency presents as described in the case above, typically in infants less than about 30 to 31 weeks of gestation but also seen at older gestational ages to infants born to diabetic mothers. Antenatal steroids reduce its incidence, and administration of exogenous surfactant to infants demonstrating evidence of the condition can be therapeutic. Listeria is an unusual cause of isolated pneumonia in the newborn, but rather presents as sepsis. The typical presentation of Listeria is a preterm infant born to a mother whose pregnancy is complicated by fever, myalgia, arthralgia, back pain, and headache similar to the symptoms of flu. A maternal history of ingestion of unpasteurized milk or milk products is helpful. Diaphragmatic hernia presents immediately after birth as severe respiratory distress due to left-sided intestinal contents (most common) transmitted across the diaphragm into the left chest. The left lung is hypoplastic, the heart is shifted to the right, and the right lung capacity is compromised. The abdomen is scaphoid due to lack of intestinal contents. Texts often describe bowel sounds heard in the chest, a finding not often noted in actual clinical practice in the child with severe respiratory distress. An H-type tracheoesophageal fistula, the rarest form of TE fistula, presents as recurrent episodes of pneumonia in early childhood. A high-index of suspicion and a contrast study will assist in its diagnosis.

Correct Answers: (see Cases 6, 11, 13, 18, 32, 33, 37, 38, and 40)

R-20:   H

R-21:   F

R-22:   E

R-23:   G

Leukemia typically presents with abnormalities of all three cells lines of the bone marrow. Thus, pallor and bruising may be seen. The CBC will also show abnormalities in the white cell line, often with blasts on the peripheral smear. Neuroblastoma can present similar to leukemia with evidence of bone marrow invasion, but classic findings of neuroblastoma include an abdominal mass and periorbital ecchymosis due to metastasis. Immune thrombocytopenic purpura presents in the 2- to 4-year-old child a few weeks after a viral illness with acute onset of petechiae and purpura, occasionally with bleeding from the gingivae or other mucous membranes. The CBC in ITP will demonstrate isolated thrombocytopenia. Children with megaloblastic anemia typically have a diet devoid of B_{12} or folate or a clinical condition (such as short gut) that inhibits absorption of these nutrients. The CBC will demonstrate isolated anemia and larger-than-normal red blood cells. Child abuse presents in myriad ways with bruising a common finding. The CBC and bleeding studies in these children typically are normal. Sickle cell disease has multiple complications with acute splenic sequestration being a life-threatening problem. The sudden onset of pallor in a sickle cell child along with the finding of a dramatically enlarged spleen is diagnostic. Rapid transfusion is required. Wiskott-Aldrich syndrome classically is described as a male child with bleeding (often from circumcision), unusual bruising, severe eczema, and frequent or unusual bacterial infections. Cystic fibrosis typically is seen in a Caucasian child with delayed stooling at birth (meconium ileus), poor growth with large and foul-smelling stools due to malabsorption, and frequent pneumonia. The malabsorption may include vitamin E deficiency which may cause anemia.

Correct Answers: (see Cases 41, 43, 48, and 49)

R-24:   A

R-25:   B

R-26:   D

R-27:   E

Obstructive sleep apnea may present in the obese child as behavioral, cognitive, cardiovascular, and growth problems. Neuropsychological and cognitive problems include attention deficit hyperactivity disorder (ADHD) or ADHD symptoms, hypersomnolence, somatization, depression, aggression, and abnormal social behaviors. Klinefelter syndrome classically is described as a male with hypogo-nadism and infertility who has an extra X chromosome upon analysis. Affected men tend to be tall and thin, and have gynecomastia, small testes, mitral valve prolapse, poor gross and fine motor skills, learning difficulties, and psychosocial problems. Primary headaches (migraines and tension headaches) are recurrent, episodic in nature, and cannot be attributed to another disorder such as a brain tumor, trauma, infection, bleeding, or medication use/abuse. Tension headache is characterized by mild to moderate diffuse headache with pain described as being tight, pressure, or band-like. In contrast, migraine is a moderate to severe, episodic focal headache often associated with nausea, vomiting, photophobia, or phonophobia; a strong familial history is often noted. The child undergoing bul-lying may report somatic complaints such as headaches, sore throat, and stomach ache when school approaches so that they can avoid the unpleasant situation, which is a form of conversion disorder. Adolescents with drug abuse present in myriad ways including decreased school performance, truancy, law involvement, accidents, and specific signs and symptoms of the abused substance. Noonan syn-drome is often referred to as the "male Turner" syndrome and is characterized by short stature, chest deformities, hypertelorism, down-slanting eyes, webbed neck, congenital heart disease, and mental retardation. Brain tumors, such as brain-stem gliomas, are relatively common in children. Presenting signs and symptoms include change in behavior along with headache, altered vision, nausea, and vom-iting. On physical examination, papilledema, sensory changes, ataxia, and gait disturbances may be seen, depending on the location of the lesion.

Correct Answers: (see Cases 29, 51, 52, 58, and 60)

R-28:   B

R-29:   D

R-30:   C

R-31:   G

Concussion is a complex process involving a decline in neurologic or cognitive function that is induced by traumatic mechanical force to the person's head, neck, or body. A football player is a prime suspect for having a concussion, but treatment with isotretinoin for acne has as its side-effects increased intracranial pressure and depression. The patient with poststreptococcal glomerulonephritis has mal-aise, generalized weakness, headache, and anorexia as well as oliguria, dark urine, hypertension, and generalized edema as clinical findings. Systemic lupus erythe-matosus presents with myriad symptoms including constitutional symptoms of fever, arthralgia, fatigue, weight loss, and dermatologic abnormalities of malar rash or photosensitivity. Among the manifestations are neuropsychiatric find-ings of seizures, psychosis, anxiety, and acute confusional states. Brain tumors, such as brainstem gliomas, are relatively common in children. Presenting signs and symptoms include change in behavior along with headache, altered vision, nausea, and vomiting. On physical examination, papilledema, sensory changes, ataxia, and gait disturbances may be seen, depending on the location of the lesion.

Subdural hematomas are less common in older children than in younger children. Chronic subdural hematoma may cause chronic emesis, seizures, hypertonicity, irritability, personality changes, inattention, poor weight gain, fever, and anemia. Bacterial meningitis is a rapidly progressive infection often caused by *Neisseria meningitides* in the adolescent population. Classic findings in teens include the triad of fever, headache, and a stiff neck; altered mental status is another often-seen finding.

Page numbers followed by *f* or *t* indicate figures or tables, respectively.